THE THIRD TEN YEARS

OF THE

WORLD HEALTH ORGANIZATION

1968–1977

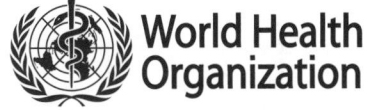

WHO Library Cataloguing-in-Publication Data

The third ten years of the World Health Organization : 1968–1977.

1.World Health Organization - history. 2.Anniversaries and special events. 3.Public health - history. I.World Health Organization.

ISBN 978 92 4 156366 6   (NLM classification: WA 11)

This book was written by Socrates Litsios, and edited and proof-read by Elisabeth Heseltine. The photo research and cover design were done by Gaël Kernen. Overall coordination on behalf of the WHO Global Health Histories project was by Thomson Prentice.

Table of contents

Foreword

The first two volumes of the official history of the World Health Organization (WHO) were published in 1958 and 1968, during the remarkable 20-year tenure of Dr Marcolino Candau as Director-General, first elected in 1953 and then re-elected three more times.

In his foreword to the first volume, Dr Candau wrote, "I believe that all those who from the outset have had faith in the Organization's aims and ideals will find in this report the justification of their hopes and evidence that tangible, even if as yet modest, results have been achieved." That volume traced the evolution of international public health, the establishment of WHO and its first 10 years of work. The range of topics was then, as now, dauntingly wide, and some of the subjects—influenza, malaria, poliomyelitis and tuberculosis—remain all too topical today. Then, as now, maternal and child health were priorities.

In his foreword to the second volume, in 1968, Dr Candau wrote, "The scientific discoveries and practical achievements of the past decade have stirred the imagination and roused our expectations for the future." He continued, "The development of WHO, and the now general recognition of the importance of health in any efforts for social and economic development, are indeed a landmark of achievement. But we cannot be satisfied and rest from our labours."

A new phrase entered the text of the second volume, 'smallpox eradication'. This occurred because, in 1958, the Eleventh World Health Assembly unanimously adopted a resolution initiating a worldwide programme for eradication of the disease. By the end of WHO's second decade, eradication campaigns were under way in dozens of countries, although there was still a long way to go.

Looking back, we can see just how important WHO's third decade actually was. By the end of it, smallpox eradication had been achieved. At almost the same time, another great landmark in the history of health was about to be established: preparations were under way for the first international conference on primary health care, in Alma-Ata. Although that meeting, in September 1978, technically falls outside the scope of this volume, it was such a major preoccupation for much of the preceding 3 years that an epilogue is devoted to it.

Dr Candau had been succeeded as Director-General in 1973 by Dr Halfdan Mahler, who would also be re-elected twice, in 1978 and in 1983. This volume then, reflects the first five of the 'Mahler years', which saw growing support for the primary health care movement. Thirty years after Alma-Ata, that movement is once again much in evidence; primary health care is again a WHO priority, in a renewed, reinvigorated form.

We are looking at and learning from the lessons of history. With the exception of this foreword and the epilogue, however, the advantages of hindsight have been firmly resisted, and this book remains a 'record of the records', drawn from contemporary reports of the activities that made up the work of WHO. Based almost exclusively on publications from that period, it offers insights into not only the Organization itself but also the political, social and economic background against which many far-reaching health decisions were made.

Understanding the history of health during the past 60 years helps us to respond to the health challenges of today. Learning from history is vital in helping shape a healthier future for everyone, especially those most in need. Sharing health knowledge inspired by history enriches global public health and benefits society at large. With these basic principles in mind, the Global Health Histories initiative was established by WHO in late 2004, with the aim of making a number of valuable contributions to this field. This volume is the first publication within the initiative.

WHO is greatly indebted to its author, Dr Socrates Litsios, an eminent health historian whose long WHO career included the period covered by this work. He has dedicated much of the past few years to the huge task of researching and writing this book. WHO also acknowledges with thanks all those, including many former and current staff, who assisted him.

This volume will be of great assistance to scholars, historians and researchers and to the many WHO staff members, past and present, who will be able to turn these pages and remember that they, too, were a part of this history. This book is dedicated to them and to my predecessors in office during those eventful years. Together, they have left a rich and challenging legacy for those of us fortunate enough to follow in their footsteps.

Dr Margaret Chan
Director-General

Geneva, 7 April 2008

Introduction

The history of WHO's first decade was published in 1958 (*1*) and that of the second decade in 1968 (*2*). It is not clear why the history of the third decade was not written in 1978 or soon thereafter, but the most likely reason is the budget cuts suffered at headquarters after the governing bodies requested that a greater percentage of funds be made available at regional and country levels. Interest in an account of subsequent decades emerged only in 2004, with the establishment of WHO's Global Health History initiative.

Had this history been written in 1978, it might have followed the style of its predecessors, in which the role of the Director-General was heavily muted. The first two histories hardly mention WHO's first two Directors-General, Dr Brock Chisholm and Dr Marcolino Candau. A decision to follow that precedent would have masked the dramatic changes introduced by WHO's third Director-General, Dr Halfdan Mahler, who took office in 1973. A more personal approach to this history therefore seemed to be called for, to capture the challenging manner in which Dr Mahler confronted the growing disparities in the world and his efforts to raise health as a priority within the wider United Nations system, especially at country level.

Arguing that health should be seen in terms of its social, economic and political dimensions, the new WHO leadership aligned itself with various governmental and nongovernmental movements that sought greater equity in health across and within countries. The plight of the poorest, most disadvantaged countries was working its way onto the agendas of the international community. There was a sense that greater, more rapid progress could be made. What was needed was responsible national and international leadership capable of amassing the necessary political will to overcome the multitude of obstacles that had hitherto blocked action. It followed, almost axiomatically, that as health is valued by all, it would attain higher priority in national and international political and economic arenas.

The early 1970s also heard new voices calling for radical changes in the conceptualization of human progress. The works of Paulo Freire, Ivan Illich and E.F. Schumacher, in particular, encouraged reconsideration of the relevance of advanced technology to the needs of individuals and communities and of how people could learn from and work with each other. In the process, the ideas of appropriate technology and a more participatory approach to learning and doing were introduced. Freire was a Brazilian adult educator, who stressed the importance of informal learning; Illich, an Austrian theologian and philosopher, critiqued modernization and its institutions; and Schumacher, a German-born economist, developed the principles of what he called 'Buddhist economics', a way of meeting local needs with local resources.

A dramatic example of what appropriate technology could accomplish was what many consider to be WHO's greatest triumph, the eradication of smallpox. Although many technical details had to be refined during this campaign, the basic idea of life-long protection with the use of a vaccine had been known for centuries.

While the virtues of appropriate technology were being extolled, there was perhaps even greater enthusiasm, and certainly more funding, for front-line science, as witnessed by the explosion of interest in the 1970s in the field of molecular biology. "The triumphs to date of molecular biology", wrote Warren Weaver, "have been largely in the field of genetics. But there is every reason to believe that molecular biology will now attack, and similarly conquer, other basic biological problems—those of immunology, of cellular growth and development (including cancer), and even some of the most basic aspects of the functioning of the central nervous system." (*3*) It was Weaver who coined the term 'molecular biology' in 1938 and who was responsible for much of the early research funding. Advances in immunology were of particular importance to the new tropical diseases programme, as immunology was believed to be the stepping stone to rapid development of new diagnostic tests and vaccines for important diseases, in particular malaria.

Strongly related to the push for more appropriate technology was the growing sense that the human resources models being promoted in developing countries were not in fact those most needed. The Christian Medical Commission, for example, which had been involved in establishing hospitals and clinics in developing countries and in training personnel for those institutions, underwent detailed review in the late 1960s. Out of this emerged the notion that perhaps developed countries had done the Third World a "disservice by exporting their system of health manpower" (*4*). Dr Candau was soon to express similar sentiments.

Meanwhile, China was totally overhauling its health system in revolutionary ways. Visitors to China reported on these developments in the western press well before the People's Republic of China was recognized by the United Nations system and WHO (e.g. *5*). Particularly striking was the training of agricultural workers to meet rural needs for environmental sanitation, health education, immunization, first aid and some aspects of primary care and post-illness follow-up. Most of these 'barefoot doctors' were peasants and were thus members of the community, rather than an extension of the Government's health system. This model was clearly a challenge to the dominant health manpower models of the developed world.

Within a few years, these revolutionary ideas and experiences had worked their way into WHO, resulting in the formulation of a new approach to health systems development, which became known as 'primary health care'. While the bureaucratic origins of primary health care and its essential features are described in Chapter 6, the reader should be aware that the underlying philosophy, which was strongly linked to both community involvement and appropriate technology, permeated much of the work of WHO during the latter part of this decade. Given its historical importance, the International Conference on Primary Health Care organized in Alma-Ata in 1978 is the subject of the Epilogue, although, strictly speaking, it falls 'outside' the decade. Even more importantly, the Declaration of Alma-Ata stands as a vision of health that has lost none of its urgency.

Like its predecessors, this account of WHO's work covers all the major programmes of the Organization. An effort was made to provide an indication of earlier initiatives, when this was particularly important. Thus, one learns of the similarity between the primary health care principles pronounced by WHO and those of the League of Nations Health Organization some 40 years earlier, a fact already noted in the 1970s. There was perhaps reason to be more optimistic in the 1970s than 40 years earlier, when war in Europe was looming, that these ideas could be translated into action. Rather than being frustrated by the lack of progress in the intervening 40 years, there was excitement in the air, engendered by optimism.

This account, being a 'record of the records', is drawn from reports of the activities that make up the work of the Organization. It is based almost exclusively on publications of that period, and no effort has been made to look forward in time to assess the successes or failures of initiatives that commenced during the third decade. Awareness of events in the intervening 40 years, however, led to an effort to provide more complete references on issues that are still of relevance today. This, it is hoped, will provide incentive for future efforts, including the histories of WHO's fourth, fifth and sixth decades.

The importance of this period in WHO's history has not been lost on historians. It clearly represented a "shift in the health paradigm", from technical approaches to specific diseases, in particular malaria, to ensuring the availability of more comprehensive services for all people (6). The commitment to reach all people was enshrined in the adoption in 1976 of the social target 'Health for All by the Year 2000'. This was a call for achieving a level of health that would permit everyone to lead a socially and economically productive life, a goal "nearer to reality" than the definition of health given in WHO's Constitution, i.e. "Health is a state of complete physical, mental and social well-being and not merely the absence of disease or infirmity" (7).

The 1970s proved to be a "heady if often stormy time for WHO" (6). It has also been judged by some to have been "a golden age of WHO and perhaps of global health in general" (8). It is hoped that both realities have been caught in this record of WHO's work.

References

1. World Health Organization. *The first ten years of the World Health Organization*. Geneva, 1958.
2. World Health Organization. *The second ten years of the World Health Organization 1958–1967*. Geneva, 1968.
3. Weaver W. *Science of change*. New York, Charles Scribner, 1970.
4. McGilvray JC. Health services and health manpower for the developing countries. *World Hospitals*, 1970, 6:1–4.
5. Sidel VW. The barefoot doctors of the People's Republic of China. *New England Journal of Medicine*, 1972, 286:1292–1300.
6. Lee K. *Historical dictionary of the World Health Organization*, Lanham, Maryland, The Scarecrow Press, 1998.
7. Howard-Jones N. The World Health Organization in historical perspective. *Perspectives in Biology and Medicine*, 1981, 24:467–482.
8. Global Health Watch. *Global Health Watch 2005–2006*. Cape Town, 2006:272. www.ghwatch.org/2005report/

CHAPTER 1

Global political, socioeconomic and institutional context

A TURBULENT DECADE

Some might imagine that an international organization concerned with the health of all the people of the world would be able to remain free from the political and economic turbulence that plagues us. This was not the case during the first 20 years of WHO's existence, nor was it so during its third decade.

In the 1970s, hardly any area of the world was free from military conflict. The Cold War was in full swing. The Middle East was caught up in yet another spiral of violence, so that the Organization spent much time and effort in evaluating the health conditions of the Arab population in the occupied Arab territories, including Palestine, an item that was addressed at length by the Health Assembly, often in a heavily acrimonious atmosphere. Military spending remained high, and major economic crises further reduced the resources that might otherwise have contributed to social and economic development. A wave of protests marked the beginning of the decade: some marched against war, others against social injustice.

The political map of the world continued to change, as new nations emerged from their colonial heritage. As each of these nations gained full rights in the United Nations, they soon became Member States of WHO, with the result that by the end of 1977 the number of Member States had risen from 126 to 197. An important development, in 1971, was recognition of the People's Republic of China as "the only legitimate representative of China to the United Nations and in all the organizations related to it" (United Nations General Assembly resolution 2758 (XXVI) and World Health Assembly resolution WHA25.1). Not all international organizations, however, recognized the exclusive rights of the People's Republic to represent China.[1]

WHO underwent considerable financial difficulties during this period. Even before the 1973 oil crisis, the Organization encountered serious budgetary problems. The reevaluation of the Swiss franc in May 1971 led to a substantial increase in the amount of United States dollars required to meet the expenditures incurred in Swiss francs. The dollar was further weakened in early 1973 when it was devalued against gold and when reevaluation of other currencies led to increased charges in United States dollars.

The energy crisis and worldwide inflation had major impacts on supply operations, resulting in higher prices for almost all commodities, slower deliveries, shortages, higher shipping costs, less frequent shipping services, a growing unwillingness of suppliers to accept small orders and an inability or unwillingness to quote firm prices for future delivery.

---

[1] As witnessed by the reservation made by the representative of the People's Republic of China to the 57th Executive Board concerning a draft resolution under consideration by the Board because "it referred to an organization in which groups and individuals belonging to the Chiang Kai Shek clique were represented" (*1*).

These and other upheavals that shook the world worked their way through the halls of the United Nations, where they resulted in the adoption of various resolutions by the General Assembly and its organs. Some specifically called upon WHO to take action of one kind or another; others invited the contributions of all the specialized agencies. Many subjects were ones that WHO had not addressed previously. These are discussed below, not only because they do not fall conveniently into any of the technical programmes covered in later chapters, but because they reflect the tensions and worries of the time.

Chemical and bacteriological weapons

General Assembly resolution 2454 (XXIII) on the question of general and complete disarmament, adopted in December 1968, requested the Secretary-General to prepare a concise report on the use of chemical and bacteriological weapons. WHO was asked to address the question of the health effects of such weapons, and the Director-General appointed a number of consultants to carry out a study.

The conclusions of this study, undertaken in 1969, were that chemical and biological weapons, even if used on a limited scale, would cause illness to a degree that would overwhelm existing health resources and facilities; their widespread use could cause lasting changes of an unpredictable nature to the human environment. The delivery of some of these agents in isolated sabotage attacks could affect large civilian targets (2). The report was addressed in particular to public health and medical authorities. It dealt with the weapons on a technical level, and efforts were made to estimate the possible effects of their use. Thus, for example, it was estimated that an attack on a city with anthrax by even a single bomber disseminating 50 kg of dried agent in a suitable aerosol form would affect an area far in excess of 20 km^2, with millions of deaths.

Certain measures could be taken with existing resources that would redound to the benefit of health and prevention, such as improving rapid detection and diagnostic facilities for air pollution and for communicable diseases, improving medical management of natural disasters and wider use of safety features in buildings and for communal water supply systems. Nevertheless, in the last analysis, "the best interests of all Member States and mankind in general will be served only through the rapid implementation of the resolutions on chemical and biological warfare adopted by the United Nations General Assembly and the World Health Assembly...."

Resolution WHA23.53, adopted in 1970 as a consequence of this study, appealed to the governments of countries that had not yet ratified the Geneva Protocol of 17 June 1925 to accede to that important and highly humane international agreement in the nearest possible future. It also called upon all medical associations and all medical workers to consider it their moral and professional duty to give every possible assistance to the international movement for the complete prohibition of chemical and bacteriological (biological) means of waging war.

In 1972, when the United Nations undertook a study on napalm and other incendiary weapons and all aspects of their possible use, WHO paid for the participation of an expert in the work of a group of consultants on the subject. That expert became the main drafter of the United Nations report, which was commended by the United Nations General Assembly (United Nations General Assembly resolution GA3076 (XXVIII)).

Human rights

Resolution 2450 (XXIII) on human rights and scientific and technological developments, also adopted in December 1968 by the United Nations General Assembly, called for studies on subjects including protection of the human personality and its physical and intellectual integrity in the light of advances in biology, medicine and biochemistry. WHO prepared a preliminary paper on the subject, while indicating to the Secretary-General in 1970 its willingness to take responsibility for preparing a document on the health aspects of human rights in the light of scientific and technological developments.

The preliminary document contained chapters on respect for the privacy of individuals in view of advances in recording and other techniques; protection of the human personality and its physical and intellectual integrity in view of advances in biology, medicine and biochemistry (genetics, tissue and organ transplantation, heart transplants, radical medical techniques in general); experiments on human subjects (in physiology, pathology and psychology, clinical testing of drugs, use of chemical additives in food and potable fluids); deterioration of the human environment; human rights aspects of the delivery of health services; mental health and nutrition.

The next paper, prepared in 1974 (*3*), briefly summarized the main situations, whether recent or long-standing, in which interventions, compulsions or restraints, performed or imposed on human beings for preventive or curative therapeutic purposes or with a view to advancing knowledge of health and disease, have implications for the rights of the individual. An important question raised by this study was what role an intergovernmental organization such as WHO should play in achieving international consensus on the point at which a medical intervention or procedure poses a threat to human rights. Until then, WHO had not enunciated any principles such as those existing in some countries. It had, however, established an internal secretariat committee to advise on research proposals involving human subjects (see Chapter 5).

This study, which dealt with a number of bioethical questions, demonstrated the limited role of WHO in fields in which moral, religious and social attitudes differ significantly from one country to another. At the same time, the study demonstrated the importance of the links between WHO and the Council for International Organizations of Medical Sciences (CIOMS) and the World Medical Association. When medical ethics was first discussed, at the fourth session of the Executive Board in 1949, it was decided that any further studies on the subject would be carried out by the World Medical Association. That Association adopted an international code of medical ethics in 1950 and continued to explore the question through its affiliates at national and international levels. The CIOMS was established jointly by WHO and UNESCO in 1949, and bioethics is one of its main long-term programmes.

The Executive Board at its fifty-fifth session, in January 1975, adopted resolution EB55.R65, which requested the Director-General to continue the studies suggested in his report, in consultation with Member States and in collaboration with the United Nations, other relevant organizations of the United Nations system and nongovernmental organizations in official relations with WHO, particularly the World Medical Association and CIOMS.

Rights of prisoners and detainees

Following adoption of United Nations General Assembly resolution 3218 (XXIX), in 1974, on torture and other cruel, inhuman or degrading treatment or punishment in relation to detention and imprisonment, WHO was called upon to outline, in close cooperation with other competent agencies, the principles of medical ethics as they relate to this subject. Two members of the Economic and Social Council, the highest body in the United Nations system responsible for coordination, urged WHO to submit a progress report on the subject "in view of the urgency of the question". The document prepared by the Director-General, entitled *Health aspects of avoidable maltreatment of prisoners and detainees*, was submitted to the Fifth United Nations Congress on the Prevention of Crime and the Treatment of Offenders and to the United Nations General Assembly at its thirtieth session, which incorporated it into its "Declaration on the prevention of all persons from being subjected to torture and other cruel, inhuman or degrading treatment or punishment" (United Nations General Assembly resolution 3452).

As a follow-up to this study, the CIOMS was asked by the Health Assembly in 1977 (resolution WHA30.32) to undertake on behalf of WHO a study on the feasibility of drawing up a code of medical ethics relevant to torture. Following publication of this study, the Executive Board in January 1978 (resolution EB61.R37) invited the CIOMS and the World Medical Association to elaborate a draft code of medical ethics relevant to the protection of persons subjected to any form of detention or imprisonment against torture and other cruel, inhuman or degrading treatment or punishment.

Economic and social consequences of the arms race and of military expenditure

This subject was addressed by the United Nations General Assembly almost annually during the decade. On the last occasion (December 1977), it adopted resolution 32/75, which expressed deep concern that, not only had the arms race not ceased, it had "continued at an alarming speed, absorbing enormous material and human resources from the economic and social development of all countries ...."

WHO was asked to contribute to the preparation of a report to be used at a special session of the General Assembly devoted to disarmament held in May–June 1978. The report focused on three themes: poverty and health, development and health, and resource needs and uses in the health sector. Each of these themes had emerged more clearly than before as a consequence of various interagency initiatives, described below.

THE SECOND DEVELOPMENT DECADE

The issues discussed above, as important as they are, played a relatively minor part in how the work of the United Nations affected that of WHO. By far the most important impact was that of social and economic development, on which the rest of this chapter concentrates, beginning with the setting of development goals in the context of the United Nation's Second Development Decade.

It was the United States President John Kennedy who proposed to the United Nations General Assembly that it should launch a development decade. Resolution 1710 (XVI), adopted in December 1961, designated that decade as the United Nations Development Decade and requested the United Nations system to "develop proposals for the intensification of action in the fields of economic and social development". The proposals included measures for assisting developing countries to establish well-conceived, integrated country plans, including, where appropriate, land reform; measures to improve the use of international institutions and instruments for furthering economic and social development; and measures to accelerate the elimination of illiteracy, hunger and disease.

By 1968, it had become evident that these objectives had not been reached. The Economic and Social Council initiated preparations for the Second Development Decade in 1966, and United Nations General Assembly resolution 2626 (XXV), adopted in October 1970, proclaimed 1 January 1971 as its starting date. On the eve of its start, Dr M.G. Candau, WHO Director-General, in his address to the Economic and Social Council, indicated that WHO was ready to support "with all the means at its disposal the objectives of the Second Development Decade". He said that the close interdependence between health and other aspects of development was a fundamental principle underlying all of WHO's work. Many health problems cannot be resolved in isolation and require parallel advances in other social and economic sectors. Similarly, development, associated with urbanization, housing, the building of roads and the construction of water works, has a strong health component.

With WHO's active involvement, specific global objectives were established in the field of health. Each developing country was called upon to formulate a coherent programme for the prevention and treatment of disease and for raising general levels of health and sanitation. Furthermore, "levels of nutrition should be improved in terms of average caloric intake and the protein content, with special emphasis being placed on the needs of vulnerable groups of population" (United Nations General Assembly resolution 2626 (XXV)).

The section that addressed human development further defined what was hoped to be achieved in the field of health:

Developing countries will establish at least a minimum programme of health facilities comprising an infrastructure of institutions, including those for medical training and research to bring basic medical services within reach of a specified proportion of their population by the end of the Decade. These will include basic health services for the protection of health. Each developing country will endeavor to provide an adequate supply of potable water to a specified proportion of its population, both urban and rural, with a view to reaching a minimum target by the end of the Decade. Efforts of the developing countries to raise their levels of health will be supported to the maximum feasible extent by developed countries, particularly through assistance in the planning of a health promotion strategy and the implementation of some of its segments, including research, training of personnel at all levels, and supply of equipment and medicines. A concerted international effort will be made to mount a world-wide campaign to eradicate by the end of the Decade, from as many countries as possible, one or more diseases that still seriously afflict people in many lands. Developed countries and international organizations will assist the developing countries in their health planning and in the establishment of health institutions.

Other aspects of health were dealt with in this section, including the adoption of agricultural and health policies in an effort to meet nutritional requirements, the supply of means for family planning and intensification of efforts to arrest the deterioration of the human environment.

Two global issues led to the creation of two new United Nations agencies early in the decade. The first was the United Nations Fund for Population Activities (UNFPA), which began operation in 1969 under the administration of the United Nations Development Programme (UNDP), until 1972, when it was raised to the same status as the UNDP and the United Nations Children's Fund (UNICEF) in recognition of the growth in its resources and in the scope of its operations. The United Nations Environment Programme (UNEP) was created in late 1972, as recommended by the United Nations Conference on the Environment (Stockholm Conference), held earlier that year.

The economic crisis greatly affected progress in achieving the goals of the Second Development Decade. In particular, the state of children's health deteriorated to such a degree that the Executive Board of UNICEF declared an emergency in 1974, and the United Nations General Assembly adopted resolution 3250 (XXIX). The mid-decade review prepared by WHO in January 1975 for the fifty-fifth session of its Executive Board portrayed the global picture of malnutrition as "alarming" (4). Declining food reserves, high inflation rates, followed by spiralling prices for staple foods, the energy crisis, shortage of fertilizers, frequent natural calamities like droughts and an ever-increasing population had all contributed to a deteriorating nutritional situation. Other setbacks noted were a worsening of the malaria situation and no improvement in the prevalence of other parasitic or sexually transmitted diseases. The picture was not, however, entirely bleak. The remarkable reduction in the prevalence of smallpox throughout the world was noted, as were favourable developments in the field of family health, particularly as related to the acceptance of family planning as part of health-care services for mothers and children.

WHO took the opportunity to identify a number of new health system trends that offered promise for the future. One was growing acceptance by governments of the use of village health auxiliaries who were locally based, locally trained and locally supervised. Another was the strengthening of WHO's coordinating role, especially at country level, where the WHO country representative was expected to assume increasing operational responsibility for assisting governments in planning, programming, managing and evaluating their health services and for directing and coordinating WHO's assistance to countries. A third trend was intensification of efforts to build national health research infrastructure. These developments and others are addressed in more detail in later chapters.

The report was also used to stress the urgency of incorporating health care as an integral part of economic and social development at national and international levels. Several obstacles were identified: lack of solid evidence of a contribution of health to economic development, poor communication between health professionals and socioeconomic planners, and the low status of public health services in overall socioeconomic planning. What was needed was strengthened planning, programming and implementation, with the application, whenever possible, of an intersectoral, interdisciplinary approach. The Organization would collaborate closely with other United Nations agencies in a multisectoral approach to solving countries' health and health-related problems. Such collaboration had been actively sought by WHO, as discussed below.

The full integration of women into development was explicitly included in the Second Development Decade. The United Nations observed 1975 as International Women's Year, and General Assembly resolution 3524, adopted in December 1975, called on the specialized agencies to "give sustained attention to the integration of women in the formulation, design and implementation of development projects and programmes". WHO contributed to the draft plan of action for International Women's Year, particularly to the chapters on health and nutrition, the family and population, and participated in the World Conference on International Women's Year in Mexico in June–July, contributing documents on the health needs of women. World Health Assembly resolution WHA28.40, adopted in 1975, recommended that particular attention be paid to protecting the health of mothers, children and working women in WHO's current activities and in establishing the Organization's Sixth General Programme of Work (see Chapter 3).

Earlier, in June 1972, WHO contributed a statement on the integration of women into development for an interregional meeting of experts convened by the United Nations, in which it approached the subject from the viewpoints of health and productivity, health problems of the labour force, employment in the health sector and employment strategies and the health sector (*5*).

UNITED NATIONS EFFORTS TO IMPROVE INTERAGENCY COORDINATION AT COUNTRY LEVEL

In parallel with the global articulation of social and economic development goals for the Second Development Decade, the United Nations undertook to improve its capacity to assist development at country level. In 1968, an important study was undertaken to create a strong central development agency within the United Nations. The 'capacity study', as it came to be known, conducted by Sir Robert Jackson and published in 1969 under the title of *A study of the capacity of the United Nations development* system (*6*), argued the case for a restructured UNDP.

It was a provocative report, which portrayed the specialized agencies of the United Nations system (of which WHO is one) as resisting any incursion onto their territory and as having become "the equivalent of principalities, free from any centralized control". The report noted, however, that the UNDP financed most of their operations; without its support, WHO and the other agencies could not hope to improve their performance at country level, which was the focus of the report. It portrayed the UNDP as "a main gear wheel, with each of the Agencies as another important wheel, all of which must mesh together if the mechanism is to function effectively ....."

The UNDP was created in 1965 by merging its predecessors, the United Nations Expanded Programme of Technical Assistance, created in 1949, and the United Nations Special Fund, created in 1958. The former channelled technical knowledge and skills to developing countries through advisors and fellowships, while the Special Fund financed more complex projects.

The Director-General, in his statement to the Inter-Agency Consultative Board in March 1970, expressed some misgivings about the study. To begin with, it gave "a terrible image of the United Nations", one that could harm the body. The image presented was one of a "machine" which had such a marked identity that no one, in effect, was in control. Furthermore, the evidence suggested that governments did not control it, and that it "is incapable of intelligently controlling itself". Dr Candau was even more concerned by the fact that the report had overlooked the past. In doing so, the diagnosis of the United Nations system had been made in a "political vacuum". No mention was made of political instability in the world or of the Cold War or of "real war in certain areas" or of decolonization, during which more than 60 countries had become independent. With respect to WHO, he expressed his unwillingness to accept the idea that no health project should be implemented if it were not an integral part of social and economic development. He considered that "there is more in the world than just this …. alleviating suffering and preventing death is part of the oath or our profession, regardless of what are the social and economic consequences of this".

Dr Candau well understood the risks of using strictly economic criteria to judge whether United Nations development funds should be used. Early in his first term as Director-General, in 1953, a funding crisis had occurred when the Expanded Programme of Technical Assistance moved away from a system in which WHO received a fixed percentage of its funds (some 20%) towards one that gave authority to local United Nations resident representatives to decide on priorities and funding. At the time, the Executive Board adopted no fewer than eight long resolutions to express its dissatisfaction with this turn of events.

During a more recent debate, provoked by decreasing funding from the UNDP, the Health Assembly in 1967 passed resolution WHA20.53, which called on Member States to take appropriate steps to draw up national health plans as part of their economic and social development plans, and requested the Director-General to intensify studies on the economic aspects of health activities, to help strengthen communication between economists and public health authorities and to accelerate the programme of training of public health administrators in national health planning, including health economics. That same Health Assembly, in resolution WHA20.52, invited WHO Member States to take any steps deemed necessary to ensure that adequate emphasis was placed on the health component in their overall plans for national socioeconomic development, and to inform the Organization about health plans to be implemented during the development decade of the 1970s.

Despite the Director-General's reservations, WHO supported the consensus that was reached at the tenth session of the UNDP Governing Council in June 1970, and subsequently by the United Nations General Assembly at its twenty-fifth session, in December of the same year (United Nations General Assembly resolution 2888 (XXV)). The consensus called for country programming based on national plans, priorities and objectives and a system of 5-year indicative planning figures for resource allocation. Key elements of the UNDP organizational structure were changed. Regional bureaux were created to act as a link between the UNDP Administrator and resident directors. While governments were recognized as having exclusive responsibility for formulating their national development plans, the input of the United Nations system would be decided in country programming by resident directors, who should be "recognized as having full over-all responsibility for the programme in the country concerned and his role in relation to the representatives of the other United Nations organizations ... should be that of leader of the team …."

The consensus differed in some important ways from the recommendations made in the 'capacity study'. While endorsing the country-centred approach of country programming, it discarded rolling indicative planning figures and the approval of programmes in order to synchronize them with each country's planning cycle. It considered that fixed, 5-year indicative planning figures made it more difficult to synchronize the work of the agencies with that of each country and might have contributed to the economic crisis that the UNDP faced in 1975, when it found itself some US$ 100 million short. Also, as pointed out by the Director-General in 1972, under the indicative planning figure system, "countries wanted to exercise complete control of the UNDP funds allotted to them" (7).

The Executive Board, at its forty-seventh session in January 1971, adopted resolution EB47.R53 which, inter alia, requested the Director-General to continue to cooperate fully in a spirit of partnership with the Administrator of the UNDP and with other appropriate agencies and organizations of the United Nations in implementing the consensus approved by the Governing Council of the UNDP. The Twenty-fourth World Health Assembly followed suit in May 1971 with a similar resolution of support (WHA24.52).

The relation between UNDP and WHO was not without problems. UNDP provided only a relatively small percentage of the funds available to WHO for technical assistance, and yet a tremendous bureaucratic effort was required to obtain and spend the funds. One WHO regional director voiced the opinion that "it was more trouble than it was worth". Nevertheless, the WHO regular budget was stabilizing, while that of the UNDP was growing, and it could be envisaged that UNDP funds would become WHO's principal source of support, as pointed out later in a memo from the Director-General to all regional directors.

The relationship between the WHO country representative and the UNDP resident representative was also an issue. While most other organizations initially agreed to locate their representatives within the office of the resident representative (paid by the UNDP), WHO refused to do so. Of greater concern, however, were the lines of communication that UNDP wished to impose on the specialized agencies. Yielding total authority to the resident representative would mean that all negotiations with countries would be managed by UNDP, something that WHO could not accept.

At issue was what WHO considered to be its prerogative as the international organization responsible for coordinating matters pertaining to health, namely the right of direct access to ministries of health. Furthermore, as stipulated in the WHO Constitution, in Article 37, "the Director-General and the staff shall not seek or receive instructions from any government or from any authority external to the Organization". WHO did, however, agree that it should inform resident representatives of all steps taken in preparation of project documents for UNDP-supported activities. UNDP, on its side, asked WHO to make a greater effort to ensure integration of health planning and activities into overall socioeconomic development efforts of the United Nations system (7).

This stimulus well suited the thinking that Dr Halfdan Mahler, the new WHO Director-General, elected in 1973, brought to the subject. At his first meeting with the Inter-Agency Consultative Board, he noted that country programming "had made WHO rethink its own approach towards technical assistance," referring to the studies on country health programming and on project systems analysis undertaken by the Organization (see Chapter 3) (8). He stressed the need to strengthen and promote the self-reliance of governments in preparing their own development plans ("... we have to be obsessive about government participation ...."). UNDP should be more aggressive in assuring a cohesive approach to the United Nations system, said he. Leadership must come from the UNDP at country and headquarters levels if the system of country programming was to reduce the tendency of each agency to go its own way. WHO was deeply committed to this approach and fully involved in preparing for the changes it involved, both in thinking and in practical approaches, he concluded. Furthermore, in introducing his annual report for 1973 to the Health Assembly, the Director-General said: "WHO has to become much more prepared psychologically to shed the last fragments of the shell of health isolationism and to be able to work together with all the other organizations of the United Nations system which are concerned about social and economic development ...." (9).

Within the year, the operational responsibilities for activities funded by UNDP were delegated to the regional directors, and new channels of communication were established to ensure that all staff in both organizations were kept adequately informed of plans.

In late 1974, UNDP undertook an internal study to explore new dimensions in technical cooperation (UNDP interoffice memorandum PRO/301/ND, 23 October 1974). A provocative internal memorandum was sent to all resident representatives that began by asking whether UNDP needed to 'redefine' its mandate. Numerous questions were asked to stimulate the resident representatives to propose changes in the way things were being done. The "increasing penetration of our preserve by the [World] Bank" might suggest that "joint financing" with the Bank would be worth exploring. The example provided was that of rural development, a subject of such importance to WHO that it is addressed separately below. Considerable attention was given to the importance of building national infrastructures as quickly as possible, "even if it means financing the establishment of such institutions or breaking them in so to speak for a certain number of years." Social infrastructure had to be addressed as well. It was also questioned whether "major areas" such as "the control of disease" were not being neglected.

As a result of this internal review, "new dimensions in technical cooperation" were introduced in 1975. While the consensus of 1970 was reaffirmed, much greater emphasis was placed on promotion of "self-reliance in developing countries by building up their productive capability and their indigenous resources and by increasing the availability of the managerial, technical, administrative and research capabilities required in the development process". Furthermore, technical cooperation "should be seen in terms of output or the results to be achieved, rather than in terms of inputs", and increased support should be given to programmes for technical cooperation among developing countries, a dimension that grew out of the debate on the 'new international economic order', as discussed below, the aim of which was to help developing countries strengthen their national capacity, such as manpower, institutions, contracting firms and procurement services, so that they in turn could assist other developing countries. While UNDP's relation with the World Bank and the importance of "social infrastructure" were mentioned in the decision of the General Assembly on this subject (United Nations General Assembly resolution 3405 (XXX), adopted in November 1975), the UNDP Administrator was requested to "give special consideration to the recruitment of experts, consultants and subcontractors from developing countries" and to "intensify ... efforts to achieve full utilization of national institutions in developing countries and the building-up of new capacities in those countries ....." (United Nations General Assembly resolution 3461 (XXX), adopted in December 1975).

The Director-General, addressing the UNDP Governing Council in June 1975, reiterated his strong support for the direction taken. WHO, he said, "is ready to accept the decisive coordinating role of a continuously strengthened UNDP. Coordination implies essentially leadership in social and economic development aimed at bringing the right solution to the right problems with the right amount and quality of resources at the right time and place .... Leadership implies also UNDP's dynamic capacity to provide a consistent stimulant for thought and action by pioneering in the solution of difficult problems and by daring to innovate in the face of conventional wisdom." It was his sincere hope "that we are moving into a new era in which technical assistance lollipops, that may taste so good but are so bad for the development teeth, become anathema and instead will yield to programmes and projects whose success or failure will be measured in their degree of impact on the growth potential for social and economic progress." (*10*)

Not all the United Nations agencies shared the Director-General's conviction. The Food and Agricultural Organization of the United Nations (FAO), the World Bank and the United Nations had come to believe that UNDP should concentrate on its role of collecting funds and ensuring that they were spent intelligently. WHO, with UNESCO and to some extent the International Labour Organization (ILO), remained convinced, however, that UNDP should take clear leadership within the United Nations system for elaborating development policies and processes and coordinating the involvement of all agencies concerned. Nevertheless, as recognized in 1976 by Mr Bradford Morse, UNDP Executive Director, important problems remained. There had not been adequate consultation for country programming, and the programmes themselves had been less than had been hoped for in the consensus. Urgent action was required to determine how joint programming could be made more useful to countries. One way proposed by WHO was the establishment of an interagency working group on government execution at UNDP headquarters (unpublished note on UNDP–agency consultations, 16–17 September 1976).

This proposal, too, met with opposition from those agencies that did not wish UNDP to become a leader in the field of development. Nevertheless, by the end of 1977, ILO and UNESCO had joined WHO as members of this working group, while the United Nations and the United Nations Industrial Development Organization (UNIDO) indicated "expressions of interest" (*11*). The Director-General stressed the role of the working group as a development forum—a role that did not exist in the United Nations system. It was intended to ensure a continuous flow of policies from WHO through UNDP to the resident representatives, thus ensuring that health concerns were adequately promoted at country level (*12*). Dr Mahler had earlier spoken on this subject in a speech at the United Nations (February 1976), where he had argued that a central policy body was needed to set broad global priorities and to arrive at a coherent, comprehensive set of common strategic approaches, both international and national, that could be extended by "formation of joint United Nations-system planning and programming teams, through secondment of staff members for the various sectoral subsystems" (unpublished statement to the second session of the Ad hoc Committee on the Restructuring of the United Nations in the Economic and Social Sectors, United Nations, New York, 13 February 1976). In that paper, he indicated that the UNDP could "undoubtedly, with the necessary political support, muster the creative energies required for this leadership role".

Despite WHO's continued support, the Director-General, 1 year later, began to express doubts about the ability of the UNDP to fulfil the role envisioned in the consensus. In a letter to Bradford Morse, written in March 1977 and copied to all agency heads, Dr Mahler asked, "are we going to do what we think has to be done, together or separately? ... Can the UNDP assume [a] central coordinating and funding role all alone?" Revealingly, he continued:

> The Consensus launched the concept of country programming as the cornerstone of the system. In practice, however, country programming—and for that matter regional programming—has not yielded the results expected. Overall policies and priorities have really not made themselves felt in the programmes; medium-term projections which have been assiduously elaborated within the governing organs of some of the agencies are not reflected in the country programmes. Where are the sectoral delineations we hoped to see? Where is the anticipated integration in the country programmes of other inputs—for instance, WHO's own regular programme, not to mention those of various funds, the banks or bilateral sources?

Addressing the Inter-Agency Consultative Board in April 1977, he noted that if the system were to move away from "the present piece-meal approach to development assistance", it was essential that the issues involved be brought to the attention of the UNDP Governing Council, the Economic and Social Council and the United Nations General Assembly. It was time that member governments defined exactly what they expected from the United Nations system, even if this made them realize the weaknesses that they themselves had contributed to the system. Only if governments could overcome their own contradictions and hesitations would it be possible to obtain support for the kind of development that was needed over the next 20–30 years, in order to close the gap between the haves and the have nots. He considered that UNDP had a clear duty to move away from being an aggregator of random experiences to become a promoter of development doctrine (*11*).

These same issues dominated the Inter-Agency Consultative Board meeting in October 1977. The UNDP Administrator said there was no clear demarcation of the responsibilities of the agencies and UNDP for development or with regard to overall contributions to and planning of technical assistance, while the Director-General noted that governments considered that they could benefit more from the system if they could deal with the United Nations family as a whole rather than individually. Dr Mahler called upon the Board to define its own attitude and strategy for making progress in the system along the lines of the new international economic order. WHO was taking steps to plan activities in the context of country socioeconomic development plans that were funded from its regular budget, to ensure a less confused and less distorted programme (*11*).

The Inter-Agency Consultative Board was unable to resolve the issues that divided the agencies. FAO, for example, took a conservative stand in the debates, stressing its near independence from UNDP resources, rules and regulations. In any case, a parallel development had radically altered the situation. The Ad Hoc Committee on the Restructuring of the Economic and Social Sectors of the United Nations System, set up at the seventh special session of the United Nations General Assembly in 1975, had prepared its report, which the Thirty-second General Assembly acted on in December 1977 (United Nations General Assembly resolution 32/197).

While UNDP country programming was still to be used as the frame of reference for operational activities carried out and financed by the organizations of the United Nations system from their own resources, overall responsibility for and coordination of operational activities for development at the country level "should be entrusted to a single official to be designated taking into account the sectors of particular interest to the countries of assignment, in consultation with and with the consent of the Government concerned". This official "should exercise team leadership and be responsible for evolving, at the country level, a multidisciplinary dimension in sectoral development assistance programmes". As for interagency coordination, the report left it to the General Assembly to consider "the establishment of a single governing body responsible for the management and control ... of United Nations operational activities for development". UNEP, UNICEF and the World Food Programme were "excluded" from this body.

Thus, the decade ended with matters very much as they had been at the beginning. New bodies and relations had to be established, a time- and resource-consuming process that did little to bolster confidence that the United Nations system was capable of taking a holistic approach to development that would fully integrate the social dimension with the economic. Nevertheless, as discussed next, a number or parallel initiatives were put forward by various organizations that kept the spirit of intersectoral coordination alive.

IMPORTANT UNITED NATIONS SYSTEM DEVELOPMENT INITIATIVES

Interagency anti-poverty rural development programme

In his address to the Board of Governors at the annual general meeting of the World Bank in Nairobi, Kenya, in September 1973, the Bank's President, Robert McNamara, proposed a strategy for rural development with an emphasis on the productivity of smallholder agriculture. He warned that official development assistance was inadequate and that over 800 million people lived in absolute poverty. In March 1975, the Bank announced that it planned to increase its assistance for agriculture and rural development greatly. *The assault on world poverty*, published several months later, examined ways in which poverty could be alleviated and outlined the programmes through which the Bank planned to help (*13*).

In 1974, the Administrative Committee on Coordination of the United Nations recommended that its organizations adjust their programmes in rural development to ensure that benefits accrued primarily to the rural poor. A task force headed by the World Bank was established in 1975, in which WHO participated. The Administrative Committee undertook a study of existing efforts in rural development, and WHO's contribution was a substantive report on health and rural development, published in late 1975 (*Health and rural development: main report*, Geneva, 1975, unpublished paper). The report subsequently served as background to the discussions held by the WHO governing bodies in 1976 on the subject (see Chapter 6).

It proved difficult to maintain the momentum of what initially seemed to be an important step in getting the various organizations concerned to work together. When, in 1976, the World Bank indicated that it would no longer be willing to serve as the lead agency, instead of selecting UNDP to take over this task, the Administrative Committee decided to rotate the responsibility on a yearly basis. On this occasion, the Director-General again stressed the importance of the programme, as it was marshalling "genuine intersectoral support for an important development activity ... for the first time". He had hoped the World Bank would continue as lead agency but supported UNDP when it became clear that the Bank would not continue in that role; when rotation of the role appeared to be receiving general support, Dr Mahler indicated that he "would support any group or agency that felt that it was capable of doing so", while noting that "in the past, the supremacy of one sector over all others had undermined rural development. That sector had been agriculture and it was worth noting that agricultural reforms had not been implemented." (*14*)

By the end of 1977, six countries had expressed interest in participating in the exercise: Bolivia, Lesotho, Liberia, Nepal, Samoa and Somalia. Dr Mahler interjected "a serious warning" at a meeting of the Administrative Committee concerning "the danger of the possible 'bureaucratization' of such exercises. It was important to understand clearly their purpose and to ensure that the countries themselves understood and appreciated these objectives." (*15*)

UNICEF's basic services approach

UNICEF, greatly concerned by the mid-decade impact of the economic and food crisis, gave urgent consideration to the question of how to improve the plight of children around the world, especially those living in the poorest countries. According to UNICEF, development was failing to reach large segments of the poor because existing services for health, education and agricultural extension were modelled on those of industrialized countries. Services rarely reached as far as the village, and, even when they did, they were usually disconnected from each other. Worse, they were often disconnected from the villagers' perceptions of their needs. As an alternative, a range of integrated basic services were proposed that would be flexible enough to be adapted by and within the community.

In 1976, the UNICEF Executive Board committed itself to the basic services approach. By this time, UNICEF and WHO were already well on the way to agreeing on an alternative approach to health care (see Chapters 6 and 15). Mr H.R. Labouisse, UNICEF Director, on the occasion of the sixty-seventh session of the Administrative Committee on Coordination, indicated that the basic services approach "would concentrate on local participation and local resources". At the same time, he expressed the wish that it would "eventually become part of a more comprehensive programme on an interagency basis" (*14*).

ILO and the basic needs approach to development

The notion of basic needs emerged in the 1970s in a variety of contexts. It was ILO, however, that made it a central theme of its programme following its 1976 World Employment Conference, where the satisfaction of basic human needs and the generation of employment had been discussed. That Conference had concluded that, if the aim of development was to make the basic necessities of life available to the majority of the population, a concentrated approach was called for that did not divert its attention to other aspects of development.

Basic needs were seen to be made up of two elements. First, they included the minimum requirements of a family for private consumption: adequate food, shelter and clothing, as well as household equipment and furniture. Second, they included essential services, such as safe drinking-water, sanitation, public health, educational and cultural facilities and public transport, somewhat along the lines of UNICEF's basic services.

The report of the Conference emphasized that a basic needs-oriented strategy "implies the participation of the people in making the decisions which affect them through organizations of their own choice" (*16*). For example, education and good health facilitate participation, and participation in turn strengthens the claim for basic material needs. Satisfaction of an absolute level of basic needs, the Conference concluded, should be placed within a broader framework, namely the fulfilment of basic human rights, which are not only ends in themselves but also contribute to the attainment of other goals. Basic needs were seen to constitute "the minimum objectives of society, not the full range of desirable attributes, many of which will inevitably take longer to attain".

GROWING DEMANDS FROM DEVELOPING COUNTRIES

In 1976, Dr Mahler stated: "The world was entering into a period where developed and developing countries would have their material interests increasingly linked in a form of international solidarity." (*17*) His optimistic view was based on the resolution adopted unanimously in September 1975 at the conclusion of the seventh special session of the United Nations General Assembly, which, in his introduction to *The work of WHO 1975*, he had characterized as a possible "turning-point in the history of the United Nations and international cooperation, since it marked a striking reversal of the previous climate of confrontation between the richer and the poorer countries" (*18*).

From the point of view of WHO, he continued, "the importance of the General Assembly's resolution cannot be overemphasized; it places the United Nations system at the centre of international cooperation and specifically calls upon WHO and its sister agencies to intensify the international effort aimed at improving health conditions in developing countries by giving priority to prevention of disease and malnutrition and by providing primary health services to the communities, including maternal and child health and family welfare."

The special session itself stemmed from earlier initiatives by various groups dedicated to improving the social and economic status of developing countries, in particular the Group of 77, which was established in 1964 when 77 developing countries signed a joint declaration issued at the end of the first session of the United Nations Conference on Trade and Development (UNCTAD). Although its membership had increased to more than 130 countries by the mid-1970s, it retained its original name because of its historical significance. As the largest Third World coalition in the United Nations, the Group of 77 aimed at enhancing the negotiating capacity of the developing countries on all major international issues addressed within the United Nations system. As discussed in Chapter 2, it played a major role in shaping WHO's approach to technical cooperation.

A major earlier milestone, one that the Director-General also lauded, was the establishment of a 'new international economic order', in a resolution adopted in December 1974 by the United Nations General Assembly (United Nations General Assembly resolution GA3201 (S-VI)). Health did not feature specifically in this resolution; its importance for WHO lay in the call for correcting inequalities and redressing existing injustices, thus making it possible "to eliminate the widening gap between the developed and the developing countries and [to] ensure steadily accelerating economic and social development and peace and justice for present and future generations".

In his addresses to three of WHO's regional committees in the autumn of 1975, Dr Mahler chose the subject 'health for all by the year 2000', to stimulate reflections on how WHO could contribute to the new international economic order, or, as he preferred to call it, a "new development order" (19). To find new ways for improving the distribution of health throughout the world, health must be considered in the broader context of its contribution to social development. To appreciate better what is implied by such development, he introduced the notion of social poverty, which he described as "a pernicious combination of unemployment and underemployment, economic poverty, scarcity of worldly goods, a low level of education, poor housing, poor sanitation, malnutrition, ill health, social apathy, and lack of the will and the initiative to make changes for the better". It was a "moral imperative of the new economic and social order that countries give health promotion its rightful place in all social and economic development."

The reawakening of interest in health promotion could be harnessed to other aspects of social development: nutrition with food production, education in health matters with individual and community self-learning in general, and protection of homes against disease vectors with a general improvement in the standard of cleanliness in the home and its surroundings. Health professionals would need to broaden their functions and apply their knowledge and skills to the most pressing social needs. Ministries of health would need to develop and support policies based on an "interlinked process—local needs giving rise to central responses and social needs giving rise to technical responses".

Dr Mahler used this occasion to introduce some of the other important ideas that marked his leadership, as discussed in subsequent chapters: strengthening of regional committees to make them the "supreme political coordinating forum for all regional health matters"; new mechanisms to ensure that bilateral and multilateral cooperation for health is channelled into programmes that conform to the country's priorities in health in such a way as to "promote national initiative rather than to smother it"; and collaboration between WHO and Member States to adapt health technology appropriate for the political, social and economic climate of each country.

References

1. *Official records of the World Health Organization*, No. 232 (EB57/SR/26). Geneva, World Health Organization, 1976.
2. *Health effects of possible use of chemical and biological weapons, report of the Director General* (EB45/18 Add.1). Geneva, World Health Organization, 1970.
3. *Health aspects of human rights in the light of scientific and technological development* (EB55/41). Geneva, World Health Organization, 1975.
4. *United Nations Second Development Decade: mid-term review and appraisal. Report of the Director-General* (EB55/44). Geneva, World Health Organization, 1975.
5. *The integration of women in development. Statement by the World Health Organization prepared for the Inter-regional Meeting of Experts on the Participation of Women in Development* (MCH/72.3). Geneva, World Health Organization, 1972.
6. *A study of the capacity of the United Nations development system*, Vol. 1 (DP/5). Geneva, United Nations, 1969.
7. *Report of the WHO representatives at the IACB meeting in New York 18–19 and 27 October 1972* (CPD/73.1). Geneva, World Health Organization, 1973.
8. *Report of the WHO representatives at the WGAFM, PWG and the IACB meetings in New York, 15–25 October 1972* (CPD/73.8). Geneva, World Health Organization, 1973.
9. The constitutional mission of the World Health Organization. *WHO Chronicle*, 1974, 28:308–311.
10. *Report of the representatives of the Director-General to the twentieth session of the Governing Council of the United Nations Development Programme, Geneva, 11–27 June 1975* (CPD/75.6). Geneva, World Health Organization, 1975.
11. *Report of the WHO representatives at the WGAFM, PWG and the IACB meetings in New York, 17–27 October 1977* (CPD/77.5). Geneva, World Health Organization, 1977.
12. *Official records of the World Health Organization*, No. 232 (EB57/SR/27). Geneva, World Health Organization, 1976.
13. World Bank. *The assault on world poverty: problems of rural development, education and health*, Baltimore, The Johns Hopkins University Press, 1975.
14. Administrative Committee on Coordination. Document coordination/SR.67.1. New York, United Nations, 1976.
15. Administrative Committee on Coordination. Document coordination/SR.69.4. New York, United Nations, 1977.
16. International Labour Office. *The basic needs approach to development: some issues regarding concepts and methodology*. Geneva, 1977.
17. *Official records of the World Health Organization*, No. 232 (EB57/SR/22). Geneva, World Health Organization, 1976.
18. *The work of WHO 1975. Official records of the World Health Organization*, No. 229. Geneva, World Health Organization, 1975.
19. Mahler H. Health for all by the year 2000. *WHO Chronicle*, 1975, 29:457–461.

CHAPTER 2

Governing bodies

All WHO's work is guided by decisions taken by its governing bodies: the World Health Assembly and the Executive Board. The Health Assembly is composed of delegates representing Member States (Members), while the Board is made up of persons designated by Members selected by the Health Assembly for that purpose. WHO's secretariat, the third element specified by WHO's Constitution, comprises the Director-General and such technical and administrative staff as the Organization may require.

The Health Assembly meets once a year, usually in May. It determines the policies of the Organization, reviews the activities of the Board and the secretariat, instructs the Board to undertake actions or studies, reviews and approves the budget, and considers recommendations bearing on health made by the United Nations in order to determine what steps should be taken by the Organization to give effect to those recommendations.

The Board acts as the executive organ of the Health Assembly, giving effect to its decisions and policies. It meets twice a year, usually in January, at its main session, and immediately after the Health Assembly, when it meets for only a few days. The Board submits to the Health Assembly for its consideration and approval a general programme of work covering a specific period. The fourth such programme covered 1967–1971 and the fifth, 1972–1977. Thus, establishment of the Sixth General Programme of Work, as discussed in Chapter 3, was an important activity in this decade. The Board can also submit advice or proposals to the Health Assembly on its own initiative.

Article 29 of the Constitution further stipulates that the Board shall exercise on behalf of the Health Assembly the powers delegated to it by that body. Article 38 provides the Board with the authority to establish such committees as are considered to be desirable to serve any purpose within the competence of the Organization.

EXECUTIVE BOARD ORGANIZATIONAL STUDY ON COORDINATION WITH THE UNITED NATIONS AND ITS SPECIALIZED AGENCIES

As spelt out in WHO's Fourth General Programme of Work (*1*), covering the period 1967–1971:

> There is a need to coordinate activities in the health field with other economic and social development activities, thus bringing into focus the importance of the health element in balanced national socio-economic development. Meanwhile, the Organization must also exercise its constitutional function as the coordinating authority on international health work and therefore collaborate closely with all those agencies, intergovernmental, governmental and non-governmental, which work in the health field.

WHO has certain obligations with respect to the United Nations and the other specialized agencies, as illustrated in part by various examples in Chapter 1. Numerous bodies, as well as mechanisms, are involved in coordinating the activities of the United Nations system as a whole. So complex had the coordination process become by the end of the 1960s that it was said that Dr Candau groaned audibly when his assistant brought in the huge stacks of papers relevant to this item when it came up for discussion during the meetings of the WHO governing bodies!

The interaction between WHO and the United Nations system represents the single most important issue of coordination, and it is continuously reviewed by both the Board and the Health Assembly. The Board had conducted an organizational study on this topic in 1960[1]. In 1967, the Twentieth World Health Assembly decided (resolution WHA20.49) that it was time for the Board to review this important subject again. The original intention was that the study would take 1 year; an extra year was added to allow the Board's working group to complete the task. Important developments within the United Nations system itself, especially the 'capacity study' described in Chapter 1, further encouraged the group to make as complete a study of the subject as possible. The final report (2) was some 120 pages long, which led one Board Member to note, when it was discussed in January 1970, that it "was the most detailed document ever produced on the United Nations".

The main conclusion of the working group was that "coordination was one of the essential techniques for achieving the Organization's basic aims" (3). Nevertheless, as several Board Members pointed out, the burden placed on the secretariat was enormous. Some 2% of the budget was estimated to be taken up by coordination. Surely, suggested one Member, simpler methods could be found for working effectively with other organizations.

The Director-General, in his response, pointed out that the Administrative Committee on Coordination had been examining ways and means of improving its own methods of work, but that it had become "increasingly difficult to discuss matters effectively" owing to the fact that it had grown from a comparatively small body to one of about 20 people. Furthermore, the United Nation's own operations had expanded considerably, particularly in the economic and social sphere. He could provide a list of subjects—population and water supply, to name but two—for which there were common areas of understanding, "of which perhaps the best was that between WHO and UNICEF".

Once it had completed its examination of the subject, the Board adopted resolution EB45.R34, which highlights the main conclusions that had emerged from the report and the discussions of the Board. To the report's conclusion that coordination was a necessity were added one on the need for the Organization to "continue to emphasize the role of health as a fundamental factor of human well-being and as an inseparable element of the development process", another on how coordination "should be so devised as to ensure maximum effectiveness without imposing excessive burdens upon the Organization" and one emphasizing that coordination at the country level "remains the key factor in the success of health

---

[1] The first such study dates back to the Second World Health Assembly, in June 1949, which asked the Board "to examine the organizational structure [of the Organization] so that the third World Health Assembly may be assisted in ensuring the administrative efficiency of the Organization and establishing general lines of policy in this respect". In 1957, the Board requested the Health Assembly to decide whether such studies might not be deferred. The Tenth Health Assembly in resolution WHA10.36 rejected that proposal and decided that they should be continued. This policy has been maintained.

development programmes". To the latter point was added the stipulation that "the major role in such coordination devolves upon the governments themselves, as only they can determine the nature and amount of external assistance from multilateral or bilateral sources to be devoted to their health needs".

The Twenty-third World Health Assembly, in May 1970, concurred with the Board's findings and conclusions in resolution WHA23.25 and requested the Director-General "to continue his participation in coordination arrangements of the United Nations system with a view to assuring the Organization's full contribution to the overall effort to attain for all peoples the full enjoyment of their economic, social and human rights".

The Board's study on coordination was followed by three further studies, which are discussed in Chapter 3: in 1975, a study of interrelations between the central technical services of WHO and programmes of direct assistance to Member States; in 1975, a study on planning for and the impact of extrabudgetary resources on WHO's programmes and policy; and, in 1977, one on WHO's role at country level, particularly the role of WHO representatives. Another important study carried out by the Board during this decade was on methods of promoting basic health services. Conducted in 1971–1973, it set the stage for the concept of primary health care, described in Chapter 6.

METHOD OF WORK

Early in the history of WHO, attempts were made to alter the frequency with which the Health Assembly met, to at least once in every 2 years instead of annually. Although this proposal was pursued throughout the 1950s, it failed to gather the necessary support. Other changes in the manner in which both bodies carried out their duties, which had been under continuous review from the first years of the Organization's existence, were explored during this decade. These covered the duration of the sessions of the Health Assembly, how the general discussions of the Assembly should be conducted, the rules of procedure to be followed and how the work of the Assembly might be conducted by committees meeting in parallel.

A number of alternatives were explored for each of these questions. With respect to the Health Assembly, the main development was the establishment of two committees (A and B) that, if necessary, could meet simultaneously. Committee A would deal mostly with programme and budget matters, while B would deal with administration, finance and legal matters. Speakers were asked to limit the length of their interventions in the committees. Technical discussions were scheduled to take place at the end of the first week, at which time neither of the committees would meet.

Another innovation was the introduction of a biennial programme and budget. The desirability of a system of biennial programming was agreed to in principle in 1969, but only in 1972 were steps taken to introduce this change. As it involved amendments to the Constitution (deletion of references to a particular budgetary period), it had to be approved by two-thirds of the Members before it could be adopted. This occurred in February 1977, and the Thirtieth World Health Assembly that year adopted resolution WHA30.20, which directed that the first biennium for which biennial budgeting could become effective was 1980–1981.

The change to a system of biennial programming was part of a broader initiative to promote long-term planning and improved evaluation, as called for in resolution WHA22.53, adopted in 1969. Although the resolution focused on improving the programming used by WHO, it noted that realistic long-term planning of WHO's programme depended on methodical health planning, formulation of a budget based on programmes and evaluation at national level. The resolution also called for the Director-General to collaborate actively in promoting the health sector aspects of the broad international strategy for the Second Development Decade and to explore further the feasibility of providing appropriate long-term financial indicators. The immediate effect of this resolution was different types of financial reports, including more detailed projections of the Organization's programme and budget.

As programme planning and budgeting became more complex, the Director-General proposed changes in the Board's and the Health Assembly's approach to reviewing the proposed programme budget, to ensure "a more active participation and involvement of the Board in the Organization's work and the programme as well as allow the Health Assembly more time for the consideration and formulation of broad programme and policy directions" (4). These proposals were judged to be in conformity with the provisions of Articles 55 and 56 of the WHO Constitution. Article 55 stipulates that the Director-General shall prepare and submit to the Board the budget estimates of the Organization, which the Board will then consider and submit to the Health Assembly with its recommendations, while Article 56 stipulates that the Health Assembly shall review and approve the budget estimates "subject to any agreement between the Organization and the United Nations".

In the process proposed and elaborated with the assistance of an ad hoc committee of the Executive Board, the Board's representative to the Health Assembly would play a more dynamic role in the Assembly's review of programme budget proposals and would then submit the programme budget, outline and explain the Board's comments and recommendations, and, with the assistance of the secretariat, answer questions on policy matters put by delegations. Furthermore, in order to encourage Assembly Members to focus their comments on policy issues, Committee A's review of the programme budget would begin with a review of the Executive Board's report, and the "review of specific technical matters" would be a separate agenda item, during which issues unrelated to policy could be discussed. These changes were introduced in 1977.

ESTABLISHING THE PROGRAMME BUDGET BEFORE RESOLUTION WHA29.48

The period chosen to illustrate this function is 1975–1977, when the demands made on the Organization multiplied in scope and complexity, as noted above. The world economy was still shaken by currency instability and high rates of inflation, which caused serious budgetary problems. Furthermore, considerable cost increases were incurred by a United

Nations-wide adjustment of professional salaries and allowances, something that was totally beyond the control of the Organization.

A brief discussion, in January 1975, about whether the Board should consider where savings might be made, led the Director-General to express the hope that "at the appropriate time the Board would be willing to discuss with the secretariat which sectors of the programme should be cut down and which enlarged, and at least to indicate which it considered to be the most important directions in which future efforts should be oriented". The secretariat, he said, "was constantly finding itself obliged to make drastic economies simply to keep abreast of current commitment, and thus there was virtually nothing left in reserve for innovation" (5).

The Board then went on to review the proposed programme budget for 1976 and 1977, in anticipation of the biennium cycle that was being implemented. In introducing this budget, the Director-General said he was "acutely aware that the document before the Board reflected the Organization's difficulties in moving from an input-oriented accountancy-type budget towards an output-oriented programme budget—and there was still a very long way to go". He had no doubt, however, that the Health Assembly's decision to move in that direction was already having positive repercussions on planning, programming and evaluation at all levels of the Organization.

The Members reacted favourably to the proposed budget, judging it to reflect the revitalized coordination role of WHO, which all accepted. They also welcomed the introduction of country health programming (see Chapter 3) as a basic pillar of the Organization's coordination role. Some indicated, however, that it was still not clear how WHO should fulfil that role. Others warned that the Organization should not generalize its approach, using the example of the national health councils that WHO was promoting widely. Instead, they proposed that "working programmes should vary depending on the country's level of development".

A new element was introduced in the 1976–1977 budget: the Director-General's Development Programme. Furthermore, considerably more attention was given than in previous years to how the Organization should evaluate its activities. The Director-General, commenting on the latter, said that. "provided there existed a will to work with evaluation as a continuous process, there would be progress.... Evaluation was a difficult matter .... It was important not to lose heart merely because the evaluation had not been sufficiently comprehensive .... A serious effort was however being made, despite problems of methodology, and he was convinced that as a result of country health programming WHO's efforts could be more effectively geared to country priorities".

The Twenty-eighth World Health Assembly, in May 1975, discussed the Board's report and adopted three related resolutions, WHA28.75, WHA28.76 and WHA28.77. Resolution WHA28.76 stated that WHO "should give increased priority to the provision of direct, immediate and adequate assistance and services to the developing countries" and that "the regular programme budget shall ensure a substantial increase, in real terms, of technical assistance and services for developing countries from 1977 to the end of the Second Development Decade". The strong link with United Nations resolutions on establishment of the new international economic order was spelt out in the introductory paragraphs. Resolutions WHA28.75 and WHA28.77 addressed assistance to developing countries.

WHA28.75 noted with satisfaction that WHO was "paying constant attention to the public health needs of the developing countries ...". It identified the main ways in which assistance was to be given:

1. assistance in establishing and strengthening national public health systems, which form an integral part of overall social and economic development;
2. assistance in training the national public health staff at all levels that is essential for providing the populations with adequate medical and sanitary care;
3. assistance in developing effective methods of disease prevention and control which should provide a scientific methodological basis for any programme to be carried out in the countries, this being a guarantee of success in disease control; and
4. the drawing up of recommendations for establishing norms and standards, including disease classification, criteria for evaluating the condition of the environment, methods of safeguarding the environment and making it healthier, the *International Pharmacopoeia*, biological preparations, etc.

Resolution WHA28.77 requested the Director-General to increase WHO's role in co-ordinating and catalysing the provision of long-term and soft credits by international financing agencies to countries planning to extend health services to their entire population and to provide technical assistance to countries in fulfilling the technical requirements of the international financing agencies.

The Director-General in his report to the Board in January 1976 (*6*) outlined the initial measures proposed to give immediate effect to the wishes of the Health Assembly. He said that the measures "should be regarded as precursors of more extensive changes to be reflected in the proposed budget for 1978/1979", which was then being prepared. Perhaps in recognition of the tendency on the part of some Member States to see WHO simply as an assistance agency, he added,

> ... it must be recognized that WHO is a permanent health organization of all countries and has to be involved in the health developments of interest in all parts of the world if it is to fulfil the important mission of helping mankind develop national global health policies and ensure the protection of future generations. It follows therefore that WHO must have the machinery, structure and staff to provide the necessary collaboration and information in support of both the coordinating and technical cooperation roles of WHO in international health work.

The measures outlined were to use newly acquired funds to augment technical cooperation in several regions and a net increase of US$ 2 million in regional allocations for 1977, to be made directly available to the countries most in need. The establishment of regional directors' development programmes was proposed, to meet special needs arising outside the conventional planning cycle.

In his introduction on this subject to the Board at its fifty-seventh session, in January 1976, the Director-General noted that, in view of the emphasis placed by resolution WHA28.76 on technical cooperation and the intent to ensure a substantial increase in such assistance and services in the coming years, an attempt had been made to establish a baseline of information that could be used for comparisons and to measure future trends. A "rather pragmatic" approach had been used to identify activities that were primarily related to technical cooperation.

The Members of the Board endorsed use of the term 'technical cooperation' in preference to 'technical assistance' and recommended that it be used uniformly by the Board, the Health Assembly, the regional committees and others throughout the Organization. The term 'assistance' "carried with it outdated connotations of donor and recipient relationships which no longer existed, and the term 'cooperation' better expressed the newer collaborative relationships between Member States and *their* health organization" (7).

RESOLUTION WHA29.48: "ONE OF THE MOST IMPORTANT POLITICAL DECISIONS IN THE HISTORY OF THE ORGANIZATION"

Nearly all the major resolutions adopted by the Health Assembly on WHO's budget are rooted in earlier discussions, in particular those of the Board's January sessions. Resolution WHA29.48 was an important exception.

The Group of 77 appeared to have decided in the interim period that the 'substantial increase' referred to in resolution WHA28.76 should be defined more precisely. In May 1976, a draft resolution was introduced by one of the members of the Group, which had "the full approval of the Group of 77". It asked the Director-General to reorient the work of the Organization with a view to ensuring that allocations from the regular programme budget for technical cooperation and provision of services reached a level of at least 60% in real terms by 1980. Four means for achieving this goal were identified: (i) cutting down on all avoidable and inessential expenditure for establishment and administration, both at headquarters and in the regional offices; (ii) streamlining professional and administrative work; (iii) phasing out projects that had outlived their usefulness; and (iv) making optimal use of the technical and administrative resources available in individual developing countries.

In justifying this request, the resolution noted "with deep concern the increasing allocation of resources of the Organization towards establishment and administrative costs", as well as expressing concern with the "widening gap between the health levels of the developed and developing countries".

The resulting discussion was tense and at time tendentious. Several representatives from outside the Group questioned the necessity for fixing a percentage: it was "undesirable", "a difficult operation", "premature", "arbitrary" and one that might "produce rigidity in programmes". The resolution appeared to show "divisions appearing in the Assembly". One speaker even suggested that adoption of such a resolution "would lead to discarding the carefully prepared Sixth General Programme of Work which the Committee had just approved". Other representatives from outside the Group questioned the reference to the 'widening gap' in terms of health levels. Resolution WHA28.76 referred to the need to "eliminate the widening gap between the developed and the developing countries" without any specific reference to "health levels".

Delegates from countries in the Group of 77 replied in various ways, some aggressively and some using the opportunity to explain carefully why they considered that further action was needed in this area. One representative expressed resentment that staff costs for 1977 had risen by nearly US$ 10 million over those for 1976 (due to the United Nations-wide salary increase, as noted earlier). Additional funds "should go towards the betterment of living conditions of the people in Member States rather than to improving the conditions of the international civil servants themselves and maintaining a top-heavy Organization". Another pointed out that the draft resolution was "the minimum acceptable".

A number of amendments were proposed. All were defeated by votes that ranged from 79 to 5 to 69 to 27. The draft resolution (resolution WHA29.48) was approved by 82 votes to none, with 26 abstentions.

The Director-General, who had remained silent during the discussion, said "that in approving the draft resolution, the Committee ... had taken one of the most important political decisions in the history of the Organization. Its capacity to respond to that decision depended on its past reputation. He had been slightly pained at the tendency to classify the activities of WHO as being on a par with those of other agencies in the United Nations system, whereas Member States had made WHO a unique organization in the whole international field". Later in his statement, he stressed the importance of underlining "the unity of purpose between the World Health Assembly, the Executive Board, Member States and the Secretariat. Such cohesion must exist between all levels of the Organization, between headquarters, regional offices and the field, and between regions. The Organization must never become a federation of six distinct regions with some vague entity at the central level as that would spell the end of WHO". He concluded by indicating how he intended to implement the resolution. First, "he welcomed the new programme budget policy reorientation ... because it reinforced his own efforts to reduce non-relevant and non-productive expenditure in WHO .... Secondly, he saw the fixed percentage of 60% as an initial target towards which the Director-General, with the full participation of the Executive Board, should work to strengthen the work of WHO .... Thirdly, the effect of the resolution must be to strengthen technical cooperation programmes at all levels of the Organization and not to fragment or weaken such technical cooperation or coordination of international health work at any one level."

Shortly after this session of the Health Assembly, the Director-General reported to WHO staff at headquarters on the significance of the resolution (Mahler H. *Director-General's address on programme budget policy to meeting of senior staff, 8 June 1976*, unpublished document). He stressed that WHO must make "much greater use of many nongovernmental organizations". He used the relation between the International Union against Tuberculosis and WHO to illustrate how a nongovernmental organization could take on greater responsibility as an "information and executive project agent". He suggested that a similar approach be taken by other programmes. For the area of primary health care and rural development, he advised: "spend as little time as possible at headquarters elaborating theory ... [and, instead] identify countries that would be interested in testing newer programme concepts...."

AFTER RESOLUTION WHA29.48

Resolution EB58.R11, adopted by the Board at its fifty-eighth session, immediately after the Twenty-ninth World Health Assembly, in May 1976, called for establishment of a programme committee of the Board that would advise the Director-General on the necessary policy and strategy to respond effectively to resolutions WHA28.75, WHA28.76 and WHA29.48 on technical cooperation with developing countries and on programme budget policy. This committee, which consisted of nine members, met for 5 days later in the year.

In his introductory comments to the committee, the Director-General emphasized "the unity of the Organization" and the need for strong political determination to "ensure that the world's social periphery got a fairer share of health resources than was presently the case...". He considered that "this was precisely what resolution WHA29.48 ... aimed at doing". The strategy that he was proposing for reorienting WHO's work "was a faithful attempt to respond to the spirit of that resolution". The word 'spirit' should be emphasized because "the mere redistribution of WHO's regular budget would not suffice in itself to bring about the change that so many Member States clearly desired". Furthermore, if the Organization "were considered as a benevolent fund, distributing money or supplies, it was doomed to speedy disintegration. If, however, it were accepted in the way its Constitutions intended, namely as *the* international coordinating authority on health matters, it had a remarkable potential for catalysing the rapid improvement of health throughout its Member States" (*8*).

The programme committee held extensive discussions on the definition of 'technical cooperation'. On the one hand, there was a need for "pragmatic identification" of technical activities for measuring progress towards the 60% target. On the other hand, in order that the WHO culture "swing" towards technical cooperation, a "guiding concept" was desirable. In the latter context, the Director-General offered an interpretation of 'technical cooperation' as meaning "activities which have a high degree of social relevance for Member States in the sense that they are directed towards defined national health goals and that they will contribute directly and significantly to the improvement of the health status of their populations through methods that they can apply now and at a cost they can afford now" and which conformed to the principle and aim of "developing national self-reliance in matters of health".

Various components of the WHO programme were reviewed. While four new programmes were judged "unequivocally" to be technical cooperation—Emergency Relief Operations, the Expanded Programme on Immunization, the Special Programme for Research and Training in Tropical Diseases (TDR) and Prevention of Blindness—there was no consensus on such basic elements as the WHO representative, which provoked the suggestion that "consideration should be given to discontinuing their activities", if that was the case. The Committee considered that the matter should be discussed by the Board as a whole.

Although at its fifty-ninth meeting, in January 1977, the Executive Board endorsed the proposals of the Director-General concerning programme budget policy (resolution EB59.R9), remnants of the tensions that had divided the Twenty-ninth World Health Assembly were still felt. One Board Member said that the report of the programme committee "had not sufficiently reflected the spirit behind the new policy". One paragraph in particular gave the impression "that it was only the Director-General who was aware of the need for a social revolution in public health". Too much emphasis had been placed on the "painful effects of the implementation of the new strategy". If WHO was "to adopt a revolutionary policy, it must be ready to take revolutionary action to implement it". Mid-way through a paragraph-by-paragraph review of the report, the Director-General reacted to these comments by observing that "he had no desire to take credit: WHO was not a personality cult organization".

The Director-General's report on policy and strategy for technical cooperation spelt out in some detail how the 60% target was to be reached. It called for a reduction in the number of established posts, both at headquarters (313 such posts) and the regional offices (an additional 50 posts), which accounted for some 84% of the total reduction (US$ 13.5 million). Because of the biennial nature of the budget, the target date of 1981 was chosen, rather than 1980 as called for in resolution WHA29.48.

The Board, in resolution EB59R9, recommended approval of this strategy, affirming that it provided a "basis for full response" to the directives of resolutions WHA28.75, WHA28.76 and WHA29.68, and urged Member States "to collaborate and make full use of their Organization for the promotion of increased, effective technical cooperation in international health work", a recommendation that the Thirtieth World Health Assembly endorsed in its resolution WHA30.30.

TECHNICAL DISCUSSIONS

In 1950, the Executive Board decided, in resolution EB6.R47, that the technical discussions of the Health Assembly should consist of thorough discussion of a few subjects, with a view to applying existing knowledge in those fields to public health administration. Two issues were initially proposed for several of the assemblies, but only one was selected for discussion. It took a decade or so before a standard approach to the technical discussions was agreed upon. Resolution WHA10.33, adopted in 1957, set down several precepts, which have been more or less agreed to over subsequent decades:

1. The objective of discussions should be to provide an opportunity for an informal exchange of views and experience.
2. The subjects should be (a) of international interest, (b) of a general character suitable for group discussions by public-health administrators and (c) clearly defined.
3. Each topic should be selected 2 years in advance by the Board.
4. Appropriate documentation should be prepared by the Secretariat and distributed about 1 year in advance to Member States.
5. Appropriate nongovernmental organizations and, through governments, national organizations should be asked to participate in preparing the discussions.
6. The Board should appoint a general chairman who is nominated by the President of the Health Assembly.

7. Group discussions should be encouraged.
8. An account of the proceedings and a report of the discussions should be submitted by the General Chairman to a plenary meeting of the Health Assembly and published later.

The subjects chosen for the decade under review were as follows:

- 1968: national and global surveillance of communicable diseases;
- 1969: application of evolving technology to meet the health needs of people;
- 1970: education for health professionals and regional aspects of a universal problem;
- 1971: mass health examinations as a public health tool;
- 1972: the contribution of health programmes to socioeconomic development;
- 1973: organization, structure and functioning of health services and modern methods of administration;
- 1974: the role of the health services in preserving or restoring the full effectiveness of the human environment in the promotion of health;
- 1975: social and health aspects of sexually transmitted diseases and the need for a better approach;
- 1976: the health aspects of human settlements; and
- 1977: the importance of national and international food and nutrition policies for health development.

The informal nature of the discussions resulted in great variation from one year to the next. Thus, the degree to which their outcomes were important for the relevant technical programmes varied according to the time taken to collect background information, the degree to which Member States chose to engage the subject both in advance and during the Health Assembly and the nature of the conclusions reached. An outstanding example of useful technical discussions were those in 1968 on national and global surveillance of communicable diseases. These contributed directly to the reform that was being undertaken at the time, as described in Chapter 9 in the section dealing with the epidemiological surveillance of communicable diseases.

JOINT UNICEF/WHO COMMITTEE ON HEALTH POLICY STUDIES

The Joint UNICEF/WHO Committee on Health Policy, composed of members of the executive boards of both organizations, was established in 1948. At its first session, it decided on the relative roles of the two organizations in UNICEF health projects: UNICEF's role was to furnish supplies and services, while WHO would study and approve plans for health programmes in which both organizations were involved. By 1967, these projects absorbed some two-thirds of UNICEF's operational budget.

New terms of reference for the Joint Committee were established in 1960. Resolution EB25.R30 set its mandate as to review periodically the overall needs of mothers and children with regard to health and to recommend suitable health programmes to the UNICEF Board. It could also consider "any other matters of joint interest" that were referred to it. This opened the door to the conduct of in-depth, comprehensive studies of needs. Furthermore, whereas in the past there had been a tendency on the part of WHO to see the Joint Committee as a vehicle for transferring guidance to UNICEF, the studies in the 1970s were truly joint undertakings, both organizations giving as well as receiving. The sessions themselves usually took place in February, following the WHO Executive Board session, and they lasted for 2 days.

At its seventeenth session, held in February 1970, the Joint Committee spent a full day reviewing the "revised global strategy of malaria eradication" with the aim of recommending future joint UNICEF/WHO assistance for antimalaria activities. At its eighteenth session, in 1971, it reviewed UNICEF/WHO assistance in education and training, while at its nineteenth session, held the next year, it addressed trachoma control. It was during this session that a member of the UNICEF secretariat made a number of suggestions for topics to be discussed at the next session, which included examination of "the extent to which existing health services were able, in terms of their orientation, coverage, quality and community relationship, to fulfil the minimum role that Member States considered desirable" (9). This proposal, as discussed below and in Chapter 6, led to a study of alternative approaches to meeting basic health needs.

In 1972, a strong drive was made inside UNICEF for negotiation and initiation of country projects in various disciplines, regardless of whether the relevant specialized agency was participating in the operation. This move, which led to UNICEF recruiting its own expertise in health, altered the manner in which the two organizations reviewed subjects. UNICEF staff now participated more actively in health-related activities, as later reflected in their full involvement in preparation for the Alma-Ata conference (see Epilogue). The first step in this direction was the selection in July 1973 of the topic 'Promising approaches to meeting basic health needs' for the next Joint Committee study by the two secretariats. This led to the historically important publication *Alternative approaches to meeting basic health needs of populations in developing countries*, which was presented to the Joint Committee at its twentieth session, in 1975 (see Chapter 6). This was followed (1975–1977) by a joint study on *Community involvement in Primary Health Care: a study of the process of community motivation and continued participation*, and *The water supply and sanitation components of Primary Health Care programmes for 1977–79* (see Chapters 6 and 12, respectively).

EXPERT ADVISORY PANELS

One of the first resolutions adopted by the Executive Board (resolution EB1.R4) approved the establishment of expert committees for various technical programmes, with members drawn from expert advisory panels. The setting up and management of expert committees and panels are governed by regulations that are periodically reviewed by the Executive Board and the Health Assembly, as mandated by Articles 18(e) and 38 of the WHO Constitution.

The Board at its fifty-third session, in January 1974, requested the Director-General to prepare a report on the subject of appointments to expert advisory panels and committees. This report was reviewed by the Board at its fifty-sixth session, in May 1975 (10).

The introduction to the report noted the necessity to "reorient these panels to allow a genuine exchange of knowledge and experience gained in various socioeconomic contexts, so as to provide wide options for ultimate selection by the Member States themselves of the most appropriate methods of solving health problems". Moreover, the Fifth General Programme of Work was based on the "composite programme needs of countries rather than on the pursuit of separate health disciplines by the Organization". What was required was a "multidisciplinary approach to the solution of problems and an adequate organizational framework within countries to accommodate the integration of such diverse expertise".

Creation of regional expert advisory panels was proposed for consideration in order to counter the "danger of global expertise becoming increasingly divorced from the needs of the vast majority of the populations of the world". These panels could deal "at closer range with regional health problems and their implications at country level". The Executive Board, in an organizational study on the interrelations between the central technical services of WHO and programmes of direct assistance to Member States, had already concluded that there was a "greater need for involvement at regional and country levels" with regard to the subjects to be studied by expert bodies and "in being more responsible in the practical applications of the technical policies elaborated" (*11*).

The report concluded that any revision of the 44 expert advisory panels "should concentrate on adapting their composition to reflect more clearly the main programme trends and priorities of WHO". The number of panel members should be kept to a minimum, and the experts should be selected on a "wider disciplinary and geographical basis". The duration of appointment need no longer be fixed at 5 years; reappointment would follow only on the basis of "a positive evaluation of services rendered". It was proposed that the age limit be abolished and every attempt made to "seek young talented experts" and to "terminate the appointments of 'inactive' members".

While the Executive Board went on to congratulate the Director-General for his reports on the subject, it considered that there was no need to alter the regulations for expert advisory panels and committees, as their basic principles remained "fundamentally sound". The discussions of the Board itself indicated a lack of consensus on certain critical changes proposed. For example, one Member was "doubtful of the value of the proposal to make the appointment of the panel members flexible and to review the lists of panels more frequently". Another Member noted that the proposal to establish regional advisory panels "might lead to a hierarchy of experts, with regional experts and world experts", while a third indicated that it ran the risk of "creating a dual system that might be to the detriment of the existing expert committees as well as of any new regional committees developed".

OUTSTANDING ISSUES

It is not the purpose of this chapter to cover all aspects of the role of the governing bodies in the work of WHO, as these bodies touch on all of WHO's work, and references to their roles are to be found throughout this book. Nevertheless, it seems fitting to conclude with a description of a short discussion that took place during the fifty-fifth session of the

Executive Board, in January 1975, that illustrates the nature of the policy issues that the Board, as befits its executive role, was asking the Organization to address.

The setting was the Board's discussion of two subjects taken together: the role of WHO in bilateral and multilateral health aid programmes, and an organizational study on planning for and the impact of extrabudgetary resources on WHO's programmes and policy. Having reviewed the Director-General's paper on the former subject (*12*), the chairman of the Executive Board's working group responsible for the organizational study noted that the group considered that a "certain number of matters" should be examined in more detail:

> ... the relationship between health, economic and social development and the plans of health ac-
> tivities in bilateral and multilateral aid; the importance of coordination, at the national level,
> between ministries of health and the bodies dealing with such aid in both donor and recipient
> countries; its coordinating role in countries where there was no WHO representative; ways of
> bringing WHO's efforts in regard to long-term planning to the situation of the bodies that rendered
> aid; and the approach to be adopted by WHO in drawing up detailed programmes, which should
> be drawn to the attention of Member countries and other organizations, including whose within
> the United Nations system. (*13*)

Other members of the Executive Board added further points, as well as indicating some of the difficulties inherent in WHO fulfilling its coordinating role fully, as called for in its Constitution.

As it was countries' responsibility to support the coordinating efforts of external donors, it was of paramount importance that each country have a "determined will" to pursue such a policy, if WHO were to play its full role in bringing together all the potentially available resources. The mechanisms that countries might use to fulfil their role should be clearly spelt out. Coordination with national staff as well as with those of bilateral and multilateral donors could put the Organization in a situation "that might prove difficult to get out of". Furthermore, the involvement of branches of a country's administration other than the health branch in implementation of programmes might prove difficult. It was essential that WHO country representatives, who would be mainly responsible for coordination, be fully tuned into headquarters' policy if they were to meet their new obligations.

To help the Organization improve links with other funding agencies, including non-governmental organizations and private donor foundations, WHO was urged to prepare its programme of work in such a way that it clearly stated its priorities and important fields of endeavour, to encourage the various organizations to allocate money for causes that WHO considered important. A certain tension can be discerned between the desire for strategies to be sensitive to the real needs of Member States and the desire to maintain a coherent set of priorities decided upon at global level by the Organization's governing bodies. These and related questions are further discussed in Chapter 3.

References

1. *Fourth General Programme of Work covering a specified period 1967–1971 inclusive. Official records of the World Health Organization*, No. 143, Annex 3. Geneva, World Health Organization, 1965.

2. *Review of the organizational study on coordination with the United Nations and the specialized agencies* (EB45/4). *Official records of the World Health Organization*, No. 181, Annex 4. Geneva, World Health Organization, 1970.

3. *Executive Board, 45th session, summary records* (EB45/SR/5). Geneva, World Health Organization, 1970.

4. *Report of the Ad Hoc Committee of the Executive Board on method of work of the Health Assembly and of the Executive Board. Official records of the World Health Organization*, No. 238, Annex 1. Geneva, World Health Organization, 1977.

5. *Official records of the World Health Organization* No. 224 (EB55/SR/4). Geneva, World Health Organization, 1975.

6. *Review of proposed programme budget for 1976–1977 (financial year 1977). Revised programme budget proposals. Report of the Director-General* (EB57/6), Appendix 1. Geneva, World Health Organization, 1976.

7. *Report on the proposed programme budget for 1976–1977 (financial year 1977). Official records of the World Health Organization*, No. 231. Geneva, World Health Organization, 1976.

8. *Report of the Programme Committee of the Executive Board. Official records of the World Health Organization*, No. 238, Appendix 1. Geneva, World Health Organization, 1977.

9. *Report of the nineteenth Joint UNICEF/WHO Committee on Health Policy* (JC19/UNICEF-WHO/MIN/72.4). Geneva, World Health Organization, 1972.

10. *Expert advisory panels. Special report by the Director-General. Official records of the World Health Organization*, No. 228, Annex 1. Geneva, World Health Organization, 1975.

11. *Organizational study on the interrelationships between the central services of WHO and programmes of direct assistance to Member States. Official records of the World Health Organization*, No. 223, Part I, Annex 7. Geneva, World Health Organization, 1975.

12. *The role of WHO in bilateral or multilateral health aid programmes* (EB55/15). Geneva, World Health Organization, 1975.

13. *Official records of the World Health Organization*, No. 224 (EB55/SR/20). Geneva, World Health Organization, 1975.

CHAPTER 3

General programme development

It may be that WHO's greatest achievements have resulted from its readiness to change, to achieve new goals, to seek new approaches and to adapt these approaches to changing world conditions. (Dr Candau on the occasion of WHO's Twenty-fifth Anniversary) (*1*).

In 1948, the First World Health Assembly established a programme in which topics were grouped by their importance. Malaria, maternal and child health, tuberculosis, venereal diseases, nutrition and environmental sanitation were assigned 'top priority', second priority was given to public health administration, third to parasitic diseases, fourth to virus diseases, fifth to mental health and sixth to other activities. To support work on these priorities, WHO set up advisory services, to be provided by regional organizations in joint actions in the field between governments and WHO. In parallel, WHO set up central technical services, comprising activities based mainly on the collection, classification, coordination and dissemination of information not directly related to field work, such as epidemiological services, health statistics and editorial and reference services. These two service departments existed until December 1958, at which time they ceased to exist as separate organizational entities, although the functional distinction remained.

As specified in the First General Programme of Work, which was approved in 1951, regional organizations were responsible for assessing national needs and requests for assistance. No sharp dividing line was drawn between the responsibilities of headquarters and those of regional organizations, however, as many headquarters services also serve governments, and many regional services depend on the ability of headquarters to estimate the extent to which a request can be met, in terms of resources of experts and knowledge (*2*). It was envisaged that efficient decentralization would lead to strengthening of regional machinery, so that many of the services provided could be planned on the spot in the light of local needs and conditions and would reach the people of the country through an agency that was close to them.

A closer look at WHO's coordinating role within the United Nations system, discussed above, showed that earlier policy decisions on how best WHO could fulfil its constitutional mandate for both coordination and technical cooperation should be reviewed. As described in Chapter 1, WHO engaged the issue of health as a component of social and economic development in a more concerted manner during the third decade, especially as it related to its programme of work. What emerged was a more decentralized approach, in which the importance of country involvement in the work of WHO through more interdisciplinary and intersectoral approaches was stressed. That goal was approached by a series of activities spread over several years.

EXECUTIVE BOARD ORGANIZATIONAL STUDY
ON THE INTERRELATIONS BETWEEN CENTRAL TECHNICAL
SERVICES AND PROGRAMMES FOR DIRECT ASSISTANCE
TO MEMBER STATES

A major organizational study, carried out by the Executive Board between 1973 and 1975, on the interrelations between WHO's central technical services and programmes in which direct assistance was provided to Member States was conducted to determine how best the Organization could discharge its constitutional duties with respect to health in its Member States and to improving world health in general (3). While it was agreed that the basic role of WHO, as defined in its Constitution, was still as fundamental to world needs as it had been when the Constitution was drafted, "the ways of achieving its goals cannot be entirely the same". The aim of the study was to determine the changes that were needed in the light of new conditions.

On the basis of a historical analysis, the Executive Board concluded that the priorities that had been identified during the first years of WHO's existence had "crystallized into distinct disciplines, self-contained and largely independent from each other and from other programme activities". Similar developments had been seen in other areas. The resulting system was "administratively simple; it facilitated the progressive elaboration of technical policies, concentrated on single-purpose projects and favoured the development of mass campaigns and eradication programmes". As these programmes were mirrored at national level, they became largely self-perpetuating, with no proper account of the evolving country situation.

In theory, the general programmes of work prepared by the Executive Board should take into account evolving situations in the regions and countries; the study showed, however, that this had not happened. Instead, the first four general programmes of work (covering the period 1951–1972) had been formulated in such broad terms that they could be taken as "*carte blanche* for almost any health activity".

A number of major conclusions and recommendations were reached:

1. The principle of the unity of conception and action within WHO remains fundamental to the Organization's policy, and its full realization is indispensable for the future success of the Organization.
2. Primary emphasis must be laid on ways and means by which the programme as a whole can be most rationally conceived and most effectively delivered.
3. Programme planning should be viewed as a joint endeavour in which national health authorities, WHO country representatives, regional committees, regional offices, the Executive Board, the World Health Assembly and WHO headquarters should all be involved.
4. The Executive Board and the World Health Assembly should establish sharper criteria for determining priorities for the Sixth General Programme of Work, so as to give more precise guidance on the achievements expected in the fields selected.

5. Collaboration with countries must take into account the fact that WHO assistance is only one facet of the total external assistance received by countries in the field of health. WHO must strengthen its advisory and coordinating roles with regard to bilateral and multilateral aid programmes in the field of health.

6. Community participation is essential if the Organization is to make adequate progress towards the attainment of its primary objective as defined in its Constitution.

The Executive Board's study effectively did away with the distinction between "central technical services" and "direct assistance to Member States", as the entire Organization would be involved in programme development, along with its governing bodies. For this to be realized, however, vastly improved communications structures—both vertically between organizational levels and horizontally within and between organizational—were needed.

The Director-General, in a presentation entitled *The constitutional mission of the World Health Organization*, which served as an introduction to his annual report in 1973, addressed some of the issues that the Board had considered in its study (*4*). To the question, "What, then, are the right priorities for WHO?" he replied:

> Among the technical criteria for selecting programme areas for WHO's involvement, I think, are that the problem must be of major public health importance, that its solution must depend on international collaboration, and, above, all, that WHO's involvement will make a significant impact on its solution.

Concerning solutions to these problems, he added:

> I think WHO's motto should be: 'Don't adopt—adapt.' Whenever possible, attempts should be made to devise simple yet effective health technologies that can be applied by auxiliary personnel to assist in meeting the needs of those hundreds and millions of people who today have no access to more sophisticated health care.
>
> And as governments will have to rely on external aid for many years, WHO should be increasingly involved in focusing international attention on priority health problems and in assisting Member countries to obtain and to use assistance that will help them in solving these problems.

These issues occupied both the governing bodies and the Secretariat throughout the decade. They are deeply intertwined, progress in one area highlighting the need for progress in all the others. Each is addressed below, beginning with the improvement of programming methods, then, improved coordination at country level, especially as regards the use of bilateral and multilateral funding, and ending with formulation of the Sixth Programme of Work, which, in effect, became a summary statement of the hopes for the future that the decade had engendered.

IMPROVED PROGRAMMING METHODS

The late 1960s witnessed the enthusiastic pursuit of more rational approaches to planning and programming, inspired no doubt by the promise offered by the power of digital computers, which was increasing dramatically from day to day. One promise was their application in setting up information systems. It was that promise which had led Dr Candau, in

1969, to transfer Dr Mahler (who had been Chief of the Tuberculosis unit up until then) to his office as a special assistant responsible for completing a study of an integrated management information system, with the expectation that he would then set up the system throughout the Organization (5). This took place in September. By the end of the year, however, it was decided that it was premature for WHO to attempt to set up such a system, and, instead, efforts were made to improve and build up the information systems serving the main administrative and programme areas of the Organization. An information users' committee was established to review all proposals made for overhauling the existing system (6).

Of more importance was the decision to clarify the responsibility for decision-making, from country level through the regional offices to headquarters, taken in that order, to generate better information for management. For that purpose, the Director-General established 'project systems analysis', with Dr Mahler as project director, reporting directly to his office.

Another finding of the study on an integrated management information system was that WHO technical assistance to countries was highly fragmented and dispersed, with considerable funding devoted to small projects with little potential for improving health status. Project systems analysis therefore initially sought methods for improving project selection, planning and management (7). Once a preliminary method had been devised for project formulation, project systems analysers worked with national personnel to solve actual country problems. After each application, the method was modified and progressively refined.

Dr Candau, in his statement to the Economic and Social Council in 1971, reported on the development of systems analytical methods, indicating that they would first be applied within the Organization and later at national level. He later proposed (see Chapter 1) "pooling the expertise available within the United Nations system" to enable a "joint approach to the formulation of development projects" (8).

From mid-1973, WHO's system analysis staff turned their attention to designing, testing and applying procedures for country health programming. An investigation into the reasons for the failure of numerous projects had indicated that it was due to inadequate political commitment to strategic objectives. Country health programming also grew in importance as a sectoral contribution to UNDP-led country programming, as noted in Chapter 1.

In a review of country programming, prepared in late 1974 by WHO for UNDP, WHO argued that the proper antecedents for a country programme "can only be effective analyses of each sector" (9). Country health programming was designed as a method for use by national health authorities to identify those of their health priorities that had intersectoral implications and the optimal tools to meet them. Such programming was portrayed as a "vehicle for medium-term planning", something that UNDP programming had not achieved. WHO's hope was that country programming would "graduate from the short-term to the longer-term approach", leading naturally to a dovetailing of country health programming into UNDP programming. For this to be realized, however, it was "imperative", in health and other sectors, that the role of sectoral programming "be formally recognized in the United Nations system and promoted in the same manner as the Consensus had promoted country programming".

As described in Chapter 1, specialized agencies representing other sectors did not look at country programming as WHO did, thus severely compromising the possibility that the United Nations system would develop a multisectoral approach to country programming in which the health sector would be fully involved.

As country health programming was a stand-alone procedure, four stages were outlined: (1) data collection, analysis and presentation; (2) situation analysis and preparation of programme proposals; (3) decisions on programme proposals and (4) continuation and integration of country health programming in the country's health structure (including project formulation and project implementation). The second stage involved 12 steps: (i) review of the information document, (ii) problem definition, (iii) identification of problem and output indicators, (iv) identification of current activities for health and health-related problems, (v) identification of current resource allocations, (vi) target setting, (vii) definition of health strategies, (viii) analysis of constraints of strategies, (ix) translation of strategies into health development programmes, (x) analysis of constraints of health development programmes, (xi) preparation of a document, and (xii) submission of the document.

At the end of 1975, an expert committee was convened to review WHO's experience with systems analysis, mostly on the basis of the experience of the project systems analysis team. Systems analysis was judged to be useful in health management in that it provided for:

- consideration of all variables, over and above the biological and technical, that affect health intervention programmes;
- a planning approach that relates input to output;
- an emphasis on quantification;
- rigour in analytical methods;
- orientation towards health problems rather than towards categories of service;
- communication with key government decision-making centres in which comparable methods are used;
- early attention to planning and priority-setting;
- improved interdisciplinary collaboration; and
- use of a wide range of analytical models and methods of considerable power.

Successful application of systems analysis, however, depends on a commitment to define objectives, set priorities and design strategies in order to make the best use of limited resources to improve health. Until such a commitment is obtained, "the application of systems analysis to directing, controlling and day-to-day administration could result in doing excellently what should not be done at all" (7).

The expert committee recognized that the systems analysis approach "had not yet become firmly rooted" and that there was no assurance "of strong and certain growth". It recommended that national authorities apply and adapt WHO's methods to current planning and administration and also evolve comprehensive strategies for raising awareness and understanding of health systems analysis, emphasizing its application to management. WHO should promote and support the adoption of systems analysis methods by national health administrations, increasing its capacity to do so by training its staff in systems concepts and methods. It should design further methods for country health programming, policy analysis and programming, incorporating suitably adapted concepts and methods and establishing appropriate procedures.

In their review, the Committee identified areas in which improved methods were required. It noted "deficiencies in epidemiological knowledge about the efficacy of health technologies", a handicap that it considered should be of "major concern to WHO and its member countries". Furthermore, "the treatment of sociopolitical data was found to be inadequate and the application of socioeconomic date inconclusive". Finally, more explicit attention should be given to "participation, particularly the participation of decision makers and consumers".

The failure of UNDP country programming to serve as an umbrella under which country health programming could evolve did not lessen WHO's commitment to the latter. A progress report prepared in October 1977 for the Programme Committee of the Executive Board, indicated that, throughout country health programming,

> strong emphasis is placed on the interaction between the health sector and other relevant sectors of the socioeconomic field, thus putting health in the broader perspective of total socioeconomic development. This is achieved by the active participation of representatives of all possible national viewpoints from all echelons of the health and related sectors. This enhances the likelihood of the health plan being understood and accepted at all important national levels, thus ensuring smooth implementation. (10)

Country health programming was first introduced in Bangladesh in 1973, and 23 other countries started using the method between 1973 and 1978. By the time the progress report was prepared, another 12 countries had indicated interest. Some difficulties had been encountered: emphasis had not always been placed on the importance of ensuring that the national team responsible for programming was multidisciplinary within the health sector and multisectoral on a national scale; furthermore, although WHO representatives played an important role in promoting country health programming, some were not fully familiar with the process.

Training workshops were organized both at headquarters and in several regions (see Chapter 4), with the participation of nationals and WHO staff members. The workshops in countries emphasized the approaches that were relevant to that country.

Country health programming was considered to have been instrumental in sensitizing countries to thinking in terms of broad programme concepts rather than isolated, fragmentary projects. Another significant result was that it gave countries the opportunity to mobilize both internal and external resources for health development.

An interregional seminar held in New Delhi, India, in early 1977, attended by national health planners and WHO staff from all six regions, staff from WHO headquarters and high-level representatives from UNDP, UNFPA, the International Bank for Reconstruction and Development and the United States Agency for International Development, recommended that research on country health programming should be promoted as "part of health services research within the framework of WHO's research programme, with a view to improving further the country health programming methodology", and that WHO should promote the inclusion of planning and management techniques in the training of all categories of health personnel (11).

With country health programming gradually taking root, WHO turned its attention to the evaluation of health programming and information systems, which had been the starting-point for subsequent developments in 1970, as described above. Provisional guidelines for programme evaluation were approved by the Programme Committee of the Executive Board at its session in November 1977. The Committee recommended that they be tested in selected WHO programmes and in countries that might be interested in applying them to their programmes (12). Testing of national guidelines was foreseen in at least one country in each region by 1978. The Committee also "strongly confirmed" the need for the new WHO information system and expressed satisfaction with the Director-General's strategy and with progress to date (13).

Another logical outcome of the decade's efforts to link WHO's programme at regional and global levels with the 'decision functions' at country level was adoption of the following procedures, as specified in resolution WHA30.23, adopted in May 1977:

- In the early stages of programme budgeting, WHO and national authorities were to collaborate in setting up programmes for cooperation, in order to attain the health goals defined in country programmes, expressed in terms of a general programme rather than as individual projects or detailed activities.
- Proposals for technical cooperation were to be be included in regional programme budgets, in the form of narrative statements supported by budgetary tables, in which the planning figures would be broken down by programme. This would facilitate the review of programmes by the respective regional committee. Country programmes would no longer be republished as an annex to the Director-General's proposed programme budget, if the material was available to delegates to the Health Assembly and members of the Board at the time of the review and approval of the WHO programme budget.
- Detailed plans of operation or work and estimated budgets for individual projects and activities planned within defined health programmes were to be drawn up later, as part of programme implementation at country level.
- Adequate information on the implementation and completion of programmes and projects and information on their progress, efficiency and effectiveness was to be made available to the delegates to the Health Assembly and members of the Executive Board for the evaluation system that was being developed in WHO.

Within the WHO Secretariat, new mechanisms were instituted to coordinate programme management. Regional programme committees were made responsible for translating the guidance on priorities received from the governing bodies and the expressed wishes of Member States into practical programmes at country and regional level. The headquarters' Programme Committee, which had been created in 1971, was now made responsible for advising on overall programme activities at headquarters, including the research component; the establishment of criteria and guiding principles for the formulation and implementation of programmes, in accordance with the policies of the Executive Board and the Health Assembly; strengthening programme information support; reviewing proposals for medium-term programmes and programme budgets, with particular attention to new technical cooperation programmes; and periodic evaluation of selected aspects of the programmes. Multidisciplinary teams were established for each of these areas. The Global Programme Committee was established in March 1977, consisting of the Director-General, the Deputy Director-General, the regional directors and the assistant directors-general, to serve as a 'top management' forum for round-table reviews of major issues in programme management for the Organization as a whole (*11*).

INCREASING BILATERAL AND MULTILATERAL FUNDING FOR HEALTH

The Fourth General Programme of Work noted that:

In the ultimate analysis it is for national health authorities to integrate all sources of aid— international, bilateral and private—for the fulfilment of stated health objectives, and for harmonizing the national and international work in the agricultural, educational, industrial and social sectors.

Nevertheless, as indicated in an Executive Board organizational study carried out in 1964–1966, WHO, as a multilateral intergovernmental organization and by its Constitution, "may be in a position, without impinging on the responsibilities of governments, to assist them in their efforts to coordinate external aid in the field of health" (*14*).

In his introduction to his annual report for 1973, the Director-General said, "I strongly believe that WHO should be increasingly involved in focusing international attention on priority health problems and in assisting Member countries to obtain and use assistance that will help them in solving these problems" (*4*). The discussions on this item during the Twenty-seventh World Health Assembly, in 1974, were not easy. The delegate for Malawi, for example, noted that "the advisory role of WHO should not be absolute", as certain countries "had eminent health consultants of their own who knew the local conditions and needs best". The delegate for Peru, following the Director-General's explanation, noted that "the advisory role proposed for WHO was for governments to use or not as they wished"; he proposed, however, that this role be "exercised through its regional organizations". Another delegate asked how WHO's advisory role would be reconciled with the country programming approach of UNDP.

Dr Mahler replied that "there should be no difficulty, as WHO was moving forward together with national bodies, and was training WHO representatives to act with nationals in the ministries of health on activities in the health sector and with all other social and economic sectors within the context of country health programming .... The Organization was engaged in studies on methods of solving various difficulties in overall coordination and, although it had been accused in the past of a high degree of isolationism, it had recently moved forward to the point where it was possible to consider its regular budget in its entirety to any country's total development effort." (*15*)

The Assembly went on to adopt resolution WHA27.29, which invited the Director-General "to study ways in which WHO could strengthen its role in the establishment of bilateral or multilateral aid programmes and priorities". This study was seen as a contribution to the Executive Board's organizational study on planning for and the impact of extrabudgetary resources on WHO's programmes and policy, which was approved at the Twenty-seventh World Health Assembly (resolution WHA27.19).

The Director-General's report reaffirmed WHO's coordination role as it had been conceived by its founders and defined in its Constitution. That role was not confined to resources under its direct control, and its role in international health was "unique" (16). As an international (as opposed to supernational) community, WHO was designed and well placed to coordinate and establish bilateral and multilateral programmes and priorities among its Members, irrespective of the source or control of funds.

In a statement to the Regional Committee for South-East Asia in 1973, Dr Mahler vividly described the implications for developed countries of a strengthened WHO role in coordination. On that occasion, he proposed the establishment of national WHO coordinating units to "mobilize national resources for WHO-coordinated studies as well as to ensure implementation of consensus decisions reached by WHO's governing bodies". He continued, "as long as the majority of developed countries are not really prepared to let WHO get under their national skins, I do not think international health coordination will receive that moral *tour de force* without which it will remain a passive game."

During the first quarter of its existence, as outlined in the Director-General's report to the Executive Board in 1975, WHO had concentrated primarily on coordinating its activities with those of the United Nations system. Its planning and coordinating efforts were largely devoted to its own budget programme and to integrated programmes financed by extrabudgetary resources under its control. Also included were cooperative programmes formulated in conjunction with other agencies, including regional economic commissions and a wide variety of governmental and nongovernmental agencies and contributors interested in health promotion. WHO's campaigns for contributions had led to the establishment of the Voluntary Fund for Health Promotion, to receive designated or undesignated contributions for health programmes and activities. Nevertheless, most international health assistance bypassed WHO and the United Nations system completely. The report noted that "this is as it should be. There is no need for such funds to flow through WHO" (16). What was disappointing, however, was that "too often there is a failure to make use of the policy and technical coordination capability of WHO in relation to such bilateral or multilateral aid programmes".

Contacts between WHO and the contributors and recipients of bilateral or multilateral assistance had been "erratic". There were examples of successful coordination, but in many instances the various parties involved had made no effort to coordinate their activities, and sometimes different donors provided conflicting technical advice or competed to provide assistance that too often ignored the real needs, priorities and resources of Member States. The health policies established by the Health Assembly failed to "find expression in national, bilateral or multilateral aid programmes". In these situations, WHO had "not been used to its full Constitutional role as the directing and coordinating authority on international health work".

The report spelled out a number of strategies for the future. First, there should be a commitment to coordination from all parties concerned. Members had to have the courage "to resist external aid for activities which have only marginal importance for the promotion of health". Staff at all levels within WHO needed a deeper understanding of WHO's coordination role, and a new type of staff member was envisaged, who had a public health capability that was "oriented to modern health management on an inservice basis".

Budgetary provisions for coordination activities had been made within various programmes proposed for 1976–1977. In addition, it was recommended, as noted in Chapter 2, that "funds for programme development be set aside at the disposal of the Director-General for the development of coordinative activities at country, regional and central echelons, for coordination of bilateral and multilateral aid, for development and coordination of health research and technology, especially in developing countries, for support of innovative or newly emerging problems and for staff development".

Promising strategies were identified for programme planning at the global level and for coordination at national, intercountry and central levels. The Smallpox Eradication Programme (see Chapter 9) was given as an example of a global programme planning approach to a major health problem the success of which rested on mobilizing resources that went far beyond those available to WHO. It was found noteworthy that the last few countries working on eradication would "not rank smallpox as a leading national health concern compared with other pressing national problems, were it not for the consensus policy on smallpox eradication arrived at by Member States". The Onchocerciasis Control Programme in the Volta River Basin Area was given as another example of a WHO activity that attracted the participation and commitment of national, bilateral and multilateral organizations (see Chapter 9).

Global programme planning required a longer-term and usually a multidisciplinary approach to health problems, which WHO was attempting to develop as part of medium-term programming. Provisional guidelines for multidisciplinary medium-term programming were drawn up and incorporated into training for programme managers. Other approaches included country health programming, as discussed above, and methods and techniques that could be used to strengthen health-care services and financing, train auxiliary health workers and develop project management and health information systems.

Special attention was given to the two-way relationship between socioeconomic development and health:

> Better health is both a cause and a result of development. Development activities have potential to raise the level of health and welfare, but they also lead to frequently unrecognized hazards to health. Good health is a prerequisite to development work, while developmental activities may themselves be enabling mechanisms for the introduction of health care services. The interrelationship between development and health is complex. WHO and its Member States, with the participation of other bilateral or multilateral organizations concerned with social and economic development must collaborate in health sector and intersectoral studies at national and regional levels. A radically new multisectoral approach to technical cooperation is required.

Specific mechanisms for coordination at national, intercountry and global levels were suggested.

At the national level, the focus was to be on strengthening the coordinating and technical capability of governments. Among the mechanisms proposed were strengthening the role of the WHO representative (considered separately below), introducing country health programming (as discussed above), creating national advisory health councils or similar structures for health policy formulation, creating WHO advisory boards (perhaps at regional level) and ensuring resource coordination for better use of external aid and to foster partnerships between national representatives and donors in the field of health.

At the intercountry level, it was proposed that the regional offices and regional committees "should take a very active role in relation to the activities of the WHO representatives, the country health programming process and the other mechanisms for coordination at national level". It was recognized that the technical advisory and coordinating capability of the regional offices should be strengthened. In this regard, it was envisaged that greater use should be made of regional expertise, possibly by creating intercountry or regional panels of multidisciplinary experts, an idea that was not met with wide agreement on the part of the Executive Board, as discussed in Chapter 2. It was also proposed, at least for the next few years, that WHO organize meetings of Member States and bilateral or multilateral donors to review present activities and formulate coordinated approaches to health problems, as had already occurred in some regions (see Chapter 4).

At the central level, it was pointed out that WHO had an "informational and promotional role to play in generating and coordinating bilateral or multilateral aid in response to the needs and priorities of Member States identified through country health programming, national and intercountry or regional coordination and advisory mechanisms, and global programme priorities and consensus policies arrived at through the forum of regional committees and the World Health Assembly". It was noted that WHO had a comprehensive programme for setting up information systems, which would support national, bilateral and multilateral health programme planning.

The Executive Board's organizational study on planning for and the impact of extrabudgetary resources on WHO's programmes and policy, carried out between 1974 and 1976, identified three major problems: (1) the inadequacy of existing resources; (2) the difficulty of planning under conditions of uncertainty; and (3) the potential impact of extrabudgetary resources and donor bias (*17*). Two recommendations were made, one on better use of extrabudgetary resources for promoting WHO global programmes, and the other for improving the coordination and technical roles of WHO at country level. For the former, it was accepted that WHO had a "leadership role to play in developing project and programme structures packaged to attract and combine multiple sources of financing". For the latter, it was agreed that WHO had a "wider role to play in relation to bilateral and multilateral health aid programmes". Specifically, "without infringing [on] the sovereignty of Member States or the integrity of bilateral arrangements, WHO must develop the capability—and Member States must use that capability—to work closely together and on a multisectoral basis to improve the planning for increased and more effective national, bilateral and multilateral health programmes."

The study was discussed by the Executive Board at its fifty-seventh session, in January 1976, and at the Twenty-ninth World Health Assembly in May of that year. No major problems were identified; however, several Executive Board members noted that the quality of WHO representatives would have to be improved if they were to play the role envisaged for them. Such improvement was not confined to the representatives alone, as suggested by one member, who noted that "the reorientation of staff would be critical".

The Director-General in his closing statement said that the "Board's study was consonant with the expectations arising out of the declaration for the establishment of a New Economic and Social Order. It was only realistic to understand that the world was entering into a period where developed and developing countries would have their material interests increasingly linked in a form of international solidarity" (*18*). He continued, "If governments were ready to place an increasing degree of confidence in WHO, the Organization could ... produce a programme reflecting the real needs of countries ... and which would be attractive to donors, or, as he preferred to term them, participants .... There was no doubt that WHO would have to fight to achieve an additional input into the health sector. The Organization had already been responsible for a considerable advance by gaining acceptance of the growing importance of health and the social sectors in socioeconomic development as a whole". He recognized that WHO staff needed a "broad comprehension of all the factors involved, including the political situation, and to have what could be called a developmental attitude".

The Health Assembly's discussion on this item took place in Committee B at the same time that Committee A was addressing the draft resolution that eventually was adopted as resolution WHA29.48 (see Chapter 2). Questions were raised about where the budgetary resources would be found for introducing the coordination and planning mechanisms and for strengthening WHO representatives' offices. Three approaches were proposed by the Secretariat: existing resources could be channelled towards mobilizing extrabudgetary resources; such resources could be used to finance activities within the regular budget; or a new mechanism could be set up, "which would not necessarily be costly since it could be in part financed by these same extrabudgetary resources". The shift of resources demanded by resolution WHA29.48 provided a clear indication, however, that more was expected of the regular budget at country level.

Although there was a difference of opinion about whether WHO should "engage in fund raising", the Board (in resolution EB57.R29) and the Health Assembly (in resolutions WHA29.31 and WHA29.32) confirmed the establishment of the Voluntary Fund for Health Promotion and requested the Director-General (a) to take particularly into account the promotion of those planned health programmes that could attract additional resources for the benefit of the developing countries; (b) to continue to develop appropriate mechanisms for attracting and coordinating an increased volume of bilateral and multilateral aid for health purposes; and (c) to continue his efforts on an interagency basis to harmonize programme budget cycles and planning and operational procedures of the major United Nations funding agencies with those applied to the regular programmes of the organizations in the United Nations system. The last point reflected the fact that the major funding agencies of the United Nations system (UNDP, UNEP, UNFPA and UNFDAC) had both different programming periods and different approaches to programme planning.

INCREASED FOCUS ON WHO'S ROLE AT COUNTRY LEVEL, PARTICULARLY THE ROLE OF THE WHO REPRESENTATIVE

As indicated earlier, it was suggested in WHO's First General Programme of Work that many services "should be planned on the spot", i.e. at country level. While this proved feasible for the large programmes of the Organization, as best exemplified by disease eradication campaigns, WHO's capacity at country level was often inadequate to meet the demands made upon it. For example, one regional director observed that the advantages of UNDP-related exercises were lost "if we are unable, through lack of qualified manpower, to implement projects".

Various recommendations for improving WHO's performance at country level were made by regional directors and by staff at headquarters. Measures "as a start towards improving our performance in the delivery of WHO's assistance programmes" were outlined in a memorandum sent by the Director-General to all regional directors in early 1975. It suggested that consideration should be given to establishing new WHO representative offices where this was indicated and that a substantial increase should be made in the resources for WHO's field establishments, including managerial and administrative personnel.

The new challenges of intersectoral programming meant that WHO representatives had to extend their working relationships to other government departments as well as keeping in touch with the representatives of multilateral and bilateral programmes. It was also envisaged that the WHO representatives should be empowered to discuss matters directly with the government's central coordinating unit or planning body, when necessary. The creation of a resource coordinating mechanism affiliated to ministries of health was also proposed, to maintain close contact with other ministries, independent health institutions and bilateral and multilateral aid representatives. In some countries, e.g. Thailand, these bodies took the form of a WHO–national coordinating committee, which received subsidies from WHO to carry out small operational research projects.

Given the attention paid to work at country level and recognition of the need to strengthen WHO's role in that respect, it was not surprising that the Executive Board discussed the subject at its fifty-eighth session, in May 1976. The working group set up to conduct the study visited 11 countries in five regions, holding consultations with national health authorities at the highest level, representatives of other economic and social sectors, WHO staff from the regional offices and representatives of WHO, other United Nations agencies and funds and other multilateral and bilateral aid agencies. The group learnt that some delegates attending the meeting of the WHO Regional Committee for Africa in 1976 saw the WHO representative as a bureaucrat who "could not be identified with technical cooperation" (19). In the 11 countries visited by the group, opinion was divided between those that favoured not only the presence of a WHO representative but also the present incumbent of that office; those that were definitely not in favour; and those that were in favour of a WHO representative but not of the present incumbent. The countries that were 'definitely not in favour' regarded the presence of a WHO representative as a "sign of dependence on the Organization".

The organizational study re-examined the role of WHO at country level "with a view to making it more efficient" (20). Topics addressed in the study were the constitutional basis of the role of WHO at country level, the evolution from the concept of technical aid or assistance to the concept of cooperation, current trends in the technical cooperation programme at country level, the need for new methods of technical cooperation, the role and functions of WHO representatives, and the repercussions of the new methods of cooperation on the structure of WHO.

Much of the review addressed issues that had been covered in earlier organizational studies. In doing so, the report reaffirmed the importance of the new methods for technical cooperation, which had matured since the early years of the decade. The issues addressed were:

- country health programming;
- an increase in the proportion of the Organization's total resources devoted to countries, in accordance with resolution WHA29.48;
- community participation in socioeconomic and health development;
- better use of national personnel in planning and implementing WHO collaborative programmes;
- national health advisory councils composed not only of representatives of ministries of health but also of other relevant ministries and national bodies;
- multidisciplinary regional expert panels;
- coordination of national, bilateral and multilateral resources for national and regional priorities;
- training of national health personnel with a view to solving local problems;
- technical cooperation among developing countries, which, in the light of the report on the subject submitted to the sixtieth session of the Executive Board and in resolution EB60.R4, could be described as a complement to current arrangements for furthering the individual and collective self-reliance of the developing world; and
- regional centres for operational research, development and training in specific programme areas, where countries would work together to solve common problems and train cadres of national personnel in self-reliance for the development of programmes in their country.

It was recognized that the redefinition of the role of WHO at country level, as outlined in the report, would have a major effect on the new relations between WHO and its Member States and also have important implications for WHO staff in countries, particularly WHO representatives. A key idea that was explored in the study was the use of national personnel in planning and implementing WHO collaborative programmes, including nominating nationals as WHO representatives. Several regions already had experience of nationals serving in a WHO capacity, and these experiences were reviewed, especially that of the African Region, from which the idea of changing the type of people appointed as WHO representatives had originated. The advantages and disadvantages of the use of nationals in this capacity were identified, but no firm conclusion was reached. The group concluded that "further experimentation should take place with the use of national personnel as WHO representatives and project managers".

The subject had been discussed during the sessions of the Board and the Health Assembly in 1977 and 1978. While the Board's report was well received, it was clear that there was no unanimous support for the idea that nationals could serve as WHO representatives. The term 'representative' was, however, judged to be inadequate, given the new responsibilities to be placed on the incumbents of this position. The Board proposed the term 'WHO coordinator', which, in the final discussion during the Health Assembly in 1978, was altered to 'WHO programme coordinator'. This person would facilitate all the functions described, and the role would therefore demand considerable technical as well as diplomatic skills.

Training in health management, especially the application of country health programming, was considered an important means of raising the qualifications of representatives and co-ordinators to the level of competence desired. Beyond that, it was essential that the regional and global organizational levels be fully supportive of this new role. Integrated country programmes required policy guidance and programme review and evaluation by regional committees. The regional programme budget should no longer be built up from a series of fragmented projects; a programme-oriented approach was needed, within which projects were identified, planned and implemented in relation to the overall programme objectives.

Regional officers should be reoriented to formulate and manage regional programmes and provide technical support for activities in countries, at the request of the representative. As part of the decentralization policy, certain functions and activities that had hitherto been the responsibility of the Organization's headquarters were transferred to the regional level in order to enhance the region's coordination role, as had already occurred with respect to managing UNDP-funded activities.

The impact of these developments at the global level remained to be seen, although certain trends were evident. Resolution WHA29.48 had led to a substantial reduction in manpower at the central level. To compensate for this reduction and, at the same time, to improve WHO's programming, it was decided to rely more on multidisciplinary programme development teams, as mentioned earlier.

The success of this new direction lay largely in the hands of the Member States, as indicated by resolution WHA31.27, adopted in May 1978 as a consequence of this study. It urged Member States to increase their participation in the work of WHO, to increase still further their already close partnership with WHO in the formulation and implementation of the Organization's policies, and to ensure that their requests for technical cooperation with the Organization conformed to the policies they had adopted at the Health Assembly.

SIXTH GENERAL PROGRAMME OF WORK

The Sixth General Programme of Work reflected the main trends in the manner in which WHO formulated its programme during the decade. In order to redress the fact that technical collaboration had "taken precedence over coordination in the evolution of the Organization's programme", the Sixth General Programme of Work proposed that programmes rather than projects be emphasized and then that the programme graduate from smaller to larger projects (*21*). When this was achieved, WHO would phase out project implementation, "giving momentum to WHO's coordinating role". National governments would take over the responsibility for current programme management.

This development was predicated on the existence of national health policies and of programmes aimed at "solving the country's most important health problems ... [which] might include major development projects where they are required and nationally acceptable". At the regional and central levels of WHO, a systematic analysis of problems identified at country level was expected to lead to "the formulation of programmes that have clearly defined, realistic purposes, whether for the support of individual national programmes or for the solution of priority regional or global health problems".

The main objectives of the Sixth General Programme of Work were grouped into six areas of concern:

- development of comprehensive health services;
- disease prevention and control;
- promotion of environmental health;
- health manpower development;
- promotion and development of biomedical and health services research; and
- programme development and support.

Two principal objectives were identified: to support health-promoting activities in the context of overall socioeconomic development and to increase collaboration with the United Nations and other international, multilateral and bilateral agencies in solving health problems and other socioeconomic problems with significant health implications.

With regard to the first principal objective, three detailed objectives were identified: (i) to collaborate in the preparation, execution and evaluation of health plans, programmes and development plans in accordance with periodically revised or confirmed health policy; (ii) to promote efficient managerial, information and evaluation systems for planning and operating health programmes and to create permanent mechanisms for health management, information and development in as many countries as possible; and (iii) to promote the integration of appropriate health components into socioeconomic development plans and social and economic activities, with a view to reducing health hazards and increasing health benefits.

With regard to the second principal objective, two detailed objectives were identified: (i) to increase international collaboration and the amount of external assistance available for health programmes, for the health component of development programmes and for development programmes with identifiable effects on health, including community water supplies and disposal of wastes, particularly in developing countries; and (ii) to plan for and provide an adequate, appropriate response to emergency situations, resulting in particular from natural disasters.

Country health programming (or an equivalent process) was considered to be the starting-point for the formulation of health development programmes and projects. Selected priorities and requests made for WHO assistance would help shape the Seventh General Programme of Work. To promote integration of health planning into overall national socioeconomic development planning, WHO would "where necessary promote effective intersectoral communication in collaboration with other multilateral and bilateral assistance agencies". The Organization would cooperate when requested in creating permanent mechanisms for health planning, programming and evaluation and provide advice on the management of programmes related to health.

To improve multilateral and bilateral collaboration, WHO would design mechanisms for coordinating international efforts and for investing resources from various sources into national or international health programmes of high priority. In doing so, it would seek to synchronize country health programming with other programme activities throughout the

United Nations system and with national development planning. The Organization would also collaborate in formulating concrete proposals to attract external financial support.

It was recognized at the time the General Programme of Work was prepared that country health programming had "not yet become sufficiently widespread for WHO to determine its programmes over the medium term in response to well-defined national needs". Nor was the Programme specific enough to define the Organization's detailed programmes. A process was envisaged in which the formulation of programmes was as detailed as the results of country health programming allowed. It was recognized that WHO could not yet assess "the value of its programme as a whole and its usefulness in solving health problems at the national, regional and global levels". A "renewed approach" was being designed for "systematic assessment of the delivery of the programme and of its ultimate impact on the health situations in the world as a whole and in individual countries".

At its twenty-ninth session, in 1976, the Health Assembly approved the Sixth General Programme of Work by adopting resolution WHA29.20. Apart from the reservations implicit in the text of the Programme, a delegate to the Health Assembly expressed concern (as quoted in Chapter 2) that resolution WHA29.48 "would lead to discarding the carefully prepared Sixth General Programme of Work", although no details were given. One probable reason for this concern was that too rapid a move of resources from the centre to the periphery would mean that, at the global level, there would be inadequate resources to ensure that the policy basis of the programme of work was well in place. This is, however, a supposition, which should be explored in subsequent volumes of this series.

References

1. *Official records of the World Health Organization*, No. 210. Geneva, World Health Organization, 1973.
2. *General Programme of Work covering a specified period. Official records of the World Health Organization*, No. 32, Annex 10. Geneva, World Health Organization, 1951.
3. *Organizational study on the interrelationships between the central services of WHO and programmes of direct assistance to Member States. Official records of the World Health Organization*, No. 223, Part I, Annex 7. Geneva, World Health Organization, 1975.
4. The constitutional mission of WHO. *WHO Chronicle*, 1974, 28:308–311.
5. *Integrated management information system (IMIS)*. Information Circular No. 88 (IC/69/88). Geneva, World Health Organization, 1969.
6. *Integrated management information system (IMIS)*. Information Circular No. 135 (IC/69/135). Geneva, World Health Organization, 1969.
7. *Application of systems analysis to health management. Report of a WHO expert committee* (WHO Technical Report Series, No. 596). Geneva, World Health Organization, 1976.
8. *Statement of Dr M.G. Candau, Director-General of the WHO to the 55th Session of the Economic and Social Council, July 1971* (DG/72.2). New York, United Nations, 1972.
9. *Review of country programming experience. Observations by the World Health Organization* (EB55/40). Geneva, World Health Organization, 1975.
10. *Progress report on country health programming, Report by the Director-General* (EB61/19). Geneva, World Health Organization, 1977.
11. *The work of WHO 1976–1977. Official records of the World Health Organization*, No. 243. Geneva, World Health Organization, 1977.

12. *Development of health programme evaluation. Report of the Programme Committee of the Executive Board* (EB61/20). Geneva, World Health Organization, 1978.

13. *Development of WHO information systems programme. Report by the Programme Committee of the Executive Board* (EB61/21). Geneva, World Health Organization, 1978.

14. *Organizational study on co-ordination at the national level in relation to the technical co-operation field programme of the Organization. Official records of the World Health Organization*, No. 157, Annex 16. Geneva, World Health Organization, 1967.

15. *Official records of the World Health Organization*, No. 218 (WHA/SR/A/9). Geneva, World Health Organization, 1974.

16. *The role of WHO in bilateral or multilateral health aid programmes. Report by the Director-General* (EB55/15). Geneva, World Health Organization, 1975.

17. *Organizational study on the planning for and impact of extrabudgetary resources on WHO's programmes and policy. Official records of the World Health Organization*, No. 231, Annex 8. Geneva, World Health Organization, 1976.

18. *Official records of the World Health Organization*, No. 232 (EB57/SR/22). Geneva, World Health Organization, 1976.

19. *Official records of the World Health Organization*, No. 239 (EB59/SR/23). Geneva, World Health Organization, 1977.

20. *Organizational study on WHO's role at the country level, particularly the role of the WHO representative. Official records of the World Health Organization*, No. 244, *Executive Board, sixty-first session,* Annex 7. Geneva, World Health Organization, 1978.

21. *Sixth General Programme of Work covering a specified period (1978–1983). Official records of the World Health Organization*, No. 233, Annex 7. Geneva, World Health Organization, 1976.

CHAPTER 4

Regional trends

Given the growing importance of regional arrangements during this decade, the Constitutional articles that pertain to this subject are relevant. The regional nature of WHO was due historically to the existence at the time of two regional bodies: the Maritime Sanitary and Quarantine Board of Egypt and the the Pan American Sanitary Bureau. Although the Regional Committee for the Eastern Mediterranean Area (and subsequently the Executive Board by its resolution EB3.R30) approved integration of the Alexandria Sanitary Bureau into that of the Regional Office of WHO, efforts to integrate the Sanitary Bureau fully at the time WHO came into being failed. Nevertheless, Article 54 indicates that such integration "shall in due course" take place.

The WHO Constitution does not fix the regional structure of the Organization. Instead, it stipulates that the Health Assembly shall from time to time define the geographical areas in which it is desirable to establish a regional organization. Having done so, the Assembly is then authorized to establish a regional organization to meet the special needs of each area. Each such organization shall be an integral part of the Organization and consist of a regional committee and a regional office.

The regional committees formulate policies on matters of an exclusively regional character. They suggest the calling of technical conferences and such additional work or investigation in health matters as in its opinion would promote the objectives of the Organization within the region, and they cooperate with the respective regional committees of the United Nations and those of other specialized agencies and with other regional international organizations having interests in common with the Organization.

While the Constitution stipulates that the head of the regional office is appointed by the Executive Board, with the agreement of the regional committee, in practice each regional director is elected by the Member countries served by the region; the Executive Board confirms that result. The staff of the regional office is appointed in a manner determined by agreement between the Director-General and the regional director.

Each WHO region has its own character. It is not the intent of this chapter, however, to cover all the activities of each region. Instead, attention is focused primarily on policies associated with the broader issues of national health services and manpower as part of national socioeconomic development, and related subjects. Events are described as in the documentation issued at the time, in order to capture the manner in which each region was striving to achieve what were essentially the same objectives but under somewhat different conditions, as dictated by the composition of their Member States. The prime sources of information include the contributions of each region to the annual report of the Organization and the reports of the regional directors to annual meetings of the regional committees.

AFRICAN REGION

The WHO Regional Office for Africa was established in 1950. During the first 10 years, when there were only two independent African countries in the Region, the Office was located in Geneva, with Europeans in charge. The number of countries in the Region rose dramatically during the 1960s, reaching 31 by 1968, and by the end of the third decade there were 39 Member States, one Associate Member and two non-Member States.

The Region had the largest number of least developed countries in the world—13 out of 25 in 1974—i.e. countries in which the per capita gross domestic product was less than US$ 100, the contribution of industry to the gross domestic produce was less than 10%, and the literacy rate was less than 20%. The economic crisis of the mid-1970s added further to the magnitude of the development challenge facing these countries, as did natural disasters, such as the prolonged drought in the countries bordering the Sahara and severe outbreaks of cholera and yellow fever.

Preparation of the Fifth Programme of Work, for the period 1973–1977, in 1969 and 1970, provided the Regional Office with the opportunity to assess the status of long-term health planning in the Member countries of the Region, then numbering 34. All 21 countries that submitted comments and recommendations noted that a socioeconomic development plan was under study; 12 countries had established planning committees, and seven were implementing their second plan. While the priority given to the health sector varied from country to country, there was general agreement that the priorities within the health sector were: training staff of all categories; improving and setting up services, particularly basic health services; communicable disease control and environmental health.

Only 12 countries provided any information on what aid they intended to request of WHO during the period concerned. This was taken as an indication that the countries of the Region had limited experience in national health planning, leading WHO to add national health planning to the list of health priorities to be addressed during the coming years.

One unfortunate consequence of the weak link between health and socioeconomic planning was discontinuation of UNDP funding in a number of countries for health programmes that had not achieved their objectives. These programmes had not been adequately reflected in the national socioeconomic plan, a criteria of some importance to UNDP. Total UNDP funding for projects in the Region thus actually fell during the early 1970s, only to pick up towards the end. UNDP's country programming, however, rarely helped to accelerate development of the health sector. Also, it was not the agency responsible for coordinating United Nations system-wide activities, as called for in the 'capacity study' (see Chapter 1), for which FAO took the leadership role in most African countries. Unfortunately, the few rural development projects in which WHO was involved proved unsatisfactory, owing to insufficient coordination among the participating agencies.

Development of human resources was understood to be the key to any progress in health in the Region. A prospective study undertaken early in the decade showed that no African country would achieve a rate of coverage of one medical officer for 1000 people by the year 2000. Only 11 could be expected to achieve one medical officer for 10 000 people, the objective set for the Second United Nations Development Decade. It was recognized that greater efforts were needed to improve the output of medical training institutions; pilot studies should be conducted on the needs for health staff; teaching of public health should be adapted to the health needs of countries; multidisciplinary training, particularly in university centres for health sciences, should be promoted; and the training of all categories of teachers should be encouraged by establishing regional centres for research and training in medical education.

The first university centre for health sciences in the African Region was established in 1970 in Yaoundé, United Republic of Cameroon. The centre aimed to provide high-quality multidisciplinary training for all members of the health team, including new concepts in the training and functions of auxiliaries. Of note is the fact that, despite "very strong pressures" to have a "French curriculum", this school was not based on any European model (*1*). In the years the followed, similar centres were established at Libreville, Gabon; Niamey, Niger; and Brazzaville, Congo.

Various meetings were organized to address the needs of different types of staff and to stimulate the involvement of high-level officials in reforming the manner in which health personnel were trained. For the first time, professors of public health were brought together to lay down minimum objectives in regard to the place of public health in medical education in the Region. Also for the first time, a meeting of deans of medical schools addressed the question of adapting curricula to African needs. At their second meeting, held in 1970, the role of medical schools in national health planning was reviewed, as was the need for integrated instruction and teacher training based on a multidisciplinary approach.

The Regional Committee itself emphasized the need for radical changes in the approach to training health personnel, finding new teaching methods and adapting course content to the realities and needs of the countries of Africa. It acknowledged the advantages of establishing demonstration and training areas, with the proviso that clear objectives be defined at the outset and evaluation carried out in order to obviate unnecessary perpetuation of activities in the area.

Study tours were organized to enable senior health officials from countries in the Region to visit several Latin American countries to observe how planning was conducted there. The value and methods of preparation of national health planning were addressed at regional technical discussions held in 1969, and health planning was featured in a workshop held in 1970. A team of five consultants helped Malawi to draw up a 15-year health plan in 1971. Planning for human resources development was the subject of a symposium held in May–June 1972, and the opportunity was taken to train teachers in educational methods in workshops for both nationals and WHO staff.

The methods of systems analysis and operational research were introduced into various projects in the Region, beginning with an analysis in Kenya to formulate a project for setting up rural health services in North-Western State of Nigeria. With UNFPA funding, the aim of this project was to conduct a demonstration project on maternal and child health and family planning. Country health programming and project formulation workshops were organized, as well as two workshops in health planning, held in 1975 and 1976, with a contribution from the United States Agency for International Development.

Despite the increased attention given to health planning, the Regional Director, Dr Alfred Quenum, in his annual report for 1975, noted that programmes unrelated to national objectives that were instigated from abroad were still being accepted by the Member countries of the Region. Countries would need the courage to refuse such offers, which further complicated an already complex development system. Similarly, countries should terminate or reorient long-standing projects that had not produced any tangible results.

In order to encourage external agencies to coordinate their activities better within countries, the Regional Office organized several conferences on health coordination and cooperation in Africa. The first, in 1973, involved five cooperating agencies and 20 countries of Central and West Africa. That in 1975, held in Yaoundé, brought together 30 countries and five national liberation movements in Africa and 26 agencies (*2*). The meeting examined means for coordinating national approaches to strengthening health services delivery and agreed to set up regional mechanisms for better coordination of the use of external aid within national priorities and resources.

At the next meeting, in 1977, held in Brazzaville, the terms of reference for a standing committee were approved, and a number of recommendations were made. The responsibilities of the committee included promoting information exchange, promoting studies of the general implications of socioeconomic development with a view to the protection and promotion of the health of African communities, encouraging the establishment in African countries of structures such as national health councils for cooperation with national planning bodies in coordinating collaboration with external agencies, and encouraging and facilitating the training of professional African national staff capable of undertaking the formulation and implementation of integrated health development programmes of a multidisciplinary and multisectoral nature. The meeting invited countries and cooperating agencies to replace the concept of 'assistance' by that of 'cooperation'. Its recommendations promoted continuous updating of country profiles and official programme statements and spelt out the duties of national health councils (*3*).

In a seminar on the training of auxiliary health personnel, held in 1971, the term 'auxiliary' was redefined in the light of the health needs of the countries and criteria such as competence, duties and supervision. The auxiliary was regarded as an essential, competent member of the health team who performs complementary, well-defined tasks within a supervisory framework, after having received adequate training adapted to his or her future responsibilities.

Reorientation of the the nursing profession from an exclusively hospital function was addressed early in the decade. A multidisciplinary study group on nursing education that met in 1973 established norms for the training and use of nurses in Africa. Particular stress was laid on the importance of social sciences for identifying and distributing available resources and the need to train all members of the health team together.

The village health committees in the Ekali pilot area in the United Republic of Cameroon were judged to be an excellent example of community organization, in which people were encouraged to get together for concerted health action. Similarly, a research project in Ghana on community involvement in solving local problems had found new approaches to strengthening health services (*4, 5*).

As awareness grew of the importance of community participation in health matters (see Chapter 6), greater attention was given to health education as part of community (health) development. The University of Ibadan, Nigeria, and the University Centre for Health Sciences, Yaoundé, were assisted in preparing course outlines and curricula for training health education specialists at undergraduate and postgraduate levels.

The Regional Committee at its twentieth session, in 1970, approved the principle of integrating into the basic health services a certain number of activities, such as sanitation, malaria control, tuberculosis control and mother and child health, which had previously been conducted independently. The integrated services should be supported by health education and an effective network of epidemiological, statistical and public health laboratory services, operated by qualified personnel and functioning in the framework of a realistic long-term plan.

As part of the efforts to strengthen health infrastructure, increasing attention was given to strengthening national epidemiological services and epidemiological surveillance, especially in relation to cholera, smallpox, yellow fever, plague and, to a lesser extent, typhus. One centre, in Nairobi, which had originally been devoted to tuberculosis, was re-adapted to help countries in the Region to establish epidemiological services, to undertake epidemiological investigations and to organize their statistical services. A centre in Abidjan, Ivory Coast, provided similar services to the French-speaking countries of the Region and also addressed the problem of yellow fever.

At the fourth interregional seminar on epidemiological surveillance of communicable diseases, held in 1972 in Nairobi, physicians, veterinary public health and animal health specialists exchanged experiences and views on common problems. The technical discussions dealt with the general method of surveillance and specific methods applicable to certain communicable diseases, including zoonoses and foodborne infections.

During its seventeenth session, in 1967, the Regional Committee decided to discontinue use of the term 'malaria pre-eradication' and to place more emphasis on setting up basic health services, a shift that UNICEF welcomed. Thus, 14 malaria pre-eradication projects in 11 countries were converted into projects for basic health services, and the two training centres (in Lagos and Lomé), which had served exclusively for training malaria workers, initiated courses for various categories of public health personnel. The fields covered by these centres were laboratory techniques, environmental health, communicable disease control, public health, health statistics and nursing; the duration of the courses ranged from 6 weeks to 3 years.

A project to control onchocerciasis in the Volta River Basin was initiated with the support of several international agencies and donor countries and with seven participating countries (see Chapter 9). Control of schistosomiasis in relation to man-made lakes was also undertaken during this decade (see Chapter 9).

In environmental health, six large-scale urban water supply and sewerage projects, financed by UNDP, proved so complex and time-consuming that they were retarding efforts to reorganize simple programmes in the rural areas where the majority of people lived. Good results in the control of communicable diseases in selected areas, by improving sanitation (housing, safe water, waste disposal and food inspection), illustrated the interdependence of public health activities. A study on the epidemiology of typhoid further underlined the importance of environmental health activities, which were increasingly being integrated into basic health services. Environmental health began to be taught in many health staff training institutions.

The first Regional expert meeting on strengthening health services, held in 1976, examined aspects of traditional medicine. Primary health care was the theme of the second meeting, in March 1977, which was prepared after dialogue with most countries of the Region.

The Regional Committee at its twenty-fifth session, in 1975, established a Regional advisory committee on biomedical research and selected, as a priority, tropical diseases, particularly schistosomiasis, filariasis, onchocerciasis, trypanosomiasis and leprosy. At its first meeting, in November 1976, the committee recommended setting up or strengthening national research councils, bringing the directory of existing centres up to date, identifying institutions likely to collaborate in the regional programme and establishing mechanisms for training research workers. At its second meeting, in December 1977, the committee defined the structures and mechanisms for establishment of a regional network of national research centres, prepared appropriate strategies for encouraging research and determined priorities, particularly with regard to the organization of comprehensive health services and maternal and child health care.

The Regional Committee at its twenty-sixth session, in 1976, adopted resolution AFR/RC26/R8, which recognized the importance of resolution WHA29.48 for the African Region and the moral obligations deriving from massive participation of African countries in the Group of 77, which had led to adoption of that historical resolution (see Chapter 2). A working group was established to make proposals on reorientation of Regional activities and corresponding reorganization of the Regional Office. The Regional Director earlier that year had reorganized the Office into multidisciplinary teams, one for each of four subregions; steps had also been taken to increase decentralization and to delegate decision-making, as far as possible, to the level at which the problem had to be solved. These changes were judged to be satisfactory by the working group. More frequent visits by Regional Office staff to countries was encouraged.

Whether national coordinators should be used, rather than WHO representatives, should be left entirely to the discretion of the Member State concerned. Should a Member State decide to have a WHO representative, the necessary consultations should be held to ensure that the right personnel were made available. Greater efforts should be made to recruit more personnel from within the Region, and those WHO personnel who appeared to lack competence and experience in international work should not be reassigned from country to country. All WHO staff working at country level should train nationals to take over their positions when they left.

REGION OF THE AMERICAS

The Pan American Health Organization (PAHO), which was created in 1902 as the Pan American Sanitary Organization, consists of a Bureau and a Directing Council, acting as WHO's Regional Office and Regional Committee, respectively.

In 1968, a special meeting of ministers of health of the Americas was convened in Buenos Aires, Argentina, to review progress in achieving the health goal specified in the 1961 Charter of Punta del Este: to increase life expectancy at birth by a minimum of 5 years and increase the ability to learn and produce by improving individual and public health (6). To attain this goal, the Charter called for the provision of adequate potable water and sewage disposal to no less than 70% of the urban and 50% of the rural population and reduction of the mortality rate of children under 5 years of age by at least one half. Other needs were to control the more serious communicable diseases; eradicate illnesses, especially malaria, for which effective techniques are available; improve nutrition; train medical and health personnel to meet at least minimum requirements; improve basic health services at national and local levels; and intensify scientific research, applying its results more fully and effectively to the prevention and cure of illness. The Charter gave prominence to the fundamental role of health activities in the economic and social development of Latin America. It encouraged Member States of the Region to make national health plans for the decade and to establish planning units in their ministries of health.

By 1968, six countries had formulated national health plans as part of economic development, and 11 countries had decided to institute planning. Governments were encouraged to increase the proportion of health projects among all the projects proposed to UNDP and UNEP; PAHO was asked to provide assistance in formulating project proposals when requested. By 1971, three countries were preparing their health activities according to UNDP country programming procedures, and seven others were participating in country planning exercises.

One outcome of the Charter of Punta del Este was establishment of the Pan American programme of health planning in Santiago, Chile, in collaboration with the Latin American Institute for Economic and Social Planning. The programme included research, training and the dissemination of information on health planning.

Early on, jointly with the Center for Development Studies of the Central University of Venezuela, PAHO designed a method for health planning (the PAHO/CENDES method) (7). Hundreds of health planners were trained in the use of this method, thus contributing to the introduction of planning into the health sector of many countries where no formal planning had existed previously. Towards the end of the 1960s, it became obvious that the method was problematic for some countries, as it was complex and called for a relatively extensive database. Its limitations led to the 'quadrennial projections system', which was designed to facilitate the coordination of external aid for health with other economic and social development programmes as well as providing a simple method that countries could use, with some adaptation, for their own health planning. The principles of the system were regarded as the point of departure for health planning, on the understanding that other techniques could be used, depending on the nature and extent of the process.

At their third special meeting, in Santiago, Chile, in October 1972, the ministers of health of the Americas prepared a 10-year health plan (8), which stressed the need to expand the coverage of health services, noting that only 63% of the total population of Latin America and the Caribbean was covered by 'basic' or 'minimal' health services. The plan recommended goals in other fields as well, for example, communicable diseases (e.g. maintaining smallpox eradication, eradicating *Aedes aegypti* from all countries and territories still infested and keeping plague under control), maternal and child health and family welfare (e.g. reducing the mortality of infants under 1 year of age by 40%), nutrition (e.g. reducing grade II and grade III protein–calorie malnutrition in children under 5 years of age by regional averages of 30% and 85%, respectively) and environmental sanitation (e.g. provision of water to 50% of the rural population).

The second group of goals set by the meeting related to the health infrastructure, consisting of human, physical and other resources. The general aims for the decade were to install a health system in each country which was adapted to that country's characteristics; to establish and expand each country's health planning as an integral part of its socioeconomic development plan; to organize systems of information, evaluation and control; to improve health statistics; to conduct systematic studies on costs and financing; to undertake research on various alternatives in sectoral policy and to define methods or techniques to increase the productivity and effectiveness of services. One aim with respect to human resources was to achieve a regional average of 8 doctors, 2 dentists, 2.2 dental auxiliaries, 4.5 nurses and 14.5 nursing auxiliaries per 10 000 inhabitants. With respect to physical resources, one objective was to create minimum comprehensive health service units, including one unit per 5000 people for scattered localities with fewer than 2000 inhabitants and health centres with comprehensive basic minimum services for localities with between 2000 and 20 000 inhabitants.

By the end of 1972, six countries were in various stages of organizing a national health system or service, and in six others agreements were concluded between ministries of public health, social security institutions and universities for the purpose of coordinating hospital building plans or providing comprehensive health services to certain population groups. Twelve countries reformulated their plans in 1974 to bring them into line with the 10-year plan of the Region.

Greater attention was given to health education, with emphasis on community participation in public health work. The technical discussions at the twenty-fifth meeting of the Regional Committee, in 1973, were devoted to "community health services and community involvement". This led to the adoption of resolution XXII, which recommended to Member governments that they assign high priority to the "formulation and implementation of programmes designed to develop in individuals a sense of responsibility for their own health and that of the community and also the ability to participate responsibly and constructively in programmes aimed at the well-being of the population". The Regional Director, Dr Abraham Horwitz, was requested to give high priority to "training of health and related personnel in health education and provide as soon as possible the necessary facilities for the implementation of training programs to meet the needs of the community". In subsequent discussions of health planning, attention was also paid to determining how to involve the community in planning and executing programmes and projects.

PAHO's activities for the development of health manpower were threefold: integration of teaching with the provision of services, educational research and development, and health manpower planning. These interrelated and complementary areas had as their final objective to extend health service coverage and improve health by making the community an integral part of the health system.

In 1968, data were collected from medical schools for a study of medical education and the teaching of preventive and social medicine, and data were collected from all public health schools for a study of their structure, functions and needs and the general characteristics of the teaching. The lack of any uniform pattern in the teaching of preventive medicine led PAHO to assist in setting up programmes at both undergraduate and graduate levels, in training professors in this field and in promoting research, especially in epidemiology and administration. Seminars were organized on the administration of medical schools for administrative personnel, and on curricula for teaching preventive medicine and public health for professors. Countries were encouraged to review their health personnel training programmes from a multidisciplinary or health standpoint in order to cater for the needs of the various services.

Priority was given to medical education early in the decade. As part of their efforts to improve medical education in the Region, PAHO, in 1967, launched a programme to provide reasonably priced textbooks for some 100 000 medical students in about 150 medical schools in Latin America. Arrangements were made to set up a revolving fund, the proceeds from the sale or rental of books being used to make the programme self-financing. New schools joined each year. The first textbooks covered biochemistry, pathology, physiology and pharmacology, and, later, textbooks were added on paediatrics and preventive and social medicine.

The acute shortage of nursing personnel at all levels led in 1972 to the establishment of programmes for training at Master's level in various clinical areas of nursing. Other activities were the elaboration of standards for nursing programmes at university level, plans for studies at higher levels of education, training of teaching personnel and instruction in curriculum construction for teaching auxiliaries who would work in rural areas. Nursing textbooks were added to those distributed through the revolving fund described above.

The nursing situation in the Region was the subject of a report submitted to the twenty-sixth meeting of the Regional Committee, in October 1974. The report reviewed the situation in 17 countries in regard to nursing personnel resources, estimates of future needs, training and absorption into the health services, and the inadequacy of the present situation in most countries. Governments were encouraged to make estimates of the nursing personnel resources required, to take the necessary steps to strengthen the nursing education system in order to prepare personnel who would, in turn, train the type and quantity of nursing manpower that were required and to adopt measures to create the positions needed in order to use graduates of all programmes.

The interrelation and coordination of the health sector with other socioeconomic sectors was the subject of two meetings held in 1975, in Colombia and Costa Rica, with the participation of educational, agricultural, labour, social security and planning agencies. A joint analysis of national health plans and programmes was made in order to determine the areas in which the interests of the various sectors conflicted or coincided. The role of international cooperation in this field was also defined. The findings of these meetings were widely disseminated, and similar cooperative efforts were encouraged in other countries.

Dr Hector Acuña, who had replaced Dr Horwitz as Regional Director for the Americas in January 1975, outlined to the Assembly that year a new 'coverage concept' that had been introduced for the proposed programme budget for 1976–1977. It called for substantive changes in traditional investment criteria, emphasizing primary health care coverage rather than large-scale construction and costly equipment. Priority was also accorded to needy populations, as called for in resolution WHA28.76.

The twenty-ninth session of the Regional Committee, in September–October 1977, took note of the final report of the fourth special meeting of ministers of health and resolved to incorporate community participation and primary health care into the policy of PAHO as strategies for extending health service coverage. It also recommended that governments renew their efforts to extend health services to underserved populations in rural and urban areas in the shortest possible time. As part of community participation, emphasis was placed on the leadership role of adolescents and young people, not only in achieving individual health and welfare, but also in protecting community health. The role of women in health services was also stressed.

The twenty-first session of the Regional Committee, in September–October 1969, stated that multinational centres were both needed and useful and encouraged PAHO to continue to establish and improve them. The Eighteenth Pan American Sanitary Conference, meeting 1 year later, approved general guidelines for the establishment and operation of such centres, which it defined as institutions or centres administered by international staff and supported to a significant degree by international funds, which provided services for all the countries of the Region or for a group in a particular area.

A number of multinational, regional centres were established in the late 1960s, and steps were taken to strengthen those already in existence. In 1967, the Caribbean Food and Nutrition Institute was established to find a regional approach to solving nutritional problems in the Caribbean. The Institute of Nutrition of Central America and Panama, which had been established in 1949 to provide specialized training and consultation in nutrition as well as conducting applied research in this field, was asked by the Regional Committee at its twentieth session, in 1968, to expand its direct responsibility to collaborate with all the countries of the continent and, where appropriate, other regions of the world.

Another important regional centre, the Pan American Zoonoses Centre, in Azul, Argentina, was established in 1968. This Centre assisted neighbouring countries in investigating and controlling zoonoses, providing laboratory services and organizing courses on the production and quality control of brucellosis vaccine, diagnosis of rabies, epidemiology, vaccine production and the care and breeding of laboratory animals. UNDP approved expansion of this Centre in 1972, and it was thus able to play a central role in controlling foot-and-mouth disease in South America.

The establishment, in 1968, in Lima, Peru, of the Pan American Sanitary Engineering and Environmental Sciences Center made it possible to meet requests for advice or more complicated aspects of environmental health. The Center provided technical assistance to all Member governments in Latin America and the Caribbean on air pollution, industrial hygiene, housing and urbanization, physical planning, water treatment, systems analysis and hydraulic resources. Countries were assisted in establishing their own information facilities as part of a regional network of collaborating centres for the exchange of information.

Later in the decade, the Pan American Centre for Human Ecology was established in Mexico, with the aims of formulating a method for addressing human health problems associated with environmental change and establishing priorities for control.

As indicated in the Charter of Punta del Este, it had been expected in 1961 that malaria would be eradicated in the Americas. This proved not to be the case; instead, smallpox was eradicated, the Americas being declared free of the disease in 1973. The demise of smallpox stimulated interest in establishing and strengthening national and regional systems of epidemiological surveillance.

Unlike the other regional offices, which established advisory bodies for research only later in the decade, PAHO already had its own advisory committee on medical research in 1962. The committee played an important role in stimulating and strengthening resources and capabilities for biomedical research in the Americas. During its 1968 session, the committee supported the decision of the Regional Director to create a department of research development and coordination and the plans made to revise and expand the regional programme. For the latter, it indicated that emphasis should be place on both biosocial and biomedical research.

An expanded programme was drawn up after the 1968 session. Three fields were selected for support: viral zoonoses, clinical medicine and regional library services. The expanded programme also provided for research and training grants, increased facilities for biomedical communication and an allocation for operations research.

Like the global Advisory Committee on Medical Research (see Chapter 5), the PAHO committee reviewed developments in the field of health research and advised the Regional Director on research topics that should be pursued. In 1971, for example, after reviewing research in agricultural and food sciences at the Institute of Nutrition of Central America and Panama, it suggested that PAHO explore practical application of the findings, using social research to expedite acceptance of new nutritional techniques and knowledge.

The PAHO advisory committee organized regular symposia to explore the status of health services development in the Region. In 1973, for example, a half day was devoted to the subject of 'medical auxiliaries'. In 1974, a symposium was held on the role of schools of public health in health care in the Americas; and in 1975, the topic of urbanization, internal migration and the spread of diseases was addressed.

SOUTH-EAST ASIA REGION

In his statement to the twenty-second Regional Committee meeting in 1969 (*9*), Dr Herat Gunaratne, the Regional Director, identified certain problems that seemed to be getting worse: the total burden of communicable diseases, the special problems of the care of mothers and children, water shortages and pollution, malnutrition, complications resulting from growing urbanization and, in some parts of the Region, explosive population growth and the overall shortage of trained manpower and education facilities. He expressed the resolve of the Region to assist further in national health planning as part of overall socio-economic plans. The Regional priorities were promotion of medical education and training of all categories of health personnel to meet the needs of integrated health services, provision of community water supplies, pursuance of the goals of malaria and smallpox eradication as part of the global WHO programme and assistance for national tuberculosis control programmes as part of general health services. In the same report, the Regional Director indicated that steps had been taken to orient administrative and technical programmes towards a country approach, as called for by the Health Assembly in its resolution WHA21.49, adopted in May 1968. That resolution stressed the importance of "sound national health plans" as a basis for WHO programmes at regional and global levels.

Dr Mahler, representing the Director-General at the 1971 session of the Regional Committee, spoke about the country approach, which he portrayed as the consequence of a "historical wind which will very much facilitate the possibility that our parochial interests of the past at various levels will be minimized" (*10*). It will "stimulate us to get the right type of integration inside our Organization". In the final analysis, however, the ability of the Organization to "deliver the goods" rested with governments. It lay with them to challenge WHO to become the type of organization they wanted it to be, "to be of real assistance at the country level. If you think it is a mediocre organization, do not put the blame on WHO. It is your organization, and it is only you who can make it into a better one".

Following the technical discussions held in 1968 on health planning, an intercountry project was established, covering various activities connected with planning. A curriculum planning committee was set up that included representatives from one national institute, the Regional Office, PAHO and the Asian Institute for Development and Planning, Bangkok, Thailand. The first annual course on the subject was given at the Institute; a health economist was recruited to assist with the course and to train general economic planners in economics, with emphasis on the health sector. Another economist was recruited in 1970 to cooperate with governments in their planning and evaluation programmes.

The Regional Director, reporting to the twenty-fifth session of the Regional Committee, in 1972, said that although some of the countries of the Region were pioneers in national development planning, health administrations still fell short of implementing plans to provide adequate health services. The lack of clear policy and failure to define programme objectives and to set quantifiable targets against which progress could be measured remained serious obstacles.

The programme on health statistics was enlarged to meet the demands of national health planning, and a statistician was added as a full member of a multidisciplinary team on this topic. At its session in 1973, the Regional Committee stressed the importance of assisting health planning units so that they could take responsibility for data analysis and the formulation of alternative approaches. Countries were encouraged to make suitable use of modern techniques, including systems analysis. An operational research seminar, the first of its kind, was held in Bangkok in 1973, where health information systems were reviewed in order to establish a more rational basis for WHO programme planning. This review led to a reorganization of the Regional Office's information and reporting systems and application of evaluation techniques in several national projects.

Several national seminars on health economics were held in 1974. These provided an opportunity for discussion of completed studies and proposals for studies of application to the health services of techniques from the social sciences (including economics), quantitative studies (including statistics and operations research), cost analyses and models of health planning and health-care delivery.

The concept of country programming as described by UNDP was widely discussed. The Regional Committee in 1971 expressed apprehension that, in view of the diminishing funds from UNDP, this approach could result in health being given lower priority. The Committee stressed that health ministries should consider the problem seriously. Country health programming was promoted as a means of strengthening the capacity of health ministries to formulate projects that would attract funding not only from UNDP but also from bilateral and multilateral sources. Projects for country health programming were formulated in three countries in 1975. UNDP financial difficulties reduced opportunities that might otherwise have materialized in this regard; for example, in 1976, UNDP made available only US$ 2.7 million of the originally planned figure of around US$ 5.8 million.

The beginning of the decade saw an increase in assistance for changing teaching methods and practice in undergraduate and postgraduate education for health personnel, accelerating the establishment of selected institutions or departments to serve as national or regional training centres and promoting group meetings for disseminating up-to-date knowledge in various fields of health. Emphasis was placed on community medicine and the preventive and social aspects of health care in all the educational programmes of the Region.

The novel project in medical education that had been started in 1963 at Baroda Medical College, India, came to an end in 1969. During that period, six teachers in various disciplines from the University of Edinburgh Medical School, Scotland, were assigned, usually for one academic year, to work in Baroda. WHO provided assistance for this exchange, financed the visits of senior short-term consultants and awarded fellowships to enable teachers from Baroda to study in Edinburgh. Books and equipment were also supplied. A total of 53 consultants and technicians participated in this teaching programme.

With the aim of setting up advanced or special medical education units in selected medical schools or departments, several interdisciplinary teams were assigned in 1969 to medical colleges to install a community approach, particularly in obstetrics, paediatrics, preventive medicine and health education. The disciplines represented in these teams were medicine, epidemiology, microbiology and nursing.

Multidisciplinary teams were also established at country and regional levels, with the organization of multidisciplinary educational meetings to promote exchanges of ideas between different categories of health workers. Numerous meetings were sponsored, including seminars and workshops on national health planning, maternal and child health, nursing, health education, health statistics, tuberculosis, plague, venereal diseases, rehydration therapy, immunology, immunization services, vesical calculus, dental health, psychiatry and community medicine.

In order to attract attention to the often neglected question of the training of medical graduates during their internship, the Regional Office assisted in organizing a seminar in 1974. The seminar recommended that interns should undergo practical training at rural health centres, their responsibilities gradually being increased so that they would be equipped to take positions of leadership at the end of their internships.

By 1975, two regional teacher-training centres had been established, with assistance from the Regional Office and UNDP, one in Sri Lanka, the other in Thailand. Both established new curricula and educational techniques. Funding was sought to set up centres in five other countries.

Assistance in nursing was concentrated on strengthening educational programmes for all categories of personnel, particularly nurse educators and administrators. Governments were helped in planning studies in both nursing and midwifery.

A guide for training all cadres of health workers in health education techniques was drawn up at a workshop held in 1968. It was recommended that health education be incorporated into the curricula of health workers and into national health plans, including programmes for training schoolteachers in health education. Research on health behaviour formed part of this effort, with emphasis on the importance of community involvement. A significant development in 1972 was the establishment of rural field practice areas in three countries to provide practical experience as part of postgraduate health education courses.

Several countries received assistance in reviewing and reorganizing health education services, especially those related to maternal and child health, family planning, nutrition, the control of disease and environmental health. Attention was paid to promoting community participation in the design, delivery and evaluation of health education services.

The potential role of voluntary health workers, including traditional medical practitioners, came under closer examination as the concept of primary health care became more widely accepted in the countries of the Region. Their preparation and the formulation of manuals and handbooks was actively pursued. Programmes for the promotion of traditional medicine included a package of research, training and service aspects. To provide supervisory links between multipurpose and voluntary health workers and primary health centres, countries were assisted in training middle-level workers (health assistants or medical assistants). An intercountry seminar was organized in 1977 to define the roles of such personnel.

The availability of additional resources from UNFPA gave a considerable stimulus to family planning programmes and led to the initiation of several new projects in the Region. Full integration of family planning into health services was a priority, and teaching materials were prepared to help countries incorporate this topic into training programmes, especially for nursing and midwifery personnel. The Regional Committee in 1971 recommended that the scope of family health programmes should be broadened so as to integrate the subject into social and economic development. Improved coordination was essential, given the increasing number of requests for assistance and the numerous agencies involved.

In 1970, a decision was taken to convert the Regional team for enteric infections into an epidemiological surveillance team, to assist in monitoring diseases selected as priorities in countries of the Region. The Regional Committee urged that more intercountry meetings be held on epidemiological surveillance of communicable diseases, in particular dengue haemorrhagic fever. Although epidemiological units and divisions were established in ministries of health, at the end of the decade it was judged that the number of diseases under surveillance and the accuracy of the data were not yet satisfactory.

The twenty-eighth session of the Regional Committee, in 1975, considered that biomedical research in the Region should be concentrated on carefully selected priorities and welcomed the proposal to establish a Regional advisory committee on medical research. The Director-General, in a letter conveying his greetings to the members of the committee, contrasted the global approach to research, as undertaken in the past by headquarters, with the new orientation, the aim of which was to meet urgent and emerging problems in developing countries. A long-range view was needed, the prime objective of which was to strengthen national self-reliance and self-sufficiency.

At its first meeting, in January 1976, the committee identified criteria for selecting priorities. Each should be of major importance in terms of its relation to the socioeconomic development of the countries of the Region and be demonstrably susceptible to solution or clarification, with a strong probability that the solution would be applied within a reasonable time and at reasonable cost. The solution or clarification of the problem should lead to the establishment or improvement of a broad national health programme destined to strengthen national or international health, involving large numbers of people. The research should lead to new scientific knowledge or adaptation of knowledge to national contexts. The problem should require Regional collaboration, taking into account, for example, variations in the frequency and distribution of the disease in different geographical areas, differences in ecological settings that influence manifestations of the disease and its response to health intervention, and the opportunity it would provide for pooling the resources of the countries of the Region for its solution.

At the second session of the committee, in August 1976, priorities were selected, and study groups were established for each field. The areas identified were: communicable diseases, nutrition, control of human fertility, environmental health, delivery of health services and a miscellaneous group, which included chronic liver diseases and liver cancer. The resurgence of malaria that year led to the inclusion of malaria as well.

A research study group that met in February 1977 explored various strategies for the delivery of health care. It concentrated on research in primary health care and on the means of obtaining information on promising developments in this field from institutions and scientists. In a seminar held several weeks earlier, the priorities for research that emerged were: extension of care-oriented systems to include educational and motivational activities; initiation of dialogue with communities and involving them in subsequent planning and execution; making higher technology available in a suitable form to the community; and stimulating 'self-help' programmes.

The committee reviewed the progress of the study groups when it met for the third time, in April 1977. It approved the recommendation made by the groups and added some topics. Thus, it recommended that consideration be given to incorporating research on vector control measures into the proposed study on dengue vaccine.[1] Given the importance of diarrhoeal diseases of children, it suggested that the acute form be included in the Special Programme for Research and Training in Tropical Diseases (TDR) in due course. In the meantime, the Regional Director was asked to establish a study group on this topic.

In 1971, the experience of the Americas with the Charter of Punta del Este led the Regional Office for South-East Asia to promote the idea of a health charter for development for the Region. The idea that it would cover all of Asia was pursued with the Regional Office for the Western Pacific, before it was abandoned for administrative reasons. The Charter for Health Development, as formulated by the Regional Office for South-East Asia, was endorsed in 1978. It affirmed the importance of health, resolved to promote health development and gave priority to:

- delivering primary health care to all underserved inhabitants of the region;
- preventing and controlling disease and pollution;
- providing safe water supplies;
- preventing nutritional deficiencies;

---

[1] In a related development, in October 1976 a group of scientists from five regions gathered in Bangkok at the collaborating centre for research on immunopathology of dengue haemorrhagic fever to plan future collaborative research in this field.

- reducing infant, child and maternal morbidity and mortality;
- developing health manpower in accordance with the needs of the people; and
- promoting regional and international collaboration in health matters.

In order to meet these objectives, it was seen necessary to:

- strengthen health planning and health information systems;
- adopt a multidisciplinary, multisectoral approach;
- emphasize prevention and promotion in health care;
- promote community self-help;
- set up an effective disease surveillance system;
- formulate strategies for water supplies;
- strengthen maternal and child health programmes;
- establish nutritional programmes appropriate to the community;
- reorient medical training so that the graduates of medical schools addressed the needs of rural residents; and
- conduct practical research on health-care delivery systems.

The Charter also recognized the relation between health and economic development. It called on the countries of the Region to become as self-reliant as possible in providing health services and to agree to devote the maximum possible resources to health development.

EUROPEAN REGION

In his annual report for 1968–69 (*11*), Dr Leo Kaprio, the Regional Director for Europe, commented that some countries had to speed up the training and education of health workers so as gradually to cover their populations with health services manned by well-trained personnel. Furthermore, central health administrations should ensure that modern medical science was applied effectively and economically for the benefit of the whole population. He characterized the current health care situation as one that was moving "from a 'handicraft' to an 'industrial' approach involving large groups of health personnel working in teams". The situation called for both long-term planning and better managerial leadership.

The work of the Regional Office reflected the responsibilities of national health administrations, and studies of health manpower and economic and planning problems were basic aspects of its work. In 1968, three long-term programmes were either under way or being planned: on cardiovascular disease, mental health of young people and the control of environmental pollution. In 1972, a long-term programme on education and training was approved by the Regional Committee.

Only 12 countries of the Region were eligible for UNDP funding, and, of these, in only three, Algeria, Morocco and Turkey, did the Regional Office maintain a sufficiently large team of experts to justify assignment of a WHO representative. Furthermore, only in Algeria did the WHO team cover a wide spectrum of public health disciplines.

Long-term planning was becoming more complex in the face of the increasing complexity of health systems. Administrators had to learn the language of economists and be versed in systems analysis, mathematical models and simulation techniques from operational research. A working group met in 1969 to study the use of computers in medicine and public health, and in that same year a seminar on the use of operational research in health services was held in Bucharest, Romania, followed by a working group in Copenhagen, Denmark. An advanced course on health planning was organized in Moscow, USSR, in 1969 and annually thereafter.

In June 1972, a working group on health planning in national development met in Stockholm, Sweden, to review the European situation and proposed that studies should be initiated to expand training in this field (*12*). Later that year, a working group on the evaluation of public health programmes stressed the role of epidemiology and the need to increase training in evaluation. Both working groups laid down guidelines for the European Conference on National Health Planning, held in Bucharest in 1974. At that meeting, health planning was described as a systematic, multidisciplinary method of dealing with health problems. It was necessary for all countries, irrespective of their politico-economic system. Each country should have a planning team, the senior members of which must be given freedom to communicate directly with ministries and with public or private enterprises. The community should be involved in planning. It recognized that planning could vary widely, from sophistication to simplicity; there was no universal blueprint. Nevertheless, a number of techniques, taken from other disciplines, were of value, including operational research, economics, statistics, social anthropology and general management science. Countries were advised to collect, assemble and make available material suitable for training health planners. WHO was seen to have an important role to play in coordinating such activities and in ensuring that national norms, standards and definitions were generally available. WHO was also seen as having a prominent role to play in helping to strengthen institutions engaged in teaching and carrying out research in health planning and evaluation, including epidemiological research.

Following the Bucharest meeting, the terms of reference for a unit of health and evaluation planning were established. The unit was to continue studies of health planning models in several European countries and to organize Regional health planning courses and a series of courses on operational research. As part of this initiative, cooperation was established with the International Institute for Applied Systems Analysis in Vienna, Austria.

Methods for estimating health personnel requirements was the theme of a symposium held in Budapest, Hungary, in October 1968. The symposium took a global approach to the problem, including its demographic, economic, administrative and educational aspects. It considered health personnel as a whole, while paying particular attention to the medical profession and to nursing. Key aspects of the educational reform required were the health team approach, application of advanced educational science to health manpower training and looking to the future. Cooperation among local, national and international professional governmental bodies would ensure that each health worker would find expression for his or her desire to serve the community. A paper presented to the nineteenth session of the Regional Committee, in 1969, concluded that WHO's most useful role was perhaps to help promote such cooperation and assist Member States to meet the challenge of health manpower and training.

A working group on trends in European nursing services, convened in December 1970, recommended that provision be made for nurses to take part in planning for health care at national, regional and local levels; that a thorough study of education for the health professions, including nurses, be undertaken, to orient it to meet the health needs of modern communities; that experiments on nursing care patterns be planned for different population groups, such as the elderly or foreign workers, and be designed in such a way that their adequacy, suitability, efficiency and effectiveness could be evaluated; that health planning as a whole should provide for research and experimentation in new ways of organizing nursing services and nursing education; and that the preparation of educational leaders and teachers of nursing should be given the highest priority. A programme of meetings and courses was launched in 1972 to address the latter need. In 1974, a planning meeting was held in Kiel, Federal Republic of Germany, to draw up plans for a programme in nursing and midwifery in Europe.

The Regional Office's long-term programme on education and training, which had been approved in 1972, was initiated in January 1975. It was to pay particular attention to communication, teacher training and continuing education, each of which was considered to be a subsystem in overall health services. Two meetings of deans, teachers and administrators of medical schools helped to clarify the priorities of the Member States in this field.

The Regional Office was made responsible for WHO's global programmes on the prevention of road traffic accidents and health care of the elderly in 1975. That same year saw the decentralization of biomedical research, which led the Regional Director to observe in his annual report of that year: "I consider that the potential provided by health services oriented research, as related to the complex health conditions of European countries, constitutes a great challenge for the Regional Office" (13).

During its twenty-fifth session, in 1975, the Regional Committee approved research on cardiovascular disease, environmental health, mental health, health manpower development, long-term care for the elderly, road traffic accidents, economic aspects of diseases, operational research, electronic data processing and health planning and programming at national level. The Regional advisory committee for medical research was given the following terms of reference:

- to assist in the coordination of national research programmes in order to improve the efficiency and cost–benefit ratio of health services in Europe;
- to identify problem areas and establish priorities, particularly for health services research;
- to promote the research components of the Regional Office's long-term programmes; and
- to make and maintain contact with research bodies in Europe.

At the second meeting of the committee, in October 1977, practical steps were outlined and planning groups were established for each of the selected research areas.

Dr Mahler, newly elected Director-General, addressing the twenty-third session of the Regional Committee, in 1973, put forward the idea that Europe "had an enormous contribution to make to the rest of the world, but had been too conservative in the past. It had exported its established methods and thus prevented many developing countries from benefiting to the full from all it had to offer. Now, however, there was a greater willingness to experiment, and this was bound to benefit the developing countries." (*14*)

Three years later, on the same occasion, he expanded on this issue by focusing on the role that the Regional Committee could play in stimulating and coordinating technical cooperation between countries (*15*). It could promote increased intercountry collaboration in areas of social relevance for the Region and could stimulate more participation by the many excellent clinical and medical institutions in the Region in research, development and genuine exchange of information, which were required to find and launch fundamental health techniques that were more appropriate than existing ones in terms of social relevance and cost.

The developed world, he continued, had nothing to lose and much to gain from cooperation with developing countries, as the solutions to many problems in those countries were of interest to more prosperous countries, as seen from the successes of the tuberculosis control and smallpox eradication programmes. The eradication of smallpox would lead to annual savings of at least US$ 1 billion to the industrial world. Furthermore, the evolution of primary health care in developing countries might well provide direct and indirect benefits for the organization of primary health care in medically affluent countries.

He concluded by suggesting that serious consideration should be given to ways of improving collaboration between the European Region and the other regions. The Regional Committee should also seek ways of encouraging its Member States to pledge bilateral aid funds, in the same spirit of cooperation, and to channel funds into the health programmes that were considered by developing countries to be socially relevant.

At the end of a long discussion on his presentation, he added that, as Europe had everything to gain from genuine international cooperation under WHO auspices, the rest of the world also stood to benefit from what the European Region could achieve, and the ways in which it got to grips with relevant techniques could serve as coherent, unfragmented models for developing countries, offering real alternatives for health development. Thus, if the European Region could agree on general health priorities and specific problems such as cancer, cardiovascular disease and the problems of the aged, the benefits for the Third World would be immense.

EASTERN MEDITERRANEAN REGION

The Regional Director, Dr A.H. Taba, in his introduction to the nineteenth session of the Regional Committee, in 1969 (*16*), said that, despite the progress that had been made during the previous 20 years, most Eastern Mediterranean countries were still in dire need of medical personnel. Furthermore, general practitioners and specialists were poorly distributed, with an inequitable concentration in urban areas. He also noted the shortage of qualified nurses and the dearth of auxiliary workers. The Region's efforts in this area, fruitful as they had been, "have but partly filled this vacuum".

Particular attention, he continued, was being given to the key issue of medical training, with growing awareness among medical educators that teaching programmes must be adapted to local conditions and that medicine should be taught in relation to the community to be served. The subject had been emphasized at each of the conferences on medical education held in Teheran, in 1962 and 1970. From 1969 on, the Region participated actively in the WHO long-term programme for teachers of medical and allied health professions (see Chapter 8).

In a position paper prepared in 1973, the Regional programme was defined as consisting of the following elements:

- continued support to health planning by Member governments, with emphasis on continuous redefinition of health manpower and teacher requirements;
- continued support to training in specific subjects, by expanding the fellowship programme and WHO-sponsored seminars, workshops and working groups in fields of priority for governments and the Organization;
- support to the programme of the regional teacher training centre that had been set up in 1972, in collaboration with Pahlavi University in Shiraz, Iran, the overall objectives of which were to promote awareness and subsequent acceptance of educational science in the education and training of health personnel (In 1975, the centre was designated as a WHO collaborating centre for health manpower development.);
- support to the creation and running of national teacher training centres;
- support for the preparation of key teachers in educational planning, in as many individual schools and training institutions as budgetary and other limitations permitted; and
- support to regional and national facilities that were likely to increase the availability of training programmes or of the teaching and learning materials that the increasing numbers of teachers required to make the most impact on their students.

In regard to the last point, a project was launched by WHO in Egypt with the objective of assisting the Centre for Educational Technology in the Health Sciences, Cairo, in applying modern educational techniques, particularly audiovisual teaching. Another promising development was an innovative approach in the small medical faculty of the Haile Sellassie I University, Addis Ababa, Ethiopia, to a rural health training project, in which every medical student underwent clerkship training as part of the design of a public health service.

Another element of support was the provision of teachers in the basic sciences, pathology and preventive and social medicine. In 1971, the exchange of professors between medical schools increased, and conferences were held on medical education in the exchange of knowledge.

A meeting was organized in June 1970 of senior national nurses and nurse–midwives in leadership positions, to discuss the nursing manpower requirements of the Region and to study how those needs could be met, including the contribution of WHO. The acute shortage of nurses in the Region led to further efforts to promote awareness among governments of the need to revise the conditions of service for qualified staff, especially to counter the trend for nurses to seek employment in other countries.

In 1975, three trends in nursing were noted. The first was initiation of an assessment of nursing care, with a view to adapting it to meet the increasing demands for nursing personnel resulting from countries' changing needs. The second was the greater extent to which the nursing systems of countries of the Region were becoming self-supporting and able to assist each other. This carried over into the third trend, which showed a decrease in the number of long-term WHO nurse advisers required and a corresponding increase in requests for fellowships and consultants to assist in more specialized nursing programmes.

In his annual report for 1972–1973 (*17*), the Regional Director described the Region as containing "an infinite variety of climatic, demographic, and topological conditions which, taken together with the different stages of development achieved in countries and even variations between districts within individual countries, result in a remarkable diversity of health problems". In an earlier report (*16*), he had indicated that, although the needs of the countries in the Region varied greatly, they had one factor in common: "their extremely rapid development (some amongst the fastest in the world)". Another determining factor was the demographic explosion in certain countries.

As a consequence of this diversity, development projects were tending to increase in size and complexity. Not only were the projects that were assisted by WHO becoming multidisciplinary, but the stake of the Organization in programmes was growing, as illustrated by the UNESCO literacy programmes and teacher-training projects and more general development projects, such as that for the Awash Valley in Ethiopia and the Lake Nasser development project in the United Arab Republic (see Chapter 9). The joint comprehensive planning exercise sponsored by UNDP in Tunisia and Lebanon was a further indication of the importance being given to comprehensive, integrated national planning by governments and the United Nations system alike.

Effective response to these many-faceted changes required a new spirit of innovation, continued the Regional Director, an understanding that transcended the traditional boundaries of health activities and a willingness to forge new associations. This led him to conclude:

- Networks of health services, a prerequisite for disease control and health programmes, increasingly required systematic establishment of technical manpower development and training programmes.
- Planning and coordination of bi- and multilateral assistance, based on countries' socioeconomic development plans, would require the establishment and implementation of efficient national planning and coordination.
- Broadening horizons and the competition for funds would lead to closer scrutiny of project proposals, with clear implications for more detailed studies of problems and proposed solutions.
- The pressure for more realistic programme planning would increase so as to narrow the gap between the planned programmes and those that were actually implemented.

UNDP country programming provided an opportunity for countries to present a framework covering 3–5 years, to ensure integrated use of UNDP and other resources that were expected to be available. Country programming called for preparation of a 'project document', which justified the project and gave the institutional framework, long- and short-term objectives, a work plan and coded budgets. In light of trends in the United Nations system to decentralize planning, operation and evaluation to country level, the number of WHO representatives was increased, as in the other WHO regions during this period, with the exception of Europe.

An interregional advanced course for WHO representatives was organized in Alexandria, Egypt, in early 1973, which covered such topics as new WHO trends and policies, especially in regard to participation in country programming and collaboration with other agencies in the field of health, changes in UNDP procedures and modern management techniques. Despite these efforts, the constraints imposed by the requirement to provide 'indicative planning figures' (see Chapter 1) made it more difficult for national health authorities to obtain the assistance required and to compete with other sectors, such as agriculture and industry, in which more easily assessable economic results had greater appeal for national planners.

By 1974, most countries in the Region had health sector plans that were part of their socioeconomic plans. Some had acquired considerable experience in the use of advanced planning techniques, while others were preparing their first sectoral plans. Still, health authorities had been slow to realize the extent to which decision-makers could be helped by being given an insight into managerial processes and by the newer techniques available. The situation was compounded by the fact that the education and training of doctors did not give them an active interest in managerial and administrative problems. Furthermore, as noted in the Regional Director's annual report for 1972–1973, too much reliance was still being placed on education and training approaches derived from other countries and too little on approaches designed to meet the needs of the country.

Four countries in the Region undertook health programming with WHO assistance during the 1976–1977 biennium. The programme in Yemen was used as the basis of the Government's first national health plan and for a structural and functional reorganization of the Ministry of Health.

Convinced of the importance of improving the administrative abilities of all senior officers of ministries and provincial health departments, the Region promoted fellowships for advanced courses in public health administration and national planning. In 1973, a seminar on modern management approaches to national health administration was organized in Cairo, at which senior health administrators from eight countries of the Region discussed the value and use of modern concepts and techniques in planning, setting up, operating and evaluating health services. To find an effective method that could be used in other countries, a management study was undertaken in Yemen to find more efficient ways of harnessing the limited resources of the existing health services.

Dr Mahler, representing the Director-General at the twenty-second session of the Regional Committee, in 1972, noted that following the golden era of the 1950s and even the 1960s, with the spectacular successes of mass disease campaigns, governments now had to face the complex task of building up a permanent structure to provide health care to their populations (18). A change in attitude had become necessary. Whereas there had been a tendency in the communicable disease campaigns to plan from the global viewpoint, now it was necessary "to start to look much more from the country upwards, through the Regional organization, to the global level—otherwise success would not be achieved". There was no magic formula for building up good, solid health-care systems; unlike the relatively easy mass campaigns, this would be a "painfully slow process".

One WHO-assisted project for health planning research, which attracted particular attention during this period, was initiated in West Azerbaijan, Iran, in early 1972. By 1973, its terms of reference were "to discover and test better ways to solve multiple health problems through an effective and efficient health delivery system". The project set up frontline health posts with two new types of primary health worker, a man to deal mainly with community health problems, environmental sanitation, surveillance of selected communicable diseases and collecting information for a population of 4000–8000, and a woman who addressed mainly personal and family health problems, particularly maternal and child health and family planning, for a population of 2000–4000. The project also included strengthening primary care at the level of the doctor or health centre to ensure continuous service, integration of essential curative components of care into preventive services and improvement of the training and management capability of district units. In the technical discussions on primary health care at the twenty-fifth session of the Regional Committee, in 1975, practical application in other countries of many of the techniques tested in West Azerbaijan was judged to be feasible (*19, 20*).

As in other WHO regions, the creation of UNFPA gave impetus to activities in family planning. Seminars were organized as early as 1970 on health aspects of human reproduction in family planning and population dynamics and on advances in the physiological, clinical and public health aspects of human reproduction.

In collaboration with other United Nations agencies, training programmes were run to prepare health personnel for planning and implementing appropriate nutrition programmes, as it was stressed that long-term policies and plans in the entire area of food and nutrition were needed to ensure lasting improvements in the nutritional status of populations. By 1977, the results of collaboration between UNICEF, FAO, UNESCO and WHO were judged to have been fruitful. Another example of effective interagency cooperation was a workshop held in Afghanistan on family health, communication and education for integrated rural development, cosponsored by FAO, ILO, UNESCO and WHO.

Interagency cooperation was also seen in assistance in health education, which was introduced into functional literacy projects that were part of the UNESCO-sponsored Arab States Functional Literacy Centre in Sirs-el-Layyan, United Arab Republic, and in the curricula of agricultural schools and of teacher training institutions in collaboration with FAO and UNESCO. Health education was also systematically introduced into family planning programmes in countries of the Region, with the assistance of WHO.

The first meeting of the Regional advisory committee on biomedical research took place in April 1976 (*21*). Two teams of high-level consultants, including several members of the WHO Executive Board, visited a number of countries to identify potential resources for research in the Region and compiled a directory of institutions involved in biomedical research. The visits confirmed the interest of governments in biomedical research, while indicating that some did not yet have an adequate overall administrative or technical infrastructure for conducting sound research.

At the second meeting, in March 1977, it was agreed that priority should continue to be given to research on health services and manpower development (*22*). It was recommended that a working paper be prepared, outlining ongoing and planned research on activities of priority to the Region and in line with the priorities of TDR (see Chapter 5). Another working paper was requested, on research manpower in the Region, with suggestions on how it could be improved. Emphasis was placed on the career structure and conditions of employment of research workers, the requirements for technicians and other middle-level personnel and ways in which WHO could cooperate in improving research manpower.

An important regional health authority, the Council of Arab Ministries of Health, was established in April 1975, its prime objective being to further advance and promote health services in all Arab countries, through health plans and institutions active in medical sciences and research. In response to a request from the Council, the Health Assembly resolved in May 1975 to include Arabic among the working languages of WHO (resolution WHA28.34).

The Region also benefited from "the generous financial support given by the more fortunate of our countries", a situation seen by the Regional Director, Dr A.H. Taba, on the occasion of the 1977 Regional Committee meeting, as "unique, perhaps for this Region, or at least occurring on a much greater scale than elsewhere in the world, and an indication of the spirit of collaboration which exists among friendly countries ...". Dr Taba singled out for particular mention the generosity of Iran, Iraq, Kuwait, Libya, Qatar, Saudi Arabia and the United Arab Emirates, which, in addition to their normal contributions to WHO, had curtailed their own demands on the Organization's budget in favour of expansion of activities in other, less favoured countries and had made substantial donations to WHO voluntary funds.

WESTERN PACIFIC REGION

With the entry of China into the United Nations system, the Western Pacific Region gained the most populated country of the world, adding further to its wide diversity. As noted by Dr Mahler in 1973, on the first occasion he had to address a regional committee in his new capacity as Director-General, there was a "richness of experience" in the Region that was "perhaps unmatched in any of the WHO regions". It was "undoubtedly a resource of great potential" if it could be properly exploited. The diversity could be made to bear fruit "through the exchange of information and ideas, and the pooling of resources both intellectual and material ... so that each Member may progress along his chosen path by deriving benefit from what is best in the community of Members." (23)

The eighteenth Regional Committee meeting, in 1968, recommended that long-term emphasis should be placed on organization and administration (including extension of health services to the periphery and improving their management); education and training; and selected programmes, such as communicable disease control, the organization of medical care, environmental health and health promotion, with particular attention to child health. Joint studies could be pursued on selected subjects of particular interest to groups of countries, for example, haemorrhagic fever, Japanese encephalitis and filariasis. Assistance was also envisaged for those Member States that were formulating national health plans, including the determination of priorities and goals in the framework of national socioeconomic development plans.

From answers to a questionnaire sent to governments in 1968 on integrated planning for health, the Regional Office learnt that 12 governments had a national planning body, and in 10 of those a health sector had been established. Ten governments expressed interest in receiving WHO assistance in this field. A Regional programme of training in health planning was established to assist ministries or directorates of health in adopting a systematic, methodological approach to the inclusion of long-range health plans in national development schemes. A course was designed in collaboration with the University of the Philippines and offered annually on subjects that included an introduction to economics, public administration, demography and sociology; a theoretical presentation of economic, physical and social development, with emphasis on national health and manpower planning; and field practice in health planning. In 1971, the Asian Institute for Economic Planning seconded a lecturer in development planning, and the course was extended to cover health planning on a wider scale than previously. In 1973, a course in Malaysia and an area course for the South Pacific replaced the regional health planning course, providing training in health planning for middle-level and local staff.

Health practice research was seen as a useful adjunct to health planning, and studies were carried out in Malaysia and the Philippines, the latter in collaboration with the University Institute of Hygiene. Operational research techniques led to alternative methods for improving the performance of rural health units.

The Regional Committee at its twenty-third meeting, in 1972, reviewed a report by the Regional Director on long-term planning in health (24). National health plans were found to be in an early stage of development, and the Regional Director was asked to continue to assist governments in increasing their own capacity for planning. The introduction of country programming by UNDP had led to preparation of a document for the Philippines, which, in 1972, was "hailed as a model". Nevertheless, despite the increased scope given to the UNDP programme, the percentage of WHO's total programme financed by UNDP pursued its downward trend, as experienced in other regions during this period.

A conference on national health planning held in 1972 revealed that national health administrators fully recognized the importance of planning their programmes in the context of national development plans. The conference recommended that development projects provide investment outlays to control health hazards associated with their operation. It suggested that countries of the Region should exchange information on planning methods and practices and provide more training in health planning. It sought the cooperation of WHO headquarters in finding a method that would be suitable for developing countries.

The first Regional seminar on health manpower planning was held in 1973, to encourage wider acceptance of the need for long-term planning. A revised health planning manual for teachers and a field manual were prepared. Systems analysis was introduced in the formulation of development projects, and country health programming was introduced in the Region in 1975.

Community health services were promoted by the adoption of comprehensive plans for the provision of WHO assistance. By 1970, projects for particular health services were grouped in a single plan of operations, the overall aim of which was to promote national health planning, to improve the coordination of national health programmes, to foster local health organizations, to make services more efficient and to encourage research in health practices.

Operational research proved to be a useful approach for improving the delivery of health services, as, even where national resources were limited, effectiveness, efficiency and greater coverage could be achieved by testing alternative approaches. Intercountry consultations were promoted for finding solutions to common problems on a regional and subregional basis.

The proposal by one government in 1967 that WHO establish a medical school in the Region, which was contrary to WHO policy, led to a closer examination of how national institutions might be strengthened to reach a standard suitable for international training. A travelling seminar organized in 1969 for deans of medical schools led to the appointment of a steering committee to study the feasibility of establishing a regional association of medical schools in order to improve cooperation and collaboration. A related development was an increase in activities to improve teaching methods in medical schools. The teaching of preventive medicine was reviewed in a regional seminar held in 1970, which also drew up guidelines for national workshops on the subject.

In 1971, the objectives of country projects in education and training assisted by the Regional Office were broadened to cover overall medical education, including the training of nurses and other health personnel. A technical advisory committee on nursing was established to provide guidelines for future assistance from the Regional Office for strengthening nursing and midwifery programmes. The committee consisted of senior nurses, public health workers and an educator from countries in the Region as well as outside experts and WHO staff.

Agreement was reached in 1972 with the Government of Australia to establish a regional teacher training centre in the University of New South Wales, Sydney. The centre was jointly funded from the regular budget of the Regional Office and UNDP. Regional Office assistance to improve basic, post-basic and postgraduate health personnel training included paedagogical methods, which were disseminated through the fellowship programme. National and intercountry workshops and other types of meetings were also held, the Regional teacher training centre providing the nucleus. With the establishment of two national teacher-training centres, in the Philippines and the Republic of Korea, in 1975, the regional programme entered into its second phase. A Master's course for health personnel education was initiated in 1976 at the University of New South Wales.

Activities in basic nursing education continued to expand, and midwifery studies were increasingly being incorporated into the nursing curriculum so that nurses could be prepared more rapidly. The use of auxiliary nurse–midwives in many situations rather than a single one became commoner as the decade progressed.

A technical advisory committee on nursing was convened in December 1973 to review the preparation and use of nursing and midwifery personnel in the Region and prepared guidelines and proposals on possible approaches to the training and use of such personnel. One conclusion was that a multidisciplinary approach should be used in all aspects of planning, implementing and organizing health-care delivery systems.

The possibility of using new types of health auxiliaries and community health aides in clinics and health centres aroused interest in time. Initially, Regional Office-assisted projects for health services development were more concerned with standardizing the duties and training of already recognized auxiliary health workers, particularly those who were to undertake many activities. A seminar in 1974 on medical assistants demonstrated the value and place of this type of worker in the health system. Several participating countries introduced new categories of assistants into their health services, the Regional Office providing advice on training programmes for these workers.

The Regional Director, Dr Francisco J. Dy, in his introductory statement to the 1977 *Work of the Region* observed, however, that, although the integrated approach to health care with multipurpose workers had "gained wider acceptance", further thought would have to be given to determine "the specific needs and hazards which apply to the family as a unit" and the priorities for dealing with them, to allow the development of "easy-to-learn techniques" to enhance the skills of the village health workers involved (*25*).

Collaboration with governments in strengthening vital and health statistics was pursued concurrently with other health activities to ensure the availability of adequate information for assessing the health conditions and needs of the population and for formulating realistic national health programmes and plans. Some of the reasons cited for the poor state of health statistical information were lack of awareness of its importance by the population and the private health sector, unfamiliarity of health personnel with the organization and use of health statistical services and the absence of health services in many remote areas. Projects were undertaken to improve the health and medical records of health centres and hospitals and to organize central health statistical units. In 1974, steps were taken to set up a health information system for use in the Region, designed to provide geographical information, socioeconomic and demographic data and information on health services and health-related activities, including epidemiological, environmental and communications data.

The integration of maternal and child health and family planning into general health services was the subject of technical discussions of the Regional Committee at its eighteenth meeting, in 1967. More technical assistance from WHO in planning, evaluating and implementing these services was recommended, with the assistance of UNICEF. WHO was also called on to assist in preparing curricula for medical and allied health professions that incorporated family planning. Activities in family planning were centred on strengthening the Regional structure for providing assistance and on preparatory work for country and intercountry activities undertaken with financing from UNFPA, which became available in 1970.

Health education was considered an essential component of all health programmes, particularly those concerned with family health. In 1973, educational materials were produced in cooperation with various experts and agencies interested in family planning, community development, education, extension work, communications and the social and economic aspects of family health. Health education was recognized as being essential for achieving community involvement and individual participation, which were crucial for successful family health care. The need for collaboration between health services and development agencies working at community level was also emphasized.

Expansion of activities on nutrition within health services and family health programmes was encouraged by setting up a small pool of national staff with the necessary technical experience in some countries and by adding Regional Office nutrition advisers to the staff of these services and programmes. Nutrition education was strengthened. Later in the decade, formulation of national food and nutrition policies and collaboration in this sphere between WHO and other organizations in the United Nations system was given more attention. Such policies were found difficult to establish, however, partly because of lack of an adequate database but also because of the difficulty of coordinating the work of the various agencies and professional disciplines (see Chapter 7).

In his introduction to *The work of the Region* in 1976, the Regional-Director noted increasing acceptance in the Region of a multidisciplinary, integrated approach to family health, as reflected in the "intensive input" districts of Malaysia, in the community-based family health programme in Bohol Province, Philippines, and in the activities of women's committees in Western Samoa. The latter was the subject of a case study by the Joint WHO/UNICEF Committee on Health Policy in 1976–1977 (see Chapter 6).

The continuing high prevalence of communicable diseases and the recurrence of epidemics drew attention to the importance of epidemiological surveillance in the Region. Recognizing that rigid quarantine measures had not been able to stop the spread of infection from country to country, the Regional Committee in 1970 endorsed the new concept adopted by WHO (see Chapter 9). The first regional courses on epidemiological surveillance and international quarantine were held in the Republic of Korea and in Fiji in 1970. The services of an intercountry communicable disease advisory team were made available. In 1971, a regional programme on health laboratory services was established. By 1974, the epidemiological services were seen to be limited by a shortage of epidemiologists, inadequate laboratory services and inadequate reliable statistical data, and the generation and exchange of epidemiological information remained minimal. As regards health laboratories, the emphasis shifted to laboratory networks at intermediate and peripheral levels, and priority was given to training staff in microbiology, basic laboratory testing, maintenance of equipment, laboratory administration, management and quality control. A Regional training course in epidemiology was organized to meet the shortage of epidemiologists, and an intercountry epidemiological surveillance project was established in 1975 to serve countries and areas in the South Pacific.

Like the other regional committees, the Western Pacific Regional Committee at its twenty-sixth session welcomed a proposal for greater involvement of the Regional Committee and the Regional Office in promoting and coordinating appropriate programmes of biomedical research, with emphasis on applied research. It endorsed the proposals of the Regional Director, which included establishment of a regional advisory committee. It also recommended that a study be undertaken of the feasibility of establishing a WHO regional centre for research and training in tropical diseases.

The Regional advisory committee on medical research held its first meeting in June 1976 and established three task forces: health services research, research in cardiovascular diseases and research in parasitic and other communicable diseases (*26*). The committee reviewed the organization and functions of the Institute for Medical Research, Kuala Lumpur, Malaysia, with a view to designating it as a WHO Regional centre for research and training in tropical diseases. At its twenty-seventh session, in September 1976, the Regional Committee approved the recommendations deriving from the feasibility study and those of the Regional advisory committee.

At its twenty-eighth session, in 1977, the Regional Committee endorsed further recommendations of the Regional advisory committee, which included establishment of a regional multidisciplinary research programme on schistosomiasis and the organization, in 1978, of a workshop on health services research and a training course on the epidemiology of cardiovascular disease.

References

1. Guilbert J-JA. *Contribution of the World Health Organization to the evolution of medical education in the African region, 1962–1972: a content analysis of policy statement documents* (HMD/STT/74.4). Geneva, World Health Organization, 1974.
2. *Conference on health coordination and cooperation in Africa. Report of the first meeting, Yaoundé, 25–26 September 1975* (AFR/PHA/159). Brazzaville, Regional Office for Africa, 1976.
3. *Conference on health coordination and cooperation in Africa. Report of the second meeting, Brazzaville, 15–16 September 1977* (AFR/PHA/188). Brazzaville, Regional Office for Africa, 1977.
4. Asante RO. Basic health services in Ghana: experiences to date and future directions. *Annals of the Belgian Society of Tropical Medicine*, 1979, 59 (Suppl):89–97.
5. Stromberg J. Education for community involvement: experiences from the BARIDEP (Ghana) Project. In: Carlaw RW, Ward WB, eds. *Primary health care—the African experience*. Oakland, California, Third Party Publishing, 1988.
6. *Special meeting of ministers of health of the Americas* (REMSA/19), Rev. 2. Washington DC, Pan American Health Organization, 1968.
7. Tejada de Rivero DA. The Pan American health planning program. *American Journal of Public Health*, 1975, 65:1052–1059.
8. *Ten-year health plan for the Americas. Final report of the III special meeting of ministers of health of the Americas* (REMSA 3/30), Washington DC, Pan American Health Organization, 1973.
9. *Twenty-first annual report of the Regional Director* (SEA/RC22/2). New Delhi, Regional Office for South-East Asia, 1969.
10. *Twenty-fourth session of the WHO Regional Committee for South-East Asia. Final report and minutes of the meetings* (SEA/RC24), Annex 2. New Delhi, Regional Office for South-East Asia, 1971.
11. *Report of the Regional Director. July 1968 to June 1969* (EUR/RC19/2). Copenhagen, Regional Office for Europe, 1969.
12. *Health planning in national development, report on a working group, Stockholm, 19–22 June 1972*. Copenhagen, Regional Office for Europe, 1972.
13. *Report of the Regional Director, July 1975 to June 1976* (EUR/RC26/2), Copenhagen, Regional Office for Europe, 1976.
14. *Regional Committee for Europe, 23rd session, minutes of the first meeting* (EUR/RC23/Min.1). Copenhagen, Regional Office for Europe, 1973.
15. *Regional Committee for Europe, 23rd session, minutes of the second meeting* (EUR/RC23/Min.2). Copenhagen, Regional Office for Europe, 1973.
16. *Annual report of the Regional Director* (EM/RC19/2). Alexandria, Regional Office for the Eastern Mediterranean, 1969.
17. *Annual report of the Regional Director* (EM/RC23/2. Alexandria, Regional Office for the Eastern Mediterranean, 1973.

18. *Regional Committee for the Eastern Mediterranean, twenty-second session, sub-committee A* (EM/RC22/Min.1). Alexandria, Regional Office for the Eastern Mediterranean, 1972.

19. *Approaches to the effective delivery of primary health care, with particular reference to the experience in West Azerbaijan, Iran* (EM/RC25A/Tech.Disc./Min.1), Alexandria, Regional Office for the Eastern Mediterranean, 1975.

20. King M, ed. *An Iranian experiment in primary health care: the West Azerbaijan project.* London, Oxford University Press, 1983.

21. *Report on the meeting of the Regional Advisory Committee on Biomedical Research, Alexandria, 6–8 April 1976* (EM/RSR/1), Alexandria, Regional Office for the Eastern Mediterranean, 1976.

22. *Report of the Regional Advisory Committee on Biomedical Research—second meeting, Alexandria, 23–26 March 1977* (EM/RSR/3), Alexandria, Regional Office for the Eastern Mediterranean, 1977.

23. *Regional Committee for the Western Pacific, twenty-fourth session, summary records of the plenary sessions*, Annex 3 (WPR/RC24/SR/1). Manila, Regional Office for the Western Pacific, 1973.

24. *Long-term planning in the field of health, including long-term financial indicators. Progress report by the Regional Director* (WPR/RC23/10), Manila, Regional Office for the Western Pacific, 1972.

25. *The work of WHO in the Western Pacific Region. Annual report of the Regional Director covering the period, 1 July 1976–30 June 1977* (WPR/RC28/3). Manila, Regional Office for the Western Pacific, 1977.

26. *Report on the meeting of the Western Pacific Region Advisory Committee on Medical Research, first session* (WPR/ACMR/76.13). Manila, Regional Office for the Western Pacific, 1976.

CHAPTER 5

Promotion and development of research

The history of the first 10 years of WHO does not include a chapter dedicated to research; it has only a short, one-page description, indicating that WHO "does not normally operate its own research institutions but uses existing national centres and institutions whose services are made available by the responsible national authorities". Much of the work undertaken at the time, especially in the fields of biological standardization, epidemiology, health statistics and nutrition, was a continuation of long-standing international programmes that had originated in the time of the League of Nations or earlier. No special effort was made to promote or coordinate research on a large scale during the period.

Matters began to change when the Eleventh World Health Assembly, in 1958, called for "a special study of the role of WHO in research and of ways in which the Organization might assist more adequately in stimulating and coordinating research and developing research personnel", the outcome of which led the Twelfth World Health Assembly, in 1959, to adopt resolution WHA12.17, which recognized that WHO had an important role to play in increasing this potential and in fostering international collaboration among scientists by stimulating, coordinating, promoting and supporting research. To this end, it decided that an advisory committee on medical research should be established to give the Director-General the necessary scientific advice on the research programme. It also agreed that provisions should be made in the regular budget to finance the medical research programme and that a special account be established to supplement the provision under the regular budget.

The objectives of the programme were fourfold: to support medical research, to provide services for research, to train research workers and to improve communication among scientists. Support of medical research was seen to consist of three activities: collaborative research, field research teams and grants to individual investigators. The provision of services consisted mainly of the creation of reference centres and preparation of reports of scientific groups, which were ad hoc groups of experts in a particular field convened to review a subject from a purely scientific point of view, to identify gaps in knowledge and to advise on needs for further research. Fellowships were made available to increase the number of persons qualified in research. The exchange of research workers contributed to promoting scientist-to-scientist communication.

The work of the Organization in this field during the second decade was recorded in two volumes, one covering the period 1958–1963 and the second 1964–1968. In the introduction to the latter, it was noted that the past few years had seen "a crystallization of the concept that medical research is a multidisciplinary function. The medical specialist and his colleague the biologist have been joined by social scientists, mathematicians, physicists, and others" (*1*). The influence of progress in data processing was noted, as was its use in mathematical and stochastic modelling.

The establishment in January 1967 of a division of research in epidemiology and communications science was described as "perhaps the most significant structural development brought about by this trend". The disciplines represented in this Division included, on the one hand, epidemiology, sociology, demography, ecology and geography and, on the other, a communications science group with biomathematics, operational research, applied mathematics, statistics and computer science. The responsibilities of the Division were to propose new methods or alternative solutions, test them in the field and adapt them to situations relevant to the Organization and to the governments of its Member States, with the techniques of a variety of disciplines. The Director-General, in a brief statement on this Division after its first year of operation, noted that such research "will be both difficult and expensive".

Another development noted in the introduction was the decision to establish a new unit at WHO headquarters, the function of which would be to promote, coordinate and carry out research in education for the health professions and assist in establishing a balanced programme on educational research. The unit would deal with such subjects as criteria for selecting students, methods for appraising students' performance, adaptation of the medical curriculum to modern needs, the effectiveness of teaching aids and the relation of medical education to national health planning.

Also noted was the establishment by the Health Assembly in 1965 of the International Agency for Research on Cancer (IARC). This Agency was set up as an autonomous body within WHO, with its seat in Lyon, France, and the objective of promoting international collaboration in cancer research.

In determining priorities, emphasis was given to problems encountered in the field, the solutions to which required new knowledge. Communicable diseases were a danger to health throughout the world and had occupied a place in WHO's programme of work from its inception. The advent of penicillin (followed shortly by a series of other antibiotics), DDT (followed by a series of new insecticides), the antimalarial drugs, isoniazid and other therapeutic substances "opened new vistas in the field of public health". The concept of 'disease eradication' was born and began to displace that of 'disease control'. A new, "perhaps over-optimistic" approach to the control of communicable diseases was taken, but it soon became clear that much more knowledge had to be acquired.

Other problems that were recognized were protein malnutrition, cardiovascular disease, cancer and other noncommunicable diseases. The environmental aspects of health and disease could not be overlooked, nor could questions related to the health aspects of population dynamics and pharmacology.

At the time, the priorities for research conducted and supported by the Organization were established by the Director-General on the basis of recommendations from the Advisory Committee on Medical Research. This Committee, composed of 18 members and a chairman, met annually at WHO headquarters to review proposals and activities. Their recommendations, as described below, had a marked effect on the evolution of the Organization's research programme.

Much of the research carried out within the different programmes is described in other chapters of this book. Long-term planning of international cooperation in cancer research and the other noncommunicable diseases is covered in Chapter 10, which describes the evolution of the policies that helped shape the research priorities of the Organization and the creation of new programmes, in particular those for research on tropical diseases and health services. First, however, accounts are given of the origin of research in epidemiology and communications science and its brief (5 years) period of existence, and the expanded programme of research, development and research training in human reproduction.

RESEARCH IN EPIDEMIOLOGY AND COMMUNICATIONS SCIENCE

The Director-General, addressing the Seventeenth World Health Assembly in 1964, indicated that the time had come for "a radical reappraisal and perhaps an equally radical extension of our efforts in health research" (2). What had been done so far was "inadequate to meet the challenge which confronts us as a result of the rapidity of scientific advance today and the growing complexity of the research problems to be solved". There was "a most urgent need for the creation of a world centre for communications and information on health research", and he called for "a comprehensive study of those problems of major importance to the world as a whole which are not likely to be explored adequately by purely national efforts".

A study was carried in which consideration was given to the "direct undertaking by WHO of basic and applied research in selected fields—a radical departure from WHO's present activities" (3). An informal meeting of scientific advisers, held in late November 1963, prepared a plan for a world health research centre, with three divisions: epidemiology, communications science and technology, and biomedical research. The proposed total staff (scientific and technical, excluding administrative and custodial) was 1273. The total budget for the first 10 years was just under US$ 300 million. It was hoped that land would be donated to the Organization, and several such offers were made in 1965.

The division of epidemiology was to conduct laboratory research and, with relevant units in WHO, to study health and disease patterns in different countries, theoretical and applied aspects of population surveys and predictive epidemiology, and selected problems of developing countries, including a laboratory for tropical communicable diseases, and to serve as a training centre for postgraduate scientists and health workers.

The division of communications science and technology was to handle information and data for WHO programmes and the other divisions; to collaborate and consult on specific problems with personnel in the other divisions; to conduct research in specific areas of mathematics, statistics and information handling, with broad reference to international problems in epidemiology, population genetics, cancer, cardiovascular disease, environmental hazards, mental health, genetic and developmental biology, mutagenic and toxic agents and integrated health planning; to serve as a focus and a link in a network of similar efforts under way on a national basis; and to serve as a research and training facility for workers in health communications.

The division of biomedical research was to study the fundamental mechanisms of induced genetic, developmental and metabolic effects and of the toxicity of chemical and biological substances and physical agents; to explore in parallel particular aspects of these mechanisms relevant to cancer and other major biomedical problems; to coordinate these efforts with research under way in other countries; and to serve as a research and training centre for postgraduate students and scientists from different countries.

The plan was presented to the Executive Board in January 1964, which asked the Director-General to provide more detailed information before a decision could be reached (resolution EB33.R22). The Seventeenth World Health Assembly in its resolution WHA17.37 in the same year requested the Director-General to continue the study in view of the desirability of applying the latest advances in communications science and technology under the aegis of WHO to improving and coordinating the worldwide exchange of information on health problems and biomedical research.

Three scientific meetings were held in 1964, one of advisers in communications science, another on biomedical research (with emphasis on the harmful effects of therapeutic agents and environmental contaminants) and the third on research in epidemiology.

The communications science group defined its subject as follows:

> Communications science refers to that body of mathematics and engineering, both theoretical and applied, which deals with the collection, transmission, codification and interpretation of physical events which human beings regard as meaningful—in other words, which carry information. (4)

It was considered that the programme in communications science "should not be developed in isolation but should be an integral part of an active biomedical research centre". Communications science was seen as important for the epidemiology and monitoring of communicable and noncommunicable diseases and conditions. In light of the recent concern about avian influenza, it is notable that an example given to illustrate what communications science had to offer was the design of "realistic and well-understood epidemic models" of arbovirus infections, with the suggestion that "an understanding of the migratory patterns of vector mosquitos or similar species could provide important predictive indicators to national health authorities".

The report of the biomedical research group (5) was short. It agreed that the problem of harmful effects of therapeutic agents and environmental contaminants was urgent and justified laboratory research in the proposed centre. The report outlined the technical requirements for such a programme of work.

The advisers on research in epidemiology had a difficult task, as they were expected to "consider the entire question anew, i.e., how epidemiological research could best contribute to the attack on world health problems, and how this could best be done within reasonable limits of finance and personnel" (6). Moreover, it was clear that to justify a 'world' centre, the problems had to have a long-term horizon and global perspective. National centres might not be guaranteed a long life, with the ups and downs of national policies. Even the example of the World Influenza Centre in England, while an acceptable model for a 'specialized field', could not be expected to address "an ever-increasing number of problems", requiring "a much broader attack". The group identified four broad functions suitable for epidemiological research: theory, methods, studies and training. Examples were given under each category, while recognizing that only when the centre was established could a final decision be made on which problems to address. The report nevertheless clearly indicated that the research centre would have to be large enough to "conduct the volume and variety of research that alone can establish its reputation as a significant centre of epidemiological research", giving as an indication of size that some 15 "senior scientists" should be appointed for long terms, with resources that would permit them to form "ten to twelve long-term groups", each group consisting of a "director, supporting professional personnel, and the specific laboratory and technical staff and facilities appropriate to the mission".

Although the Director-General in his introductory statement to the Eighteenth World Health Assembly in May 1965 indicated "that the creation of the proposed Centre is a logical and unavoidable step in the evolution of WHO", when the item was discussed it quickly became evident that he would be frustrated in his desire. With few exceptions, one delegate after another questioned the wisdom of engaging in such an ambitious project. Various reasons were given. Some questioned the comparable advantage of a centralized centre as opposed to a series of regional centres. Others questioned its cost. Almost all rejected the need for a biomedical laboratory facility, noting that, when needed, existing ones could be used. As a result, resolution WHA18.43 stated that research in these areas could best be undertaken within an international research programme, collaborating with and upgrading regional and national institutions, with early attention to the control of communicable diseases, monitoring adverse reactions to drugs and environmental contaminants. Establishment of a world health research centre required further study and consideration, and the Director-General should "develop WHO research activities and services in epidemiology and the application of communications sciences and the system of reference centres as a step for the extension of WHO activities in the field of health research".

Instead of a world health research centre, three programmes came into being: the IARC in 1965 (see above and Chapter 10), an international system for monitoring adverse reactions to drugs (see Chapter 11) and the Division of Research in Epidemiology and Communications Science, which came into existence officially in January 1967 but became fully operational only in mid-1968.

Research in epidemiology and communications science was conducted by 26 scientists, almost equally divided between epidemiology and communications science. The Division was made responsible for conducting field, theoretical and multidisciplinary epidemiological studies; devising and applying methods to describe differences and variations in humans and their environment and their relations; devising and testing mathematical models; designing and applying new and existing operational research, epidemiological, mathematical, ecological, behavioural and computer-based techniques, singly or in combination, to problems of public health; and consulting with and assisting other divisions of WHO and other organizations in using these techniques and skills.

Within 1 year, five main areas of research had been defined: the organization and strategy of health services, the epidemiology of high-risk groups, the health effects of urbanization, the epidemiology of disappearing diseases and mathematical models of disease processes. Research on the organization and strategy of health services was the main operational sector of the programme, as, through this line of study, it was hoped to devise a method for bringing epidemiological research to bear on the structure of health services, facilitate decision-making at various administrative levels and ensure effective use of limited resources. The second area of research, the epidemiology of high-risk groups, was seen as having wide implications for the operation of health services. Several activities were initiated. First, the suitability of different urban sub-areas for predicting the disease experience of their inhabitants was examined from the epidemiological, geographical and sociological view-points. A second line of enquiry was an examination of the practicability and cost–effectiveness of screening procedures, to help in formulating certain programmes. An initial study of myocardial infarct and cerebrovascular accidents was started in 1969 in Yugoslavia.

Research on the health effects of urbanization followed two interrelated approaches. A group of epidemiologists, geographers and sociologists reviewed a number of areas where large-scale primary migrations from rural to large urban areas were in progress and undertook a longitudinal study of a sample of migrant families during part of their adaptation phase. A pilot field study was undertaken in Iran in 1969 in the cities of Isfahan and Teheran. In the same context, data from studies on the effects of urbanization on health in countries in Asia, northern and western Africa, Latin America and Europe was collected and, in some cases, supplemented.

In the fourth area of research—on the epidemiology of disappearing diseases—a joint study on malaria was undertaken, on the basis of epidemiological, immunological and mathematical descriptions of the patterns of prevalence, distribution and transmission of malaria in populations living in savanna areas of Nigeria. Work on the mathematical theory of disease processes covered studies of communicable and noncommunicable diseases, including those genetically based. In the studies on communicable diseases, for example, estimation of the latency and the infectious and incubation periods of certain diseases was completed in 1969, with a new computerized approach based on mathematical theory.

By the end of 1970, the concept of 'planning for health' was identified as a suitable objective around which to focus the activities of the Division. This was taken to mean assuring the knowledge, skills and methods necessary for planning for health in the overall context of social, economic and environmental planning (to include but not be limited to planning for the provision of health services). A substantive report on the activities of the Division (7), presented to the Executive Board at its forty-seventh session in January 1971, outlined three main conceptual areas, "diverse in their subject matter but all closely related to the central theme" of planning for health:

- the organization and strategy of health services, covering the organizational problems of public health decision-making at an operational level;
- scientific studies of single diseases with well-defined mechanisms, for which the population dynamics could be described in some detail; and
- scientific studies of complicated multifactorial problems, with special emphasis on human ecology.

As a first major step in gaining an understanding of the operational aspects of planning, a field project was started in July 1970 in Colombia, conducted jointly by the Colombian Government, PAHO and WHO. One of its purposes was to ascertain what data on health were being used for planning and decision-making and to indicate the type of data that would provide the optimum grounds on which to base decisions. Colombia was chosen for this study because two approaches for gathering planning data were used, one based on the PAHO/CENDES approach (see Chapter 4) and the other on a national health survey conducted by the Colombian Ministry of Health and the Colombian Association of Medical

Schools. The national health survey (*8*) was sponsored by the Milbank Memorial Fund and had taken several years to plan and carry out. Some 10 000 homes were visited and 50 000 individuals interviewed, of whom 5000 were examined clinically. It was the first survey of its kind to be carried out in a developing country. Both approaches were judged to be costly and inadequate from several points of view, including the lack of any epidemiological analyses of the health problems faced by the Colombian population.

An example of work on the control of a single disease was an investigation into the epidemiology and control of malaria in the African savanna, which was conducted in conjunction with programmes for malaria eradication, immunology and vector control. Data collection was initiated in late 1970, and a model was constructed to permit quantitative description of the factors involved in malaria transmission. The Director-General was to note in a talk on the limitations of economics in health planning at the Colloque sur l'Economie de la Santé, Coppet, Switzerland, in 1975 that the model prepared for this project was the first success obtained in "fitting an epidemiological model for malaria to an actual group of villages". The model was later described in a WHO publication (*9*).

An example of a complicated problem associated with human ecology was the project involving comparative ecological studies of certain diseases borne by small mammals in Iran. The approach involved understanding the dynamics of the reservoir and the vector, the relation of the reservoir to the ecological zone in which the vector lived and the contacts between humans and the reservoir. By 1971, the zoonotic agents identified included *Rickettsia sibiricus*, *Coxiella burnetii*, Sindbis, West Nile and Crimean haemorrhagic fever viruses, and *Franscisella tularensis*.

Dr Mahler, introducing the work of the Division of Research in Epidemiology and Communications Science to the Executive Board in January 1971 in his capacity as Assistant Director-General, indicated that the Director-General had been somewhat concerned in 1970 when it became apparent that independent projects were easier to set up than interdependent ones. The reviews that were undertaken suggested that perhaps the Division had taken on more than it could immediately handle, and that it should endeavour to concentrate on a unifying theme, out of which emerged that of 'planning for health'.

Replying to questions about the basic philosophy of the Division and the link between its work and the Organization's other operational activities, he indicated that national health administrators considered "that there was an acute need for 'planning tools'". The Organization had been under constant pressure to assist governments in making the best possible use of their planning techniques. Courses and seminars had been organized, but these had not been altogether satisfactory. What was needed was "an improved kind of planning philosophy, so that governments could be assisted with a technique commensurate with their particular situation". Governments had to develop their own abilities to analyse political, economic and social constraints in their countries, as the Organization would never have either the obligation or the possibility of doing so adequately. Throughout 1970, efforts had been made to bring about a "continuous dialogue" between the Division on Research in Epidemiology and Communications Science, the Division of the Organization of Health Services and the Division of Family Health. It was also around this time, as described in Chapters 3 and 4, that country health programming was initiated under Dr Mahler's leadership.

New projects were reported to the Executive Board at its forty-ninth session, in January 1972. A study had begun in West Azerbaijan, Iran, on the basis of the experience gained in Colombia, to demonstrate the feasibility of achieving more rapid results in health planning (see Chapter 4). Another major effort was a study of health interventions in the Netherlands and the USSR, including the possible benefits of investment in mass health screening by developed countries. Dr Mahler took the occasion to indicate that application of mathematics and systems analysis to WHO's programme was no easy task but was being pursued with great determination.

In August 1972, the Division of Research in Epidemiology and Communications Science was merged with the Division of the Organization of Health Services, to create the Division of Strengthening of Health Services. The existing units for research in epidemiology, communications science, behavioural sciences, ecology, operational research, mathematics, statistics, numerical analysis, community health services and nursing were disestablished.

At the end of the discussion by the Twenty-sixth World Health Assembly on research in epidemiology and communications science, the Director-General observed:

> There was a tendency to believe that mathematical gymnastics would provide health care to people. They would not. And it is important to note that WHO had never believed that they would. Managerial methodologies could only accelerate the delivery of health care if there was a strong political and social will to provide such care. As has been pointed out, unless there was at all levels in Member States the will to provide such care an operational research project would serve no purpose; in fact it might do more harm than good. (*10*)

In its resolution WHA26.43, the Health Assembly took note of the reorganization of the Division of Research in Epidemiology and Communications Science, commenting that the programme was being more "clearly focused on the analysis of the health delivery systems with the ultimate goal of increasing their efficiency and effectiveness", and requested the Director-General to present the programme "as an integral part of the overall WHO programme in biomedical and medicosocial research".

EXPANDED PROGRAMME OF RESEARCH, DEVELOPMENT AND RESEARCH TRAINING IN HUMAN REPRODUCTION

Strong opposition from several Member States in the early 1950s had prevented WHO from entering the field of population studies in any significant way. At the time, there was only one project on family planning, and it was concerned with the 'rhythm method'. Only in the early 1960s did the Organization begin to address the subject seriously, when it began to promote research on human reproduction.

The Director-General, in his presentation in August 1962 to the fourth World Congress on Fertility and Sterility, emphasized that the biology of certain aspects of human reproduction had not been thoroughly studied and was less well understood than other aspects of medical science. Clearly, the importance of many medical, biological, social, cultural and economic factors in human reproduction made it a major public health problem. In 1963, the first scientific group on human reproduction met, and 14 such meetings were convened over the next 6 years.

Scientific knowledge on the biology of human reproduction and the medical aspects of fertility control was recognized as being insufficient on at least two occasions by the governing bodies (resolutions WHA18.49 and WHA19.43) in the mid-1960s. Further impetus for research in this field was given by the United Nations Population Commission in April 1965, which attached high priority to research on fertility.

From its inception, the programme addressed a wide range of problems and interests. Initially, the focus was on infertility, fetal development, early growth and methods of fertility regulation. By 1969, the programme had been broadened to include administrative and public health research as it related to health problems of reproduction, including family planning. Epidemiological studies were initiated, as were investigations of clinical and physiological problems.

The Advisory Committee on Medical Research, at its meeting in 1969, congratulated the Organization on the orientation of its research programme and on the extent to which it had been implemented. Following a review of the report of the Scientific Group on Developments in Fertility Control, the Advisory Committee recommended that research be initiated to determine the biosocial factors that influence motivation and the failure or non-use of fertility control. In 1970, it considered the question of setting up WHO laboratories and training institutes for various uses, including studies of the biology of human reproduction.

In his address to the Twenty-third World Health Assembly, in May 1970, the Director-General noted:

> While we know quite a lot about the short-term and medium-term effects of various contraceptive methods, we know less about the long-term consequences, particularly those which may affect our descendants. We must therefore push further ahead with clinical, physiological, psychological and biological research. As I see it, the gaps that remain to be filled offer, for the Second Development Decade, an inspiring opportunity for cooperation between international governmental organizations and private bodies concerned with public welfare. (*11*)

In June 1970, WHO convened a meeting of agencies concerned with promoting and supporting research in human reproduction, including national medical research councils, technical assistance agencies, family planning departments and private foundations. The picture that emerged from this meeting was somewhat disquieting: little progress had been made during the previous 5 years, and the state of knowledge about reproductive processes remained inadequate and incomplete. An intensified research effort was needed at the fundamental, clinical, pharmacological and epidemiological levels. Research to find new methods of fertility control was needed, and the assistance in this field was insufficient. The meeting recommended that a feasibility study be carried out to establish a planning strategy for further research in human reproduction and particularly in fertility control. WHO was asked to undertake the study, focusing on the potential input that might be made by WHO to expanding research efforts in this field. One of the agencies present, the Swedish International Development Authority, provided the funds for the study.

The feasibility study involved consultations with scientists and research administrators and visits to more than 70 research institutions in 25 countries. Scientists from institutions in many countries assisted in the study, in planning sessions in Geneva and in assessing research institutions during the site visits. Objectives were defined and priority areas identified, with several interrelated mechanisms for research promotion, including task forces, research and training centres, a network of clinical research centres, improved documentation and expansion of such programmes as the provision of chemicals and spare parts to scientists, assistance in research training, consultations and publications. A framework for implementation of the programme was outlined, which included setting up an advisory group of outstanding scientists who would meet two or three times a year to review and make recommendations to WHO on research priorities, research strategy and allocation of resources; and formulation of a procedure for scientific assessment of research projects and long-term evaluation of the Programme as a whole.

The Expanded Programme of Research in Human Reproduction was initiated in 1972, and over US$ 4.5 million were pledged for its first year. The overall objective of the Programme was to increase understanding of human reproduction in order to find a variety of safe, acceptable, effective methods for regulating human reproduction. Other areas of research addressed problems such as the factors affecting reproductive health and disease; alternative ways of providing related health services, particularly family planning; the interrelations between health, health services and population dynamics; and promotion of national research expertise.

By 1974, the Programme had established nine multidisciplinary, multinational task forces for collaborative research and development in areas such as contraceptive drugs for men; devices that can be placed in the vagina, cervix or uterus that have an antifertility effect either through their physical presence or by releasing steroids; new injectable contraceptive preparations; prostaglandins for the termination of pregnancy or the induction of menses; immunological methods of fertility regulation; new approaches to occlusion of fallopian tubes; and improved techniques for the prediction or detection of ovulation for couples wishing to practise the rhythm method (*12*).

The Advisory Committee on Medical Research reviewed the Programme in depth in 1974 (*13*). Their discussion brought out the complexity of the issues involved, areas of human reproductive biology in which there were still large gaps in knowledge and other areas, such as male and female infertility and pregnancy wastage. More research was needed on the effects of environmental factors during pregnancy on the mother, on maternal–fetal relationships and on fetal growth and development. The Committee considered that increased emphasis should be placed on research on services and motivation for fertility regulation, in close relation to national family planning programmes. It commended the involvement of social scientists in specifying new methods for WHO's programme of research.

The Programme expanded steadily during the decade. It continued to attract voluntary funding from a number of countries, particularly Norway and Sweden. By 1977, total funding amounted to some US$ 12 million annually. At that time, the subjects of research were: the health rationale for family planning; assessment, improvement and development of fertility regulating methods; service delivery of fertility regulating methods; infertility; diseases of pregnancy and fetal disorders; and resources for research in human reproduction. Further details on the service aspects of family planning, including 'service research' are given in Chapter 7.

FURTHER INTENSIFICATION OF WHO'S
RESEARCH PROGRAMME

The Director-General, in his introduction to *The work of WHO 1971* (*14*), recalled that 10 years earlier he had indicated that the best hope for the future of the world's health lay in an intensification of medical research. That was even clearer at present. Technical problems were being encountered that called for new knowledge. Without such knowledge, the progress that had been made by many countries in their fight against disease would be slowed down and, in some areas, might even be halted. It was evident, he concluded, that if the world was to solve its most pressing problems in the foreseeable future, increased funds would have to be set aside for an expanded programme of research, at both national and international levels.

During the Twenty-fifth World Health Assembly, in May 1972, several delegates introduced a resolution that called on the Director-General to prepare proposals for long-term WHO activities in medical research. One of the sponsoring delegates noted that the purpose of the draft resolution "was not to promote the development of large research centres. WHO was in a unique position to coordinate work in the various countries and could so so very effectively, as it had shown through the International Agency for Research on Cancer". After a relatively brief discussion, resolution WHA25.60 was adopted, which called on WHO to intensify activities in the field of biomedical research. The Director-General was requested to prepare proposals for long-term activities in this area.

The Advisory Committee on Medical Research reviewed this subject at its fourteenth session, in June 1972 (*15*). Owing to shortage of time, it discussed only certain aspects of the subject. It expressed its satisfaction at the continued progress of WHO in stimulating and supporting sound research in carefully established priority areas and recommended programmes that would bring together research workers at meetings and conferences and permit visits of scientists to other laboratories, so that knowledge and experience could be shared to the benefit of all. It indicated that WHO should play a role in establishing guidelines for priorities in biomedical research and help in exchanges of experience between national bodies responsible for organizing such research. Also, WHO could play a supporting role in research programmes at national, university and institutional levels, helping them to be more effective in meeting community health needs.

An interim report on WHO's role in the design and coordination of biomedical research (*16*) was prepared for consideration by the Executive Board at its fifty-first session, in January 1973. The report was primarily historical, noting that WHO activities in the field of medical research stemmed from Article 2(n) of the Constitution, which states that one of the functions of WHO is "to promote and conduct research in the field of health". Guiding principles established in 1949 by the Second World Health Assembly stated that priority should be given to research that directly related to the programmes of WHO and that the Organization should support such research in existing institutions, rather than establishing international research institutions under its own auspices. The decision taken in 1958 that had led to the creation of the Advisory Committee on Medical Research was described, as was the decision taken in 1965 against creation of a world health research centre. No recommendations, as such, were made; however, it was indicated that, following the meeting of the Board which requested the Director-General to continue the study, a review would be carried out by former members of the Advisory Committee and other consultants. This was scheduled for February 1973.

One delegate to the Twenty-sixth World Health Assembly, in May 1973, proposed that an ad hoc body of the Health Assembly be set up to study WHO's biomedical research policies, trends and projects and help in setting priorities. Dr Candau strongly rejected this proposal, indicating that "the research programme should be evolved at the scientific level" (17) and should be protected by the Advisory Committee on Medical Research. The Board should review the programme, and the Health Assembly would be given any information it needed. "The intervention of politics would lead to very serious difficulties in the implementation of the programme", he concluded. The resolution adopted, WHA26.42, requested the Director-General to continue the study and to present a full report to the Twenty-seventh World Health Assembly, which should include the recommendations of the Advisory Committee and "suggestions on the means to be adopted in order to enable the Executive Board and the Health Assembly to follow more closely the evolution of those programmes". It should be appreciated that previously the reports of the Advisory Committee were restricted for use only by the Director-General.

The Director-General also used his response to the discussion to illustrate an area in which WHO could "stimulate research in fields not of interest to the rich countries though extremely important to the developing countries". He chose the problems of the parasitic diseases, naming onchocerciasis, trypanosomiasis, schistosomiasis and filariasis. Perhaps the seeds of the TDR programme were already being planted on this occasion.

The matter was discussed by the Advisory Committee during its fifteenth session, in June 1973. The Committee emphasized that WHO's research programme should concentrate on solving problems not covered by national efforts, particularly those that cut across national boundaries or could not be investigated satisfactorily without international cooperation or assistance. For developing countries, research on nutrition and communicable diseases (particularly parasitic diseases) should remain high priorities. The cooperation of national agencies should be sought, to enable WHO to maintain an up-to-date, comprehensive record of research under way in various parts of the world. In view of the success of the WHO research and training centres, the principle behind them should be extended to all fields, as appropriate, including operational research. Greater provision should be made for peer review of decisions on individual projects before their approval, and technical documents should be made available as widely as possible for research workers.

A more substantive report was prepared by the Director-General for the consideration of the fifty-third session of the Executive Board, held in January 1974 (12). Coordination and collaborative research involving national institutions and research workers in various countries was identified as "by far" the "largest type of activity in the WHO research programme". Member States were called on to help the Organization in its task of "identifying those institutions and workers willing and capable of forwarding WHO's research programme through collaborative efforts". This was of particular importance with respect to developed countries, "which have the financial, material and manpower resources needed to carry out advanced types of research".

The report indicated that the priorities corresponded to those given in the Fifth General Programme of Work, i.e. strengthening health services, increasing manpower, disease prevention and control and promotion of environmental health. The areas for research support were derived from discussions at the Health Assembly, the Board, the Advisory Committee on Medical Research, scientific groups, informal meetings of research workers and expert advisory panels and committees. For the purpose of the report, however, some general considerations were in order.

The need to conduct research of an applied, operational type on strengthening health services had become evident. The main problems included tapping community resources and goodwill and harnessing the often limited capacity and capability of health services staff to maximum effect. Effective methods for achieving these aims remained to be elaborated. The Director-General therefore proposed to intensify research on this problem, including operational research, particularly in developing countries. A minimum of 3–5 years would be required before useful results could be expected from such research.

Perhaps the greatest need, especially in developing countries, was training of research workers. The means available to WHO (fellowships and grants) should be supplemented in order to increase WHO's contribution in this field, by:

- increasing the number of short training courses, workshops and seminars conducted by technical units and regional offices in selected fields;
- extending WHO research and training centres to cover additional activities;
- obtaining additional support from developed countries for research training in developing countries; and
- encouraging prominent research scientists to spend sabbatical leaves and part of their academic year in institutions in developing countries.

During the discussion on the subject at the fifty-third session of the Executive Board, in January 1974, the Deputy Director-General, Dr Thomas Lambo, who had been designated by the Director-General to address this area, noted that the "most pressing need" that had emerged from the study so far was the "development of research resources and potentials in the developing countries". Among the health problems facing these countries, parasitic diseases were selected to provide "the model for basic and applied research in centres of excellence, since it was thought that the research potential established thereby could be applied to almost any other class of biomedical and public health problem that might require attention in the future" (*18*).

Following a relatively brief discussion, the Executive Board adopted resolution EB53.R36, transmitting the Director-General's report and comments on it to the Health Assembly, with a recommendation that the Chairman or other designated members of the Board should attend the sessions of the Advisory Committee and that the Chairman of the Advisory Committee or other members should attend stipulated sessions of the Executive Board and the Health Assembly. With respect to the work of the Advisory Committee itself, the Director-General's report made it clear that it was of "great importance that complete candour continue to operate". The Committee had been established as an advisory group to the Director-General. It had been free to make candid technical appraisals and recommendations on research activities in closed sessions, which for the most part had been reflected in its reports.

The Twenty-seventh World Health Assembly, in May 1974, discussed the subject at length. Its first major decision was adoption of resolution WHA27.52, which recognized that the tropical parasitic diseases were one of the main obstacles to improving the level of health and socioeconomic development in countries of the tropical and subtropical zones and that WHO should intensify its activities in this field, seeking extrabudgetary resources on a wider scale. (Subsequent developments in this programme are described below.) Having dealt with the priority of tropical parasitic diseases, the Health Assembly returned to the more general issue of biomedical research. Although one delegate indicated that the Director-General's report had not specified the "ways in which WHO should undertake its research programme", nor had it indicated "the criterion for the selection of those areas of research", the Health Assembly did approve (resolution WHA27.61) the proposals of the Director-General to increase international cooperation and coordination of biomedical re-search through medical research councils and similar national bodies and other institutions, and to promote and initiate research in developing countries, particularly with respect to diseases of importance in those areas. The Health Assembly also welcomed the proposal for greater involvement of the regional offices in research, under the technical guidance of headquarters. All Member States and voluntary agencies were called on to contribute to the Voluntary Fund for Health Promotion for research activities and to assist the Organization in other ways to promote its research programme.

The Advisory Committee on Medical Research at its sixteenth session, in June 1974, noted the need for greater involvement of the regional offices in the research activities of WHO and suggested that small regional committees, possibly including some members of the Advisory Committee, be set up to provide a more continuous link with research in the regions (13). It reaffirmed the important function of WHO in coordinating and stimulating biomedical research through bilateral and multilateral arrangements, as well as it own role in helping in the selection of the most promising areas of research and in suggesting prior-ities for long-term programmes.

In a brief discussion during the fifty-fifth session of the Executive Board, in January 1975, about the proposed programme budget for 1976–1977 for research promotion and development, the Director-General observed that the Organization had perhaps erred in the past in failing to involve the regions in the research programme (19). A statement prepared by the secretariat on the research included in the Board's organizational study, which was also discussed during the session, stated that research had opened "an immense field of interest and activity, thereby renewing and broadening its technical responsibility. How-ever, this new vigorous interest permitted a further degree of isolation from the regional programmes of direct assistance to governments" (20). The same report indicated that "WHO does not run any research set-up of its own (IARC excepted)".

An underlying concern was establishing and maintaining a "continuing link between research and the services". It was hoped that by establishing regional advisory committees and mobilizing regional expertise, WHO in its advisory and coordinating role would help "in avoiding the difficulties that tended to exist between the research and the services com-munities at country level". It was in this context that the idea of creating regional expert panels was proposed (see Chapter 2). When asked how these measures would be funded, the Director-General replied that the development programme for 1975 and part of 1976 would mobilize US$ 10–20 million dollars annually in such a way that the measures in question would be supported by outside resources. Resolution EB55.R35 was adopted, which endorsed the greater involvement of the Advisory Committee, the regional committees and regional offices in the research activities of the Organization.

With approval of the Sixth General Programme of Work by the Twenty-ninth World Health Assembly in 1976 (resolution WHA29.20), the aim of WHO's work in this area was reformulated as being to promote and collaborate in the design and coordination of biomedical research, including health services research, with the objectives of identifying research priorities, strengthening national research capabilities and promoting international coordination of research, especially with respect to problems of major importance to WHO and to promote application and proper transfer of existing and new scientific knowledge and research methods to serve as the basis for the development of comprehensive national health services.

The Advisory Committee at its eighteenth session, in June 1976, reaffirmed the criteria endorsed by the Director-General for selecting priorities for WHO research:

- the magnitude of the problem, especially in developing countries;
- the suitability of the problem for international collaborative research coordinated by WHO;
- the priority of the problem as perceived by countries themselves;
- the relevance of the problem to the socioeconomic development of Member States;
- the probability of finding solutions (or important clarifications) and the feasibility of applying them nationally, taking into account the time and costs required;
- the availability of manpower, facilities and funds to carry out the research in order to ensure as far as possible the achievement of significant results;
- the involvement of the countries themselves, especially their scientific communities and facilities, in the research to be undertaken, preferably where the problem exists, so as to upgrade national research capabilities;
- the level of research being carried out, both nationally and internationally, to solve the problem;
- the benefits that would accrue from application of the results of successful research, especially in developing countries; and
- the potential usefulness of the results of the research in solving other problems.

As indicated in Chapter 4, each of the regions except the Americas, which already had its own advisory body on research, established a regional advisory committee on research as a consequence of the decisions taken by the Executive Board and Health Assembly. Members of the global Advisory Committee on Medical Research were deeply involved in assisting the regions in this process. Mechanisms were established to coordinate the activities of these committees with national research needs and programmes, as well as with WHO's global research. It was envisaged that such coordination would be assured through close collaboration with national medical research councils or analogous bodies, with the

Advisory Committee and with headquarters and regional research committees. It was the Director-General's hope that a significant increase in WHO's research activities would stem from greater involvement in research by the regions.

Not all Executive Board members or Health Assembly delegates were fully convinced of the direction proposed by the Organization. With regard to the policy of decentralization, the USSR delegate to the Twenty-ninth World Health Assembly noted that "it was important to avoid the extremes and the mistake of decentralizing science". Concerning the central role given to the Advisory Committee, the Israeli delegate to that Health Assembly pointed out that "it had to be remembered that specialists were not always the best persons to assess the needs of countries". Or, as the USSR member of the Board put it, at the fifty-ninth session in January 1977, "from their Olympian heights, Nobel Prize winners sometimes failed to appreciate the relationship between science and public health or were not aware of all the possibilities afforded by science". These concerns possibly grew out of the fact that health services research had not developed as rapidly as had been hoped, as discussed below.

Despite these reservations, the Thirtieth World Health Assembly adopted resolution WHA30.40, which noted "with satisfaction the orientation of WHO's research promoting and coordinating activities in conformity with the Sixth General Programme of Work". It endorsed the research policy guidelines outlined, with particular attention to:

- the role of WHO in strengthening national research capability, promoting international cooperation and ensuring the appropriate transfer of existing and new scientific knowledge to those who need it;
- the emphasis on greater regional involvement in research, with the active participation of regional advisory committees on medical research;
- the setting of research goals and priorities in the regions in response to the expressed needs of Member States;
- the concept of special programmes for research and training in major mission-oriented programmes of the Organization; and
- keeping an appropriate balance between biomedical and health services research.

The need to strengthen research development and coordinating mechanisms was confirmed, with emphasis on:

- close coordination between the regional and the global advisory committees on medical research in the long-term planning and implementation of the WHO research programme;
- collaboration with medical research councils or analogous national research bodies to ensure effective coordination of national, regional and global research programmes;
- use of research promotion mechanisms, such as scientific working groups, to ensure broad participation of the scientific community in planning, implementing and evaluating WHO's research programmes;

- increased technical cooperation with and between research institutions of Member countries to carry out collaborative research and training and improve communication among scientists;
- strengthened research into efficient use of resources in health-care delivery systems, especially nationally and regionally;
- a broader base of advice and support for health services research, by extending the membership of the Advisory Committee on Medical Research and related committees and the WHO collaborating centres to include representatives of social, management and other sciences;
- an increased number of collaborating centres for health services research and strengthening of this research; and
- a balanced geographical distribution of collaborating centres for biomedical and health services research.

TROPICAL DISEASES RESEARCH PROGRAMME

In his introduction to *The work of WHO 1973*, the Director-General indicated that WHO's approach to the control of parasitic diseases had "as yet been somewhat piecemeal", with the exception of malaria. The main problem was the many gaps in fundamental research on host–parasite relations, the multiplicity of factors that modify the incidence and severity of the diseases, the lack of persons with the diagnostic competence required and of technical resources, and the unsatisfactory nature of the environmental measures and chemotherapeutic agents then available. A much more aggressive attack was needed. He expressed the hope that it would be possible "to establish centres in the countries where there are major public health problems to carry out the necessary fundamental and applied research on which to base comprehensive programmes" (*21*).

The adoption of resolution WHA27.52 by the Twenty-seventh World Health Assembly, in May 1974, as noted above, opened the way for WHO to further expand activities in this area. The Advisory Committee on Medical Research discussed the subject extensively at its sixteenth session, in June of that year (*22*). It recommended that the objectives of an expanded WHO programme for research and training in tropical communicable diseases should be:

- application of modern biomedical concepts and methods to find new approaches to the prevention, diagnosis and treatment of tropical communicable diseases;
- creation of expertise in the relevant biomedical sciences in developing countries, the initial emphasis being on Africa but, on the basis of the experience grained, extended to other regions as rapidly as available resources allowed;
- provision of research training in developing countries, in close cooperation with universities and allied institutions, and improving the career opportunities for research workers; and
- instigation of studies on the demographic and socioeconomic impacts of these diseases and of disease control measures against them.

The Advisory Committee affirmed that financing for the expanded programme could not be covered by the regular budget of WHO, and it recommended that the Director-General approach governmental and private granting agencies to obtain the necessary support. WHO was the only organization that could coordinate efforts internationally and raise funds to improve facilities for research and to recruit research workers; it had unique knowledge of problems on a global scale, a capacity to override national and political barriers, the prestige and ability to persuade people to work for and collaborate with it, experience in evolving flexible organizational methods of administration with minimal bureaucratic control and proven success in setting up regional research and training centres, as already noted in the 1973 report of the Committee.

In July 1974, a team from WHO and the Advisory Committee visited Zambia to explore the possibility of establishing a clinical laboratory research institute at N'dola Central Hospital. At that time, a three-part programme was envisaged, involving:

- designation of a network of WHO research and training centres, by strengthening university and research institutions in which research and training were already under way or could be started;
- creation of WHO regional multidisciplinary institutes for research and training, the first of which would serve as a strong link in the network serving East, Central and South Africa; and
- organization of project groups to plan, coordinate and implement research on vaccines and effective chemotherapeutic or prophylactic measures for parasitic and other tropical diseases. The research would be carried out in the African network of laboratories and in appropriate laboratories elsewhere in the world.

The Advisory Committee emphasized that whatever institute was selected initially, it should have access to good clinical and epidemiological facilities and should establish its postgraduate training programme in association with the universities of the region. It envisaged that the programme would bring new concepts from such disciplines as immunology, molecular and cell biology, biochemistry and genetics to bear on problems at the most sophisticated level of knowledge and expertise. These disciplines would be brought together for a multidisciplinary but goal-oriented attack on parasitic and other tropical communicable diseases. The Institute of Nutrition of Central America and Panama was indicated as providing a "valuable model" for the expanded programme.

A planning group that met late in 1974 recommended malaria, schistosomiasis, filarial infections, leprosy, trypanosomiasis and leishmaniasis as priorities. Organization of project teams to formulate and guide activities on each disease was recommended, as was setting up a network of research and training centres and collaborating laboratories with a focus on Africa south of the Sahara but linked to institutions with similar interests in other developing and in developed countries. It was estimated that the recurrent cost of the proposed approach might be in the order of US$ 15 million per annum but that the projects might have to be tailored "to use whatever funds became available".

The Special Programme was announced in a circular issued on 7 January 1975. Two main goals were indicated: to develop, through biomedical research (combining laboratory, clinical and epidemiological research), new methods for preventing, diagnosing and treating the main communicable diseases, especially parasitic infections, in developing countries of the tropical and subtropical zones; and to train scientists and technicians in the disciplines and techniques relevant to improving research on and methods of control of these diseases.

The six diseases selected were seen to hold together as a group from the point of view of research; advances in one might open up new approaches for another. Thus, the development of a vaccine for leprosy could point the way to vaccines against others of the six diseases. Leishmaniasis, although less important numerically as a disease, was included, as the parasite was readily handled in the laboratory and there were exceptional opportunities to study the relation between this parasite and certain cells of the body. This kind of research could lead to better drugs not only for leishmaniasis but also for leprosy, trypanosomiasis and malaria, in which the same body cells are involved. Malnutrition was seen as a major factor in all these diseases, and its effect on severity and on the effectiveness of remedies would also be studied.

Concern was expressed during the fifty-fifth session of the Executive Board, in January 1975, regarding the concentrated effort being proposed for Africa. Replying to some of the points raised, the Director-General indicated that the Organization "had faced very considerable problems internally as well as externally in its efforts to move forward in the field of biomedical research .... The difficulties were greater when the attempt was made to take a broad-based, cohesive approach to the problems". He shared the concern expressed by some Members that the Organization, by concentrating on one centre in Africa, risked setting up "yet another kind of biomedical research effort to try to attack parasitic diseases". What was needed in this regard was "to see the totality of the problem in its relation to the social and economic sectors". The problem had to be approached

> horizontally, in all its ramifications, rather than treated in isolation. Such an approach presented a tremendous challenge to the Organization ... the effort being made should not only be at headquarters level; it should also be made at country level, and it was of great importance that individual governments should set up their own mechanism ... to identify the problems. He did not think that kind of approach would lead to fragmentation, since this particular programme needed to decentralize in order to achieve better productivity" (*19*).

To conduct this large programme, two parallel systems of organization were proposed, task forces and networks, with which WHO had experience and success, especially in the field of human reproduction, as noted above.

A meeting of heads of agencies was held in October 1975, with the cosponsorship of UNDP. Sixteen countries, three United Nations agencies and four intergovernmental organizations were represented, as well as three foundations and one centre. The meeting considered the objectives of the programme, the mechanisms proposed to achieve the objectives and its scope. Questions were raised, particularly as regards the setting up of an international research centre at N'dola. It had been hoped that the meeting would generate sufficient funds to allow the programme to start activities on each of the diseases selected. As it was, enough funds were pledged to continue planning and pilot operations.

An informal discussion was organized in May 1976, to outline plans for training, for strengthening research institutions in tropical countries and for associating research institutions in tropical and nontropical countries by incorporating them as centres within the Special Programme's network. It was emphasized that research and training should pertain to practical problems encountered by community health services. For this purpose, creation of peripheral units based on existing health-care facilities such as rural health centres and clinics was proposed. Peripheral units would be linked to large centres within the network.

A working group on organization and finance for the Special Programme met in July and December 1976. It proposed an organizational structure and made a number of recommendations for funding, as follows:

- The administrative bodies should include representatives from all three groups of participants: the participating countries where tropical diseases constitute serious health problems, contributing governments and agencies that make financial donations to the Programme, and sponsoring agencies (then UNDP and WHO).
- The World Bank should be invited to consider setting up and managing a tropical diseases fund, which could receive financial donations to the Special Programme.
- A scientific and technical advisory committee should be established to provide an overall scientific assessment of the plans and progress made by the scientific working groups.
- A joint coordinating board should be established to coordinate the interests and responsibilities of the parties cooperating in the Special Programme.

The review of this group was favourable. The notion of one central research centre had been replaced by a network of research activities to be managed and directed by the Special Programme. It agreed that the Programme had a sound technical foundation and should begin large-scale operations in 1977, for which a total of some US$ 7.5 million had been pledged. WHO's contribution was agreed upon, in the order of US$ 1 million per year. When all contributions were added up at the end of the year, US$ 11.5 million had been made available for 1977.

The Executive Board at its fifty-ninth session, in January 1977, in resolution EB59.R31, decided to establish a Special Account for Research and Training in Tropical Diseases as a sub-account of the Voluntary Fund for Health Promotion and requested that the Director-General continue to cooperate with UNDP, cosponsor of the Special Programme, and the World Bank, particularly with regard to further financing of the Programme.

In 1977, the planning phase of the Special Programme changed to a preparatory phase of organization and pilot activities, leading to full operation of projects. The main task was to establish new groups, that on the immunology of leprosy serving as a model. Groups on chemotherapy for leprosy and on malaria met for the first time. Further developments are described in Chapter 9.

HEALTH SERVICES RESEARCH

In the WHO publication describing the medical research programme from 1964 to 1968, a relatively short chapter is dedicated to public health practice (*1*). This was subdivided into sections: public health administration, organization of medical care, maternal and child health, health education, nursing, occupational health, mental health, dental health, radiation health and health laboratory services. Concerning public health administration, it was noted that "the development of operational research in the field of public health administration has been very slow and, to a certain extent, rather disappointing. The most important single reason for this lack of progress is the fact that operational research is usually outside the competence and experience of health administrators". It was noted, however, that the need for this kind of research was increasingly being felt, as reflected in the many activities of the regional offices in this domain (see Chapter 4).

Although the proposals for a world health research centre had not explicitly mentioned health services research, several of the subjects described fell into that area. For example, in the description of the work of the proposed division of epidemiology, there was a brief section on 'health economics', in which theoretical (mathematical models) and field studies on the economics of health were proposed. It envisaged "long-term studies on interrelationships, and their changes, of health and disease and social and economic problems" (23). Similarly, the scientific advisers on communications sciences identified 'health planning' as one activity for the centre (24).

The Division of Research in Epidemiology and Communications Science, as described above, did initiate research projects in health planning which included an element on the organization of health services. Furthermore, health services research of one kind or another was being undertaken at the beginning of the 1970s in many other programmes, yet the Polish delegate to the Twenty-third World Health Assembly, in May 1970, concluded that not enough attention had been given to "to research on the organization of community health services" (11). Research of that kind had been allocated only 2% of the intensified research budget. He introduced a draft resolution (adopted as WHA23.49), requesting the Director-General to review the WHO research programme in this field and to report at an unspecified time to the Health Assembly. When asked to clarify the kind of research he had in mind, he replied that what was wanted was a comparison of health services organization in countries at various levels of economic development and with different social structures, with the aim of presenting some conclusions about the models that would give the best results under given conditions.

Further impetus was given to the subject with the adoption in 1971 by the Twenty-fourth World Health Assembly (resolution WHA24.58) of the Fifth General Programme of Work, covering the period 1973–1977, which mentioned a number of fields and topics that merited attention, including:

> Research is an intrinsic component of most WHO programmes. While research in various biomedical fields, such as biological standardization, immunology, genetics and human reproduction will not be neglected, increasing emphasis will be laid on research in planning for health, on the organization of community health services and on the education of health personnel.

As called for in resolution WHA23.49, the subject was reviewed by the secretariat and then presented to the Twenty-fifth World Health Assembly, in 1972 (24). Four areas were noted as deserving "greater emphasis": studies on the economics of health; studies on manpower resources and development, especially with rationalization of manpower requirements and projections; community participation; and selection, specification and standardization of procedures and techniques used by more and less skilled personnel using more and less sophisticated equipment in the health services. While noting that much research had been conducted in recent years, the report concluded that WHO had "not yet assumed a major role in coordinating the application of research results to public health practice".

The Polish delegate to the Twenty-fifth World Health Assembly drew on this last sentence to suggest that the "Director-General might be requested to present a comprehensive programme of research in the organization of community health systems for discussion at the next Health Assembly". Dr Mahler, who had introduced the subject in his capacity as Assistant Director-General, had qualified it as a "difficult" one for various reasons, including "the realization that the solutions for the development of community health services would not be pleasant in that they would involve a painful redistribution of resources, concentrating them no longer on privileged groups as in the past, but on the rural populations, whose need was greatest". WHO's ability to help its Member States "would depend on their allowing it to take part in their research" (25).

Following a lengthy discussion, during which delegates provided information on research being conducted in their countries and commented on various aspects of such research, including difficulties and the possible role that WHO might play in assisting them, resolution WHA25.17 was adopted, indicating "a need to elaborate a proper strategy of research development in the organization of community health services" and that WHO "should play a leading role in the coordination of international research on the organization of community health services". The Director-General was called on to submit to a future Health Assembly a comprehensive, long-term WHO research programme on systems of health-care organization at local and country levels. One delegate requested that a specific Health Assembly be designated for submission of the report, but this was stated to be impossible, as the Director-General "did not know at what time he would be able to submit the comprehensive long-term programme referred to". The Polish delegate to the Twenty-sixth World Health Assembly managed to include in resolution WHA26.35 another request to the Director-General for a report on a comprehensive long-term research programme on systems of health care organization at local and country levels, this time with no response from the Director-General.

Both the Advisory Committee on Medical Research and the governing bodies, in their discussions of WHO's role in research development and coordination during the period 1973–1976, raised the difficulty of moving ahead in health services research, despite the passage of resolutions calling for action. The Advisory Committee, for example, at its fifteenth session, in 1973, indicated that "the diversity of national health systems itself affords invaluable research data of a kind WHO is uniquely qualified to collate in synoptic fashion to serve as the foundation of such studies. More use should be made of the comparative effectiveness of the different national approaches and systems of health care in their broadest sense" (26). At the same time, it recognized that the level of analysis that could be applied to such information was limited by financial strictures.

There was a brief exchange in January 1974 between the Colombian member of the Executive Board and the Director-General concerning the role of health services research, which shed further light on the thinking of Dr Mahler on this subject. After noting that WHO action should be solidly based on research and qualifying the project initiated by the Division of Research in Epidemiology and Communications Science and supported by

Colombia, WHO and PAHO as "successful", the Colombian Board member noted that research programmes also required "careful planning if there was not to be duplication of work and waste of scarce resources that might have been better employed in direct public health work". Dr Mahler replied:

> If a problem that was so full of social, economic, and political constraints were to be successfully tackled, there was need for total confidence between the government and the Organization. If that confidence were lacking, all that would result would be an academic study, which risked producing a negative impact because it was not placed in the context of any national health service system. The reason why WHO had failed with so many of its pilot projects in this area was that the projects had been outside the mainstream of government priorities. WHO would be able to make little progress in the field unless governments were prepared to take it into their confidence. (27)

In Dr Mahler's first address the Advisory Committee as Director-General (June 1974), he challenged the Committee to indicate which fields of medical research (including operational research, systems analysis and health-care delivery research) WHO should sponsor. The Committee gave a partial response:

> WHO should now begin to develop activities in the field of positive health promotion, including the definition of criteria for the assessment of desirable physical and mental performances, and the institution of community-based model programmes to achieve them. It was recommended that such programmes should employ management techniques involving operational research, systems analysis, and evaluation procedures. The need for collaboration with social scientists in formulating such research activities was stressed. (13)

On the next occasion (June 1975), the Director-General outlined the challenges that were facing WHO, one of which was the "untouched or neglected fields of research within the priority programme areas of WHO, such as the delivery of health services, educational techniques and other aspects of manpower development and training" (28). In its review of the programme for strengthening health services, the Advisory Committee endorsed the importance of research "in this relatively neglected field". Such research had "some unique characteristics". Research had to take into account the population's health status, work output and resources and the country's political, social, ecological and historical background. Furthermore, extensive, detailed knowledge was required of the wide range of solutions and techniques for modifying or changing health systems that could be adapted to the unique conditions of each country. Greater involvement of decision-makers and service staff in the studies was required to ensure that applicable findings were followed by appropriate public health action.

The Chairman of the Advisory Committee at its next session, in June 1976, expressed some frustration at having no actual projects to review, noting that the subject had been discussed in one form or another during the three previous sessions. On this occasion, the Committee recognized that health services research was the "next programme challenge" to be faced by WHO. It recommended that a planning group, with adequate representation from all regions and including a full-time secretary, should be established in the Organization to set up a framework for a special programme in health services research.

Meanwhile, concern was being expressed by both the Executive Board and the Health Assembly about the relation between health services research and biomedical research. The

Finnish Executive Board member at the fifty-seventh session (January 1976), for example, indicated that it would be a "misuse of words to maintain that the meaning of 'biomedical' could be extended to include such subjects as epidemiology, policy analysis and evaluation, health services research, systems analysis, operational research and health economics" (*29*). Furthermore, the inclusion of health services research into what he called 'health research' had implications for the membership and terms of reference of the Advisory Committee. At the moment, not more than two or three members were interested in that subject. He also noted "a certain distortion of emphasis in WHO research inputs, most of which went to a single very large programme financed from extrabudgetary resources", a distortion that resulted "from the biases of the contributors, which were Member States".

The Director-General, replying to these concerns, said that

> it was clear that [the Advisory Committee] had not yet been able to put the Organization on the right track with regard to 'systems research', the problem there being to find the necessary scientific potential in the world. In that respect, he also blamed governments, since this type of research would never reach the productive phase unless governments were willing to make use of the results that were intimately linked with the political decision-making process; otherwise the results would remain purely academic and would not produce the kind of methodology that would enable WHO to make the requisite recommendations to Member States .... He would welcome recommendations from Member States for [Advisory Committee] membership of scientists with a broad overview of both the managerial and biomedical services. He trusted, above all, that the regional advisory committees on medical research would provide the input for the global [Advisory Committee] on that very issue. (*29*)

The Executive Board went on to adopt resolution EB57.R32, which requested the Director-General to "give consideration to measures to broaden the areas of expertise represented by the membership of the [Advisory Committee on Medical Research] so as to reflect the increasing importance of health services research within biomedical research".

The representative of the Advisory Committee to the Twenty-ninth World Health Assembly, in May 1976, responding to the questions of many delegates concerning the place of health services research in biomedical research, reported that the Committee had debated the topic extensively at its session in June 1975, had welcomed inclusion of such research and had recognized the close relation with biomedical research as such. Nevertheless, the general feeling had been that health services research, which was a science midway between medical research and sociology, was at an earlier stage of evolution than strictly medical research. Accordingly, while the Committee welcomed extension of the concept and would do its best to provide assistance, it intended to proceed with caution so as not to detract from its well-established basis of action (*30*). On that occasion, resolution WHA29.64 was adopted, which confirmed the need for a comprehensive, long-term programme of biomedical and health services research.

In his reply at the fifty-ninth session of the Executive Board in January 1977 to members who expressed doubt about the ability of the Advisory Committee to move ahead in this area, the Director-General said that "unless prestige were attached to public health research, WHO goals would not be achieved. The Nobel Prize Committee should consider the basic goal-oriented research, the controlled clinical trials, the epidemiological community research, the operations systems analytical approaches, and the experiments with all the components, that finally lead to a health care delivery system in which the poor villager benefited from basic research" (*31*). He concluded that only the promise of intellectual satisfaction and the possibility of international recognition would attract young people to carry out the necessary research.

The sentiment was expressed at regional level that the global level was too remote from the ground to play an important role in this field. The advisory committee on medical research at the Regional Office for the Western Pacific rejected the idea of a health services research programme at WHO headquarters. because such a programme had to be "attuned to the particularities and peculiarities of national and even subnational groupings" (*32*). While welcoming the idea of a global programme, it would be a "compendium of regional and national programmes characterized by uniformity in things like format, statistics, and so forth, but by plurality at the periphery in terms of the sorts of problems that need to be attacked".

Shortly before and after the Thirtieth World Health Assembly, which adopted resolution WHA30.40 (see above), steps were taken to develop a 'global programme'. In late April 1977, a consultation on health systems research was held, involving WHO staff at headquarters and in the regional offices who were responsible for strengthening health services. The notion of 'health services research' had been extended to 'health systems research' in order to include consideration of organizations and actions "external to the conventional health services, but which nevertheless profoundly affect health service development and health" (*33*). The report of this consultation was considered by a group consisting of several members of the Advisory Committee, eight temporary advisers and WHO staff in different programmes, including nutrition and vector biology and control, that met in June. The difference between 'health systems research' and 'health services research' was not addressed; however, the meeting concluded that WHO should have a "special programme in health services research" and outlined the form that such a programme might take and how information from such research could be collected and analysed (*34*). Their recommendations were considered at the nineteenth session of the Advisory Committee the following week.

The Committee reaffirmed the "urgent need for a major increase in health services research" (*35*) and discussed the requirements in areas such as nutrition, maternal and child health, family planning, primary health care, immunization, community water supplies and health manpower development and the need for research on how to introduce the knowledge gained from biomedical research into health services practice. They stressed that high priority should be given to coordinating health services research within WHO, for the "common purpose of improving the health services", concluding that funds and training facilities were needed "to develop competent health services research manpower and to support health services research projects in the countries".

They recommended "immediate formation by the Director-General within WHO of a planning group with adequate representation from the regions and a full-time secretariat to formulate a special programme in health services research". Once the group had assessed current activities and identified priorities, it should devise a plan of action, identify training needs and prepare background material for a meeting of donor agencies, to be convened by the Director-General to seek funds for implementing the programme. A decentralized programme was envisioned, the global functions of which might include mobilization of extrabudgetary resources, improving methods, interregional communication and coordination and dissemination of information. In the meantime, it was judged important that existing technical programmes strengthen their efforts "immediately".

The recommendations of the Advisory Committee were presented to the sixty-first session of the Executive Board, in January 1978. The report (*36*) noted that the recommendations were being implemented gradually and that the new health services research programme would result from work that was being pursued in the regions and from close collaboration between countries and the Organization's regional offices and headquarters. Emphasis would be given to setting up institutions in countries and training a cadre of national research workers who would have competence in and commitment to health services research, improving the quality of health services research and mobilizing resources for health services research in countries.

The Advisory Committee established a subcommittee on health services research, which, at its first meeting in late 1978, formulated the following definition:

> Health services research is the systematic study of the means by which basic medical knowledge and other relevant health knowledge is brought to bear on the promotion of health in individuals and communities under a given set of existing conditions. (*37*)

ETHICAL ASPECTS OF MEDICAL RESEARCH

In 1967, in response to increasing concern by scientists and national administrators about moral and ethical problems related to investigations on human subjects, the Director-General established a secretariat committee on research involving human subjects to study and advise on the subject. All projects that had implications for human experimentation were reviewed by this committee. On the basis of advice from the Advisory Committee in 1975, the committee's clearance was required for all WHO-sponsored research involving human subjects.

WHO issued a report of a study, entitled *Health aspects of human rights with special reference to development in biology and medicine* (*38*), which was discussed by the Executive Board in January 1975 and published by WHO in early 1976. The Advisory Committee at its seventeenth session, in 1975, addressed WHO's position on research involving human subjects and recommended that the existing documentation on WHO clearance be reformulated to avoid unwarranted hampering of clinical research. It also recommended that consultant groups be convened to discuss topics such as radiation safety, psychological testing, the use of placebos and the protection of minors and others unable to provide informed consent.

An international conference was convened in March 1976 on the role of the individual and the community in research on and the development and use of biologicals. The conference was cosponsored by the World Medical Association, the International Association of Biological Standardization, the Council for International Organizations of Medical Sciences (CIOMS), the United States Public Health Services and WHO (see Chapter 1 for further information on the CIOMS).

A number of conferences were sponsored by WHO and organized by the CIOMS on the ethical aspects of medicine and health care, and increased attention was given to the subject by the governing bodies in 1976 and 1977. Resolution WHA29.64, adopted by the Twenty-ninth World Health Assembly in 1976, referred to the importance of "information, methodological and ethical problems", which would grow with further evolution of biomedical and health services research, and asked that WHO's comprehensive report on research include "possible ethical" recommendations.

In March 1977, a WHO expert committee on the use of ionizing radiation and radionuclides on human beings for medical research, training and nonmedical purposes examined the ethical implications of this subject, classified research projects according to the radiation dose delivered and the risks involved, and recommended that all research projects involving radiation should be reviewed by ethical review committees.

In December 1977, WHO cosponsored the eleventh CIOMS round-table conference on trends and prospects in drug research and development, at which the ethical aspects of drug development were discussed.

WHO and the global and regional advisory committees on medical research collaborated with the CIOMS in 1977 to examine ethical review procedures in various countries, with the goal of preparing guidelines for ethical review committees and setting flexible criteria for the review of research projects, taking into consideration regional and local differences.

References

1. *The medical research programme of the World Health Organization 1964–1968. Report of the Director-General*. Geneva, World Health Organization, 1969.
2. *Official records of the World Health Organization*, No. 136. Geneva, World Health Organization, 1964.
3. *Medical research programme. Report of scientific advisers on special development of international health and biomedical research. Note by the Director-General* (EB33/27). Geneva, World Health Organization, 1964.
4. *Meeting of scientific advisers on work in communication science in the proposed world health research centre. Official records of the World Health Organization*, No. 140, Appendix 1. Geneva, World Health Organization, 1965.
5. *Meeting of scientific advisers on biomedical research in the proposed world health research centre: harmful effects of therapeutic agents and environmental contaminants. Official records of the World Health Organization*, No. 140, Appendix 2. Geneva, World Health Organization, 1965.
6. *Meeting of scientific advisers on research in epidemiology in the proposed world health research centre. Official records of the World Health Organization*, No. 140, Appendix 3. Geneva, World Health Organization, 1965.
7. *Activities of the division of research in epidemiology and communication science. Official records of the World Health Organization*, No. 190, Appendix 11. Geneva, World Health Organization, 1971.
8. Badgley RF, ed. Social science and health planning: culture, disease and health services in Colombia. *Milbank Memorial Fund Quarterly*, 1968, 46(2), Part 2.
9. Molineaux L, Gramiccia G. *The Garki project: research on the epidemiology and control of malaria in the Sudan savanna of West Africa*. Geneva, World Health Organization, 1980.

10. *Official records of the World Health Organization*, No. 209 (WHA26/SR/A/11). Geneva, World Health Organization, 1973.

11. *Official records of the World Health Organization*, No. 185 (WHA23/SR/A/14). Geneva, World Health Organization, 1970.

12. *WHO's role in the development and coordination of biomedical research. Report by the Director-General* (EB53/5, Appendix II). Geneva, World Health Organization, 1974.

13. *Report to the Director-General. Advisory Committee on Medical Research, sixteenth session* (ACMR16/74.15). Geneva, World Health Organization, 1974.

14. *The work of WHO 1971. Official records of the World Health Organization*, No. 197. Geneva, World Health Organization, 1971.

15. *Report to the Director-General.* Advisory Committee on Medical Research, fourteenth session (ACMR14/72.14). Geneva, World Health Organization, 1972.

16. *WHO's role in the development and coordination of biomedical research. Interim report by the Director-General* (EB51/6), Geneva, World Health Organization, 1973.

17. *Official records of the World Health Organization*, No. 210 (WHA26/SR/A/5). Geneva, World Health Organization, 1973.

18. *Official records of the World Health Organization*, No. 218 (WHA27/SR/A/2). Geneva, World Health Organization, 1974.

19. *Official records of the World Health Organization*, No. 224 (EB55/SR/14). Geneva, World Health Organization, 1975.

20. *Organizational study on the interrelationships between the central services of WHO and programmes of direct assistance to Member States. Official records of the World Health Organization*, No. 223, Part I, Annex 7. Geneva, World Health Organization, 1975.

21. *The work of WHO 1973. Official records of the World Health Organization*, No. 213. Geneva, World Health Organization, 1973.

22. *WHO's role in the development and coordination of biomedical research. Progress report by the Director-General* (EB55/8, Appendix 1). Geneva, World Health Organization, 1975.

23. *Report of scientific advisers on special development of international health and biomedical research. Note by the Director-General* (EB33/27, Appendix, Annex 1). Geneva, World Health Organization, 1964.

24. *Meeting of scientific advisers on work in communications science in the proposed world health research centre, Geneva, 1–3 July 1964* (EB35/13, Annex 1). Geneva, World Health Organization, 1965.

25. *Official records of the World Health Organization*, No. 202 (WHA55/SR/A/2). Geneva, World Health Organization, 1972.

26. *Report to the Director-General. Advisory Committee on Medical Research, fifteenth session* (ACMR15/73.11). Geneva, World Health Organization, 1973.

27. *Executive Board, 53rd session* (EB53/SR/6 Rev.1). Geneva, World Health Organization, 1974.

28. *Report to the Director-General. Advisory Committee on Medical Research, seventeenth session* (ACMR17/75.14). Geneva, World Health Organization, 1975.

29. *Official records of the World Health Organization*, No. 232 (EB57/SR/19). Geneva, World Health Organization, 1976.

30. *Official records of the World Health Organization*, No. 234 (WHA29/SR/A/18). Geneva, World Health Organization, 1976.

31. *Official records of the World Health Organization*, No. 239 (EB59/SR/17). Geneva, World Health Organization, 1977.

32. Inside view: *WHO Chronicle* interviews two ACMR members. *WHO Chronicle*, 1977, 31:327–334.

33. *Health systems research. Advisory Committee on Medical Research, nineteenth session* (ACMR19/77.INF.DOC./1). Geneva, World Health Organization, 1977.

34. *Consultation on health services research. Report and recommendations. Advisory Committee on Medical Research, nineteenth session* (ACMR19/77.8). Geneva, World Health Organization, 1977.

35. *Report to the Director-General. Advisory Committee on Medical Research, nineteenth session* (ACMR19/77.14). Geneva, World Health Organization, 1977.

36. *Development and coordination of biomedical and health services research. Report by the Director-General* (EB61/23). Geneva, World Health Organization, 1978.

37. *WHO efforts in health services research. Progress report June 1978 to May 1979* (HSR/79.1). Geneva, World Health Organization, 1979.

38. *Health aspects of human rights with special reference to development in biology and medicine.* Geneva, World Health Organization, 1976.

CHAPTER 6

Strengthening health services

As indicated in the Introduction, the 1970s witnessed a dramatic resurgence of interest in improving the health services available to underserved populations.[1] This time, strengthening communities' role in both health promotion and achieving broader developmental goals, such as improved nutrition, housing and education, were stressed. Community participation and intersectoral collaboration combined with improved coverage of health services were the main features of what came to be known as the 'primary health care' approach.

FROM BASIC HEALTH SERVICES TO PRIMARY HEALTH CARE

The basic health services model had been articulated by the WHO expert committee responsible for public health administration at its second session, in 1953 (*1*). The model included maternal and child health, communicable disease control, environmental sanitation, maintenance of records for statistical purposes, health education of the public, public health nursing and medical care, the extent varying with the needs of the area and access to large hospitals.

When, in the mid-1960s, UNICEF sought "technical guidance" from WHO on planning and setting up such services, it was given in the form of "broad principles based on experience gained from field activities jointly assisted by UNICEF and WHO" (*1*). The basic health services were defined as "a network of coordinated peripheral and intermediate health units with a central administration capable of performing effectively a selected group of functions essential to the health of an area, and assuring the availability of competent professional and auxiliary personnel to perform these functions". The auxiliary personnel identified were nurse auxiliaries, sanitary assistants and sanitary health aids.

Various statements issued by the secretariat indicated that the basic health services model was not working well. The Director-General, in his introduction to *The work of WHO 1967* (*3*), observed that "the development of the essential basic health services continues to be slow and difficult, mainly because of the financial obstacles encountered by many governments and the shortage of trained personnel". Two years later, he pointed out that "our greatest shortcoming still relates to the development of sound health infrastructures on which these countries can build the facilities required for the protection and promotion of the health of their citizens" (*4*). The following year, at the forty-seventh session of the Executive Board in 1971, the subject chosen was methods of promoting the development of basic health services. This gave the Organization an opportunity to review the subject and to devise new approaches.

---

[1] Such interest manifested itself in the work of the League of Nations Health Organization in the 1930s under the guise of rural reconstruction. Twenty years later, similar concerns were addressed during formulation of the basic health services approach.

One year later, Dr Mahler, in his capacity as Assistant Director-General, introduced a working paper prepared by the secretariat for the forty-ninth session of the Executive Board session, which indicated that the basic health services "were more often an objective than a reality". He noted that the paper contained "the bitter comment that when such services were needed, countries could not afford them, and when they could afford them they no longer needed them" (5). He expressed his belief that "there were sufficient financial and intellectual resources available in the world to meet the basic health aspirations of all peoples" and suggested that "there was a need for an aggressive plan for worldwide action to improve this unsatisfactory situation", action which "required a high sense of social responsibility and political will on the part of governments in both developed and developing countries".

The working paper (6), although maintaining the definition of basic health services, adopted a markedly different tone from that of the 1965 paper. It was much more realistic concerning the degree to which basic health services had been developed and less dogmatic about what needed to be done. "Trial areas" were called for, as well as health manpower adapted to both the financial and the socioeconomic realities of a country.

In a parallel development, a senior UNICEF official told the nineteenth session of the Joint UNICEF/WHO Committee on Health Policy, that met in February 1972, that UNICEF considered it "important to examine the extent to which existing health services were able, in terms of their orientation, coverage, quality and community relationship, to fulfil the minimum role that Member States considered desirable" (7). He concluded by noting that "it was important to consider whether the two agencies were able to assist in the most effective way in increasing the coverage of health services in a manner consistent with national objectives and resources". No decision was taken on this matter; it remained on the agenda for consideration at a later date, as described below.

The Executive Board established a working group in January 1972 to continue its critical review, and the group presented its results to the Board at its fifty-first session, in 1973. This report (8) differed even more markedly from the WHO report 2 years previously. Its tone was more dramatic; the picture presented of the current status of the health services was more alarming than had been indicated earlier. Its key conclusion was that the basic health services approach had failed and that a "major crisis" was "on the point of development", which must be faced at once. The crisis was reflected in the "widespread dissatisfaction of populations" for reasons that included "a feeling of helplessness on the part of the consumer, who feels (rightly or wrongly) that the health services and the personnel within them are progressing along an uncontrolled path of their own which may be satisfying to the health professional but which is not what is wanted by the consumer."

Five principles dominated the final report of the Executive Board's organizational study. The first was that, while the problem of establishing 'health services' (the notion of 'basic' having been dropped) was essentially a national affair, it should be possible to structure responsibilities to give "greater emphasis to consumer preferences". Secondly, "outputs" should be seen in terms of "the final return to the individual in health status and in service"; the needs of health personnel as such should be dealt with separately. Thirdly, to overcome the current fragmentary nature of the health services, they "must be taken as a whole, public and private; national and international; curative and preventive; peripheral, intermediate and central". Fourthly, the performance of the health services should be judged on the basis of health status, operational factors (e.g. coverage and use), accepted technology, cost and consumer approval. Lastly, considering it improbable that an international model or 'standard' would be developed, "each country will have to possess the national ability to consider its own position (problems and resources), assess the alternatives available to it, decide upon its resource allocation and priorities, and implement its own decisions".

The first of three suggestions on the role of WHO programmes was dedicated to "world health conscience". It was indicated that WHO could be used not only as a forum to express ideas or dissatisfactions but also as a mechanism to point out directions in which Member States should go, concluding that "it is more than useful to have a conscience; it is essential".

Although the working group had drafted a resolution for consideration by the Executive Board at its session in January 1973, agreement could not be reached, and the matter was passed on to the Twenty-sixth World Health Assembly, which met in May 1973. In introducing the working group's report to the Health Assembly, the Executive Board's representative noted:

> It had been impossible to reach agreement on what was meant by basic health services. The study had therefore dealt with the development of health services as a continuing process .... The Board ... felt that it should lay down the following principles: the health services should make the people whom they serve feel that that they belong to them and are not imposed on them; the health services should be judged by how they benefit the individual; they should be seen as a whole; and criteria should be laid down for the evaluation of their development and performance. (*9*)

A draft resolution was introduced by the Executive Board member who had chaired the organizational study. She underlined the fact that the study was

> no more than a beginning. An immense task lay ahead; not only to assess the real situation, particularly so far as concerned the primary health services at the peripheral level, but also to try to coordinate under a common plan the often scattered and disparate health facilities and resources that might be funded by the State, by local authorities, by private persons or institutions, and by bilateral or multilateral assistance. A holistic approach was essential if great disasters later in the century were to be averted. (*9*)

The resolution adopted (WHA26.35) drew the attention of Member States to the findings, conclusions and recommendations of the study and listed a series of recommendations for action by the Director-General, beginning with programmes that would assist countries in extending their health-care systems to their entire population, especially to meet the needs of those groups that have clearly insufficient health services. It also requested him to report to the Executive Board "on the steps to be taken for the implementation of the conclusions and recommendations of the study and their impact on future programmes of the Organization".

A related development was the decision by WHO and UNICEF in July 1973 to explore "promising approaches to meeting basic health needs". This responded to the request made during the nineteenth session of the Joint UNICEF/WHO Committee on Health Policy (see above) that the two organizations study the most effective ways of assisting countries in increasing the coverage of their health services. Approaches were sought that met (not necessarily all) three criteria that had been derived from the Board's study. The approach should be effective and efficient in meeting the basic health needs of populations "that are not usually covered by adequate health services", ensure adequate coverage and "can, on the whole, be applied within five, or, at most, ten years in a country of extremely limited resources". In a letter signed by Dr Pierre Dorolle, Deputy-Director General, and dated 25 July 1973, the regional offices were asked "to take a fresh look at existing problems and at alternative approaches to their solution".[2]

At a meeting of WHO and UNICEF staff held in October 1973, it was agreed that

> the study should be multi-sectoral and not only medically oriented or limited to the mandate of health departments, since resources benefitting health can be harnessed from various sources both within and without the Government, such as measures which can be taken through channels outside the traditional health structure. (Note for the record on a meeting of the Joint WHO/UNICEF Committee on Health Policy Studies, UNICEF HQ, 23 October 1973)

The Director-General, in his annual report on the work of WHO for 1973 (*10*), indicated that a turning-point in the life of the Organization might have been reached, with the unequivocal admission that "the most signal failure of WHO as well as of Member States has undoubtedly been their inability to promote the development of basic health services and to improve their coverage and utilization". As there were few models to demonstrate that primary health care can be brought to villages at reasonable cost and in a technically and socially acceptable manner, it was urgent that WHO find countries that were willing and able to set up systems of primary health care and demonstrate their effectiveness. The title of this report, when published in the *WHO chronicle*, was 'An international health conscience' (*11*).

The Board's study showed that WHO had a role to play in "selectively encouraging and participating in national endeavours for health service development". WHO would attempt to follow the approaches outlined in the study at all levels of the Organization. The strategy that had evolved in 1973 would be "followed in selected countries ready for intensive and continued health service development". In each, a health programme would be set up by the ministry of health, with the assistance of the Organization, in which the problems and objectives would be presented in a "holistic and intersectoral way" (*12*).

Although the study of the Executive Board had come to an end, the USSR delegate to the Twenty-seventh World Health Assembly, in May 1974, introduced a resolution (WHA27.44) that requested WHO "to assist governments to direct their health service programmes towards their major health objectives" and asked the Director-General to report to the fifty-fifth session of the Board and the Twenty-eighth World Health Assembly on the steps that could be taken by WHO to further implementation of this and the related resolutions referred to. The request of the USSR delegate that an international conference be held to consider the subject of national health services was not supported by the Board on this occasion.[3]

---

[2] Dr Dorolle was Deputy Director-General of WHO from 1950 to late 1973, when Dr Tom Lambo, who had been an Assistant Director General, took over.

[3] Although the planning for this conference, which took place in 1978, was related to the issues covered in this chapter, it is described separately in the Epilogue. The reader might wish to read that section first, especially as it highlights conceptual difficulties surrounding primary health care.

Following the Twenty-seventh World Health Assembly, a meeting of regional advisers on community health services was held in Geneva to review problems, discuss new research findings and new managerial approaches (in particular that of country health programming), and agree on future action to be taken by WHO. Staff involved in both health manpower development and family health participated. Dr Mahler referred to WHO's inability to learn from failures and said that change was necessary if "we want to keep our credibility among the countries to be able to assist them effectively", that ways should be found of achieving proper coordination between headquarters, the regions and field projects, and that "dialogue is one of the concrete mechanisms whereby we can ensure that a cohesive policy is created and then implemented at all levels". It was agreed that a change of attitude among WHO staff was needed. Programmes should not be imposed upon countries, and greater sensitivity to cultural background, local conditions and real needs was required.

Progress in the study of alternative approaches was reviewed on this occasion. Three factors were seen as affecting the success of a programme: community involvement, emphasis on auxiliary staff or community health workers and teamwork, with permanent supervision and support from the intermediate echelons to the periphery. Also, the training of physicians should be reoriented and adapted to the needs of the community.

For a brief period during the second half of 1974, the division dealing with strengthening of health services at headquarters studied the possibility of a programme for community involvement in primary health care. One example was a project on community involvement in solving local health problems initiated in the Kintampo region of Ghana (see Chapter 4). This idea was dropped; instead, in the report presented to the Board in January 1975 in response to resolution WHA27.44, community involvement was identified as one of the critical features of primary health care (13). This report argued that the "resources available to the community" should be brought into "harmony" with "the resources available to the health services". For this to happen, "a radical departure from conventional health services approach is required", one that built new services "out of a series of peripheral structures that are designed for the context they are to serve". The design should adapt primary health care to the life of the population; involve the local population; place maximum reliance on available community resources while remaining within cost limits; provide an integrated approach of prevention, cure and promotion for both the community and the individual; ensure that interventions were undertaken at the most peripheral practicable level of the health services by workers basically trained for the activity; designate other echelons of service to support needs at the peripheral level; and be fully integrated with the services of the other sectors involved in community development.

The Board adopted resolution EB55.R16, which requested the Director-General to set up a programme for primary health care in the light of the discussions of the Executive Board, his consultations with Member States and other relevant agencies and the conclusions of the meeting of an ad hoc group of the Executive Board to be held before the Twenty-eighth World Health Assembly. The chairman of this group, introducing its report to the Health Assembly, said that the group recognized that primary health care had to take into account local community development plans. Concerning the most suitable personnel to be used, "there was no single solution to the mixture of skills required for the provision of health care in different countries; what was meant by 'doctor', a 'nurse' or a 'health auxiliary' would vary not only according to countries but also according to the stage of development of the health care system of any particular country". A "radical change of approach would be needed in many countries if health services were to be built from the primary care level up rather than from the top" (*14*).

The Joint UNICEF/WHO Committee on Health Policy, meeting in February 1975, recommended that WHO and UNICEF "adopt an action programme aimed at extending primary health care to populations in developing countries, particularly to those which are now inadequately provided with such care, such as rural and remote populations, slum dwellers, and nomads" (*15*). Positive steps should be taken to "inform, educate, and orient" all staff, as such a programme required "detailed awareness and understanding" as well as "an organizational adaptation to respond to the new challenges".

Two publications on primary health care had become available: *Alternative approaches to meeting basic health needs of populations in developing countries* (*16*) and *Health by the people* (*17*). The Joint UNICEF/WHO Committee recommended that the organizations continue to study not only the innovations described in the first publication but also those occurring in various parts of the world. The two organizations "should record and monitor them; learn from them; evaluate them; make their results widely available; assist them when necessary; adapt them; build upon them; and encourage similar endeavors, even though some may present some risk in the sense that their favourable outcome is not clearly predictable" (*18*). Soon thereafter, the two organizations agreed that more knowledge was required about successful community-based development activities. Therefore, an agreement was reached to ask the twenty-first Joint UNICEF/WHO Committee to review and analyse examples of community participation that were considered to have improved health and the general standard of living. The results of this study are described below. In May, as well, the UNICEF Executive Board endorsed the alternative approaches, adopted its principles as UNICEF policy and initiated worldwide action to implement its recommendations.

The Twenty-eighth World Health Assembly adopted resolution WHA28.88, which requested the Director-General to "promote and assist in the development of primary health care activities with the active participation of different socioeconomic sectors, and through the use of different entry points, e.g. national development planning, and rural and other intersectoral development activities". The content of this resolution underwent considerable discussion and compromise before it was agreed to. Two drafts were presented at the beginning of the discussion, one from the Board's ad hoc group and the other from several socialist countries. The latter introduced several new elements, in particular the need for medically qualified personnel working under the supervision of higher levels and all "subordinate to local health authorities and state authorities", and "an international meeting or conference under WHO auspices to exchange experience on the development of national health services". A number of delegates pointed out that this draft went beyond the subject under discussion, namely primary health care. The last point was accepted, but the idea of a conference was maintained. The Executive Board was instructed to consider and determine at its fifty-seventh session the date, place and concrete programme for such a conference. It was this request that led to the Alma-Ata Conference, which took place in September 1978, as described in the Epilogue.

In October 1975, an informal meeting of representatives from UNDP, UNICEF, the World Bank and WHO was held in New York on primary health care. The meeting's purpose was to achieve consensus for interagency action under a common policy and to extend the dialogue to other interested organizations and funding agencies. The principles of primary health care were endorsed by all those present. The World Bank stated that the primary health care approach was fully in line with the Bank's policies, while noting that its implementation might require a large amount of resources. The UNDP found the timing to be propitious, as the funding cycle covering the period 1977–1981 was beginning. The meeting concluded that a broad approach to health development was required; community-based primary health care seemed to contain the principles of success. It considered that the knowledge available was sufficient to implement primary health care nationally or subnationally, without pilot or demonstration projects.

In notes prepared after the meeting for distribution to field personnel of the participating agencies (*19*), a list of "implications within a national context" was presented, which further defined what implementation of primary health care entailed:

1. Merging concerns at grass-roots level

    The needs to be met and the development to be promoted are largely dictated by the specific socio-cultural–economic realities of each community. They cannot be dictated from above .... Community 'development' committees and community 'health' development committees should be one and the same committee.

2. Multisectoral support of primary health care

    Self-reliance at grass-roots level does not imply that self-sufficiency is possible. It is precisely because most communities of the developing world do not have sufficient resources or technical know-how to be self-reliant that full multisectoral support is a necessity.

3. Special role of the health sector

    Rather than being a single-sector service delivered from above, the health sector will need to find ways to organize its activities so as to enhance the merging of concerns at the grass-roots level as well as to encourage wider intersectoral support.

4. Multisectoral planning for primary health care

    The means chosen by communities, sub-districts and districts to promote health through intersectoral activities will need to be reflected in all sector plans to the degree that these activities require the expenditure of national resources controlled by the individual sectors.

5. International agencies at country level

    The Resident Representative of the UNDP already accepts a coordinating role in relation to the WHO representative, the representative of FAO, etc. This function would become of even more crucial importance as health proposals would no longer be restricted to the generally accepted health sector and would need to be ultimately linked with other sectors and other levels of government.

Progress was reported to the fifty-seventh session of the Executive Board, in January 1976, and to the Twenty-ninth World Health Assembly, in May of that year. Much of the discussion concerned the place and timing of the conference (see Epilogue). A consultation between headquarters and the regional offices had been held in Geneva in June 1975 to work out the global WHO strategy in collaboration with UNICEF. Agreement was reached on the primary health care approach, the role of the Organization in promoting and supporting primary health care and a global plan of action.

Resolution WHA28.88 was favourably received by each of the regional committees of WHO. Regional focal points were designated and regional primary health-care teams formed. Working groups were established at headquarters to prepare technical guidelines for primary health care under the direction of a newly established steering committee. Other activities were undertaken in staff development and training and in interagency and country-level promotion of the primary health care approach. Country-level activities centred around organizing what was called a 'national dialogue', which was expected to involve the government health ministry; other sectors, including planning, rural development and education; nongovernmental organizations; the health professions; and consumer and village representatives. The purpose of the dialogue was to examine the present national health system and make proposals for change, taking into account the principles of promotion of national health services and primary health care. Both WHO and UNICEF were prepared to support governments in organizing such dialogue.

The papers presented to the Twenty-ninth World Health Assembly introduced two new themes: primary health care and rural development, and primary health care and appropriate technology. Motivation for the former was largely due to the initiative of the Administrative Committee on Coordination of the United Nations on rural development (see Chapter 1). Various steps were outlined for promoting interagency cooperation and actions, including multiagency task forces, pooling the human resources of the agencies and joint training.

The Director-General was asked to establish a programme of health technology for primary health care and rural development and to promote and conduct research on new technologies that were both appropriate and effective. Resolution WHA29.74 incorporated the latter recommendations, adding a request that the Director-General "stimulate health manpower training institutions to intensify their efforts for promoting and strengthening their roles" in the appropriate technology programme. As for primary health care and rural development, the resolution requested the Director-General "to take appropriate steps to ensure that WHO takes an active part, jointly with other international agencies, in supporting national planning of rural development aimed at the relief of poverty and to improvement of the quality of life". Owing to the difficulties encountered in promoting interagency cooperation, described in Chapter 1, little progress was made.

In the absence of support from a broad-based interagency approach to national development, WHO's partnership with UNICEF was even more appreciated, as noted in numerous resolutions. At the international level, the community of nongovernmental organizations involved in promoting primary health care stimulated developments that might not otherwise have occurred. In June 1976, these organizations established a joint planning exercise for primary health care. Its initial membership consisted of the Christian Medical Commission, the International Union against Tuberculosis, the League of Red Cross Societies,

International Cooperation for Socio-economic Development, the International Planned Parenthood Federation and the International Federation of Anti-leprosy Associations. Earlier, the Christian Medical Commission had helped to identify important projects, which were were described in the publication *Health by the people* (*17*), and stimulated national dialogue in countries in which they worked. These and other nongovernmental organizations (see Epilogue) played important roles in ensuring the success of the Alma-Ata Conference.

A programme on health technology in primary health care was established in January 1976 with the aims of promoting the use of health technology appropriate to the needs and resources of each country, to reduce the dependence of these countries on imported or inappropriate technologies and to ensure that they become self-reliant and self-sufficient in this domain. A consultation held that same month with appropriate technology groups and interested agencies of the United Nations system identified priorities in a number of areas. With respect to immunization and prevention, for example, the priorities were: elimination of syringes for vaccinations, simplification of vaccination with bacillus Calmette-Guérin (BCG), a more efficient principle for powering jet injectors and a visual indicator of vaccine deterioration. In the area of education and training, the priorities were for a simple front projector for colour microfiches; production, distribution and use of low-cost visual aids; and alternative training methods for diagnosis and treatment in developing countries. Other areas considered were environmental health and management of health services.

A contractual agreement was concluded with the Appropriate Health Resources and Technologies Action Group in London, England, for establishment of a clearing house for information on health technology. Later in 1977, plans were formulated for country activities, including intercountry workshops, identification of study areas to explore problem identification and the design and field testing of techniques, and a study of problems in the acceptance of new technology and its production, marketing and evaluation.

The twenty-first meeting of the Joint UNICEF/WHO Committee on Health Policy, in early 1977, reviewed a report on community involvement in primary health care (*20*), which contained nine case studies describing the activities of different peoples involved in community development. The cases reflected a broad spectrum of social, cultural, economic and political structures and conditions in a variety of geographical settings. The recommendations called on WHO and UNICEF to continue work in this area and to collaborate with countries in finding methods for identifying community human, economic and material resources that could contribute to local primary health care activities. They should assist in appropriate training programmes to form local leadership for primary health care and encourage and assist governments to provide appropriate support to communities involved in their primary health care and development projects. The report was well received by the Committee, which incorporated the recommendations in its report (*21*), and the sixtieth session of the Executive Board, in May 1977, also supported the recommendations (resolution EB60.R1).

By the end of the decade, 17 countries in the African Region had accepted the primary health care approach. In the South-East Asia Region, eight countries had integrated primary health care projects into basic health services. Seven countries in the Eastern Mediterranean Region expressed interest in the approach, and many Member States in the Western Pacific

Region initiated primary health care programmes, with emphasis on training health-care workers.

Primary health care also had an impact in developed countries. In the European Region, four issues emerged: the relation between social services and health services, the rapid increase in the cost of health services, the role of outpatient treatment and health centres and the functions of professionals involved in primary care. Many of these issues were the subject of a symposium organized by WHO and the New York Academy of Sciences, on primary health care for industrialized countries, held in New York City in December 1977 (22). (See Epilogue for further information on regional activities related to primary health care.)

TRADITIONAL MEDICINE

The first paper on primary health care (13), introduced to the Board in January 1975, called for harmonization of services organized by the government with those traditionally available to people, such as traditional birth attendants and herbalists. The Chinese delegate to the Board underlined the importance of this aspect of primary health care, indicating that "such medicine should be fully developed so as to strengthen basic health care" (23). Renewed interest in traditional medicine in the People's Republic of China had started in the late 1940s, but only with its entry into WHO was the subject introduced into the discussions of WHO's governing bodies (e.g. 24). Several Member States enquired about follow-up action in this area, particularly with regard to the promotion and development of their respective traditional and indigenous systems of medicine. A small group consultation was held, and in January 1976 the subject was considered by the Board. The following actions were proposed:

- collect all available data on traditional healers and indigenous systems of medicine, including the results of surveys and research, studies of traditional practices and training programmes for traditional healers and indigenous practitioners;
- analyse the information to determine the relevance of traditional healing to the primary health care of populations;
- study, in the field, existing systems of traditional or indigenous medicine in each region;
- suggest the main directions for action, especially the training of traditional healers and their use in the health system; and
- suggest further action by Member States and the WHO secretariat.

An interdivisional working group was formed at headquarters to coordinate these activities, and the regions initiated training programmes for practitioners of traditional medicine, including traditional birth attendants, and orientation courses for physicians, nurses, midwives and other health workers. The regional office representatives concerned with traditional medicine met in October 1976 and proposed the following programme objectives: to foster a realistic approach to traditional medicine, in order to promote and further contribute to health care; to explore the merits of traditional medicine in the light of modern science, in order to maximize the useful and effective practices and discourage harmful ones; and to promote the integration of proven valuable knowledge and skills in traditional and scientific medicine.

The Thirtieth World Health Assembly, in 1977, requested (resolution WHA30.49) the Director-General to assist Member States in organizing educational and research activities and to award fellowships for training in research techniques, for studies of health-care systems and for investigating the technical procedures related to traditional and indigenous systems of medicine. Later that year, a study tour on traditional medicine in China was organized, during which 29 participants from developing countries studied how China had harnessed the legacy of traditional medicine to the needs of its vast rural population and had combined the traditional Chinese system with western medicine.

A meeting held at the end of 1977 of expert representatives of the major systems of traditional medicine recommended that WHO "use all the possible resources at its command to continue to promote and develop traditional medicine" (25). Specifically, the Organization should promote the formulation and declaration of national policies for encouraging, supporting and developing traditional systems of medicine indigenous to Member States. The elements of such a policy should include legal recognition of traditional medicine and its integration into comprehensive national health-care systems, including primary health care. The Organization should establish a committee of experts to advise on the promotion and development of traditional medicine, monitor and coordinate research and evaluate programmes for re-planning and the proper reorientation of strategies.

THE WIDER HEALTH SYSTEM: PLANNING, MANAGEMENT AND FINANCING

At the beginning of the decade, the Organization was providing assistance to more than 70 countries in health planning and public health administration. This subject was among the first to be reported on in the annual report of the programme. As noted by the Director-General in 1968, it was "axiomatic that any improvement in the health of a people depends on an integrated approach to preventive and curative services", and "these services can best be effectively developed within the framework of a comprehensive health plan". WHO was accordingly "substantially increasing its assistance to countries engaged in working out long-term plans for the building up of their national health services" (3). The emphasis given to health planning is reflected in the work of all the WHO regional offices, as summarized in Chapter 4. By promoting health planning as an integral part of overall national socio-economic planning, it was hoped that national budgets for health would increase and the nature of services provided would be more in keeping with the social and economic needs of the population, especially those in greatest need.

The late 1960s also saw interest in applying various managerial methods, especially operational research and systems analysis, that had been used over the past few decades by industrial businesses and national military establishments. Numerous activities were undertaken in all the regions to promote and apply these methods, as briefly touched upon in Chapters 4 and 5. A consultation of experts on research in public health practice was convened in December 1968 to review activities in this field. A number of priorities were identified: manpower, including studies of personnel use, such as the optimal mix of doctors, nurses and other health professionals in different health services but especially in health centres; organization, such as studying the advantages of separate provisions for medical care of the sick and personal preventive care, as opposed to integrated health care; and cost, e.g. cost–effectiveness and cost–benefit studies. Within the Organization's programme of research in public health practice, support was provided in 1969 for three studies of community health, in Brazil, Hungary and the United Arab Republic. The methods used in these and other studies were described in a publication, *Health practice research and formalized managerial methods (26)*. A protocol was designed for conducting research to evaluate primary health centres as a means of protecting and furthering health in developing countries (*27*). Although the protocol was not used, the document provides an extensive, valuable review of the history of health centres and previous evaluation efforts.

The PAHO advisory committee on medical research at its seventh session in 1968 endorsed the potential value of operational research and suggested that the techniques of control and evaluation be built into future PAHO research programmes to the extent possible. A symposium on application of systems analysis to health services was held in June 1971. While it was agreed that systems analysis had a role in decision-making in health administration, especially in planning and evaluation, "its role will continue to be largely experimental until it is understood, accepted and supported by health administrators in their day-to-day decision-making in the broad field of health" (*28*).

A joint ILO/WHO committee met in 1970 to consider the subject of personal health care and social security. Speaking on behalf of the Director-General, Dr Mahler indicated that it seemed "timely to develop a concerted approach to the planning, administration, and financing of personal health services". The committee recommended that studies be carried out to determine the approximate levels of development of national economies and basic health services suitable and appropriate for extension of social security systems for the delivery of personal health care. The range of services envisaged for such systems included health promotion, personal preventive services, family planning (where relevant), ambulatory medical care, hospital care (including outpatient services), medical rehabilitation, long-term care (where relevant), diagnostic facilities, therapeutic facilities and medical supplies. Studies should continue on alternative methods of organizing personal health services and determining suitable methods for fostering the coordination of such services with other social services (*29*).

A WHO expert committee was convened in 1971 to consider the organization of local and intermediate health administrations. The committee noted (*30*) that regionalization of services was a means of providing "comprehensive health care to a community or group of communities. It concerns local and intermediate health services, and implies that health care and support are distributed through resources strategically located in the area of the community or communities served". Additional studies were called for. The importance of modern principles and techniques of administrative and personnel management was stressed.

The advantages of centralization as opposed to decentralization were explored on this occasion. While centralization ensured the distribution of personal medical care and public health services of even quality throughout the regional system, its distribution was not affected significantly by variation in regional resources and financial structures. When centralization was interpreted bureaucratically, there was a tendency towards rigidity and uniformity. Decentralized systems were in close contact with the consumer, and decisions on health services were strongly influenced by the consumer's needs and demands. Its main disadvantage lay in the different social and economic conditions of local communities. As a result, substantial subsidies were required to maintain uniformity in the quality and distribution of services. Also, dependence on local resources (particularly manpower) and local solutions to problems could lead to a certain mediocrity and to an inability to withstand local political and other influences and pressures.

This committee encouraged further research on application of managerial and behavioural sciences to health administration. Several topics were identified, including: the behaviour of the providers of health services towards the recipients, human relationships within the administrative and organizational structure and the functional and economic organization and management of health services. WHO, it was noted, was well placed to collate and disseminate information obtained from these studies as well as to foster research in these areas (*30*).

Perhaps the most compact statement on this subject, as it was understood in the 'pre-primary health care' period in WHO, emerged during the Twenty-third World Health Assembly, in 1970, following the introduction by the USSR of a resolution entitled 'Basic principles for the development of national health services'. A statement had been identified as desirable in paragraph 5 of WHO's Fourth General Programme of Work (*31*). After a relatively brief discussion, during which some problems of terminology were cited and changes proposed, the resolution was revised and accepted (WHA23.61). This resolution stated that "among the most effective principles for the establishment and development of national health systems are those which have been confirmed by experience in a number of countries". These included:

- proclamation of the responsibility of the State and society for the protection of health of the population, to be based on a complex of economic and social measures which directly or indirectly promote the attainment of the highest possible level of health, through the establishment of a nationwide system of health services based on a general national plan and local planning, and through the rational and efficient use, for the needs of the health services, of all forces and resources that society at the given stage of its development is able to allocate for those purposes;
- the administration of rational training of national health personnel at all levels as a basis for the successful functioning of any health system, and the recognition by all medical workers of their high degree of social responsibility to society;
- the development of health services primarily on the basis of extensive measures to foster the preventive approach both for the community and the individual, which will require the integration of curative and preventive services in all medical and health establishments and services, emphasizing the protection of the health of mothers and children, who embody the future of every country and of the whole of mankind, and

the establishment of effective control over the condition of the environment as a
source of health and life to 'present and future generations';

- the provision for the whole population of the country of the highest possible level of
  skilled, universally available preventive and curative medical care, without financial
  or other impediments, by setting up an appropriate system of curative, preventive and
  rehabilitative services;

- the extensive application in every country of the results of progress in world medical
  research and public health practice, with a view to ensuring conditions that will make
  it possible to obtain maximum effectiveness from all health measures taken; and

- health education of the public and participation of wide sections of the population in
  carrying out all public health programmes, as an expression of the personal and collective responsibility of all members of society for protecting human health.

A report on various approaches to national health planning was published in 1972 (*32*),
with examples from India and the USSR, and outlining the Swedish approach to regional
planning, the method designed by PAHO and the Centre for Development Studies of the
Central University of Venezuela, health planning in the United States, health manpower
planning in various developing countries and what was termed "the pragmatic approach"
used in less developed countries. The authors concluded, "health administrators in a country
or area will wish to make their own choice from the variety of planning processes available".
Having made that choice, they can then give "proportionate weight ... to the political, technical, and administrative aspects of health planning for a particular time and place". A
working group sponsored by the Regional Office for Europe that met in June 1972 to review
progress in health planning in national development, concluded that the studies and research
undertaken by institutes, agencies and groups on health planning and health services research relevant to health planning should be reviewed, and this was undertaken later in the
decade.

In 1973, the technical discussions of the Health Assembly were on the organization,
structure and functioning of health services and on modern methods of administrative
management (*33*). Various ways in which WHO could contribute in this area were identified, including: the provision of teams to advise and help national personnel to apply
managerial methods; assistance in managerial training and associated research and development; dissemination of information; and support for initiating international cooperation
in research and comparative studies of management problems. Regional meetings on this
subject followed.

Also in 1973, an interregional seminar on health economics was held. Although WHO
had already collected and made available authoritative information in this area, the seminar
suggested that the Organization "consider providing assistance to countries needing economic expertise in health programming, in health services development, and in the establishment of health economics departments in colleges and planning institutions" (*34*).

The usefulness of health services development institutes was explored in several countries. Seen as health research and development organs of ministries of health, the objective
of such institutes was to promote community health by gradual, adaptive change. Their
sphere of interest covered technology, organizational patterns, allocation of resources,

managerial control of services, adaptation of training to service requirements, education techniques and operational and other applied research (*35*). With the support of the Swedish International Development Cooperation Agency and the Danish International Development Agency, institutes were established in Iran and Indonesia in 1974. The former was regarded as a mechanism for bringing together different ministries, local authorities, organizations and universities to deal with common problems. Its first major activity was the West Azerbaijan project, described in Chapters 4 and 5. In Indonesia, the programme included research with epidemiological and operational methods into the structure and functioning of district and provincial health services and hospitals.

After a 'project systems analysis' (see Chapter 3), an expert committee, meeting in 1975, recommended that WHO establish an "international partnership" to promote the application of systems analysis in national public administration (*36*), the eventual objective being "to achieve an interdisciplinary advisory and technical support capacity that can be provided to countries for intersectoral analysis and policy and strategy design. It was suggested that pooled funding might be sought from programme-oriented organizations as well as regional and bilateral development agencies and from the private sector". Systems analysis had been used in a number of projects on health services, including one in Malaysia to set up a rural health service in a land development area, one in the Philippines for medical care development in Rizal Province, and one in Thailand for health services in Chonburi Province and establishment of a provincial health planning system.

A WHO study group met in November 1977 to discuss the financing of health services. It reviewed approaches to improving the financing of health activities and methods of collecting the necessary data (*37*). Case studies from developing countries, provided as background material for the meeting, showed that information of sufficient reliability could be collected and analysed at modest cost. It was suggested that such studies could make important contributions to health planning. For example, they could be used to quantify the gap between the resources that could reasonably be expected for the health sector and those necessary to achieve the country's medium-term policies. Quantifying the gap could help countries to assess the type of (appropriate) techniques that could be used to match the resources obtainable to the resources needed. Surveys of financing could focus attention on alternative ways of finding further resources for the health sector and could provide data to ensure equitable allocation of resources.

The study group recommended that WHO promote the principles and methods described, cooperate with interested countries in carrying out surveys, collaborate with research institutions to encourage research in this area and collect information on low-cost techniques for analysing the financing of health services.

ORGANIZATION OF MEDICAL CARE AND REHABILITATION

The hospital had been seen as the node in regionalization of health services during previous decades. An expert committee, meeting in 1956, portrayed the hospital as an integral part of social and medical organization, the function of which was to provide complete health care, both curative and preventive, with outpatient services for the family in its home environment; the hospital should also be a centre for training health workers and for biosocial research (*38*). In 1967, another expert committee on hospital administration found it necessary to define the hospital "in more practical terms ... as an institution that provides in-patient accommodation for medical and nursing care" (*39*). Depending on its level of development, such an institution "may also participate in the education and training of health personnel and carry out medical, epidemiological, social, and organizational research". While the hospital was no longer being promoted as a pivotal institution in community health services and primary health care, the need for well-designed hospitals functioning within a well- planned regional system did not lose its importance. The Organization was increasingly asked to advise on the planning of hospital services, their equipment and maintenance and the architectural design of hospitals.

A supplement to the *Fourth report of the world health situation* (*40*), published in 1972, contained a review of the organization of hospital services. An even more extensive review was prepared in 1973, which covered hospital laws and administration, organization, systems and general trends in organization. The content of this report was based on replies received from 52 Member States to a questionnaire devised and issued by WHO consultants.

In 1974, a comprehensive study of the planning, programming, design and architecture of hospitals and other health-care facilities in developing countries was undertaken by WHO. The first in a series of five sets of guidelines resulting from this study was published in 1976, entitled *Approaches to planning and design of health care facilities in developing areas* (*41*).

The main report of a WHO international collaborative study on the use of medical care, in which the Organization had been formally involved since 1967, was completed in 1975 and published in 1977 (*42*). The study involved 12 areas in seven countries, and the results covered population groups representing more than 15 million people. The aim was to answer questions about the health-care needs of populations, the organization, resources and use of health services, factors influencing patterns of use and some methodological problems. The Organization, considering that the main study report was too detailed and voluminous to be immediately useful, encouraged some of the study collaborators to prepare a volume that highlighted the key findings. This appeared in the form of a public health report in 1977 (*43*).

Medical rehabilitation was addressed by an expert committee in 1968. The meeting defined relevant terms, stressed the importance of arriving at a classification of disabilities and gathering statistical data and information on them, outlined various forms that the organization of medical rehabilitation services might take, conceptualized the functions and training of an ideal rehabilitation team, and listed projects it considered suitable for research No specific role for WHO was recommended.

An interregional seminar on planning, organization and administration of medical rehabilitation services was held in New Delhi, India, in September 1972, followed by an informal consultation in 1973, when the role and programme of WHO in this field were discussed. Further discussions with various United Nations agencies and selected experts led to the drafting of an operational plan for WHO activities in disability prevention and rehabilitation in 1974. Geriatrics was considered to form a specific part of such a programme. In 1976, the Health Assembly resolved (resolution WHA29.68) that the WHO policy on disability prevention and rehabilitation be oriented to:

- the promotion of effective measures for preventing disability;
- encouragement of the application of effective approaches and appropriate techniques to prevent disability, while integrating disability prevention and rehabilitation into health programmes at all levels, including primary health care;
- emphasis on those problems of disability that can be solved most efficiently and effectively and in a manner acceptable to populations; and
- inclusion of training in appropriate methods for preventing disability and for rehabilitation into the curricula for all relevant health manpower.

References

1. *Methodology of planning an integrated health programme for rural areas. Second report of the expert committee on public-health administration* (WHO Technical Report Series, No. 83). Geneva, World Health Organization, 1954.
2. *Basic health services. Joint UNICEF/WHO Committee on Health Policy, fourteenth session* (JC14/UNICEF/WHO/2.65). Geneva, World Health Organization, 1970.
3. *The work of WHO 1967. Official records of the World Health Organization*, No. 164. Geneva, World Health Organization, 1967.
4. *The work of WHO 1969. Official records of the World Health Organization*, No. 180. Geneva, World Health Organization, 1969.
5. *Executive Board, 49th session, summary records* (EB49/SR/14 Rev.1). Geneva, World Health Organization, 1972.
6. *Organizational study of the Executive Board on methods of promoting the development of basic health services. Background documentation* (EB49/WP/6). Geneva, World Health Organization, 1972.
7. *Joint UNICEF/WHO Committee on Health Policy. Nineteenth session.* (JC19/UNICEF- WHO/MIN/72.4). Geneva, World Health Organization, 1972.
8. *Organizational study on methods of promoting the development of basic health services. Official records of the World Health Organization*, No. 206, Annex 11. Geneva, World Health Organization, 1973.
9. *Official records of the World Health Organization*, No. 210 (WHA26/SR/B/4, WHA26/SR/B/5). Geneva, World Health Organization, 1973.
10. *The work of WHO 1973. Official records of the World Health Organization*, No. 213. Geneva, World Health Organization, 1973.
11. Mahler H. An international health conscience. *WHO Chronicle*, 1974, 28:207–211.
12. *Report of the World Health Organization in 1973: analytic summary* (PCO/74.1). New York, United Nations, Economic and Social Council, 1974.
13. *Organizational study of the Executive Board on methods of promoting the development of basic health services. Background documentation* (EB49/WP/6), Geneva, World Health Organization, 1972.
14. *Official Records of the World Health Organization*, No. 227 (WHA28/SR/A/19). Geneva, World Health Organization, 1975.

15. *Joint UNICEF/WHO Committee on Health Policy: report on the twentieth session. Official Records of the World Health Organization*, No. 228, Annex 2. Geneva, World Health Organization, 1975.
16. Djukanovic V, Mach EP, eds. *Alternative approaches to meeting basic health needs of populations in developing countries*. Geneva, World Health Organization, 1975.
17. Newell KW, ed. *Health by the people*. Geneva, World Health Organization, 1975.
18. *Joint UNICEF/WHO Committee on Health Policy: report on the twentieth session. Official records of the World Health Organization*, No. 228, Annex 2. Geneva, World Health Organization, 1975.
19. *World Bank/WHO health sector review, 9–10 October 1975. Note for the record* (CPD/76.1). Geneva, World Health Organization, 1976.
20. *Report for the 1977 Joint UNICEF–WHO Committee on Health Policy. Community involvement in primary health care: a study of the process of community motivation and continued participation* (JC21/UNICEF WHO/77.2). Geneva, World Health Organization, 1977.
21. *Joint UNICEF/WHO Committee on Health Policy: report on the twenty-first session. Official records of the World Health Organization*, No. 242, Annex 1. Geneva, World Health Organization, 1977.
22. Burrell CD, Sheps CG, eds. Primary health care in industrialized nations. *Annals of the New York Academy of Sciences*, 1978, 310.
23. *Official records of the World Health Organization*, No. 224 (EB55/SR/6). Geneva, World Health Organization, 1975.
24. Croizier RC. Traditional medicine in communist China: science, communism and cultural nationalism. *China Quarterly*, July–September 1965, 1–27.
25. *The promotion and development of traditional medicine. Report of a WHO meeting* (WHO Technical Report Series, No. 622). Geneva, World Health Organization, 1978.
26. *Health practice research and formalized managerial methods* (WHO Public Health Paper No. 51). Geneva, World Health Organization, 1973.
27. *Evaluation of community health centres* (WHO Public Health Paper No. 48). Geneva, World Health Organization, 1972.
28. *Advisory Committee on Medical Research. Report to the Director*. Washington DC, Pan American Health Organization, 1971.
29. *Personal health care and social security. Report of a joint ILO/WHO committee* (WHO Technical Report Series, No. 480). Geneva, World Health Organization, 1971.
30. *Local and intermediate health administration. Report of a WHO expert committee* (WHO Technical Report Series, No. 499). Geneva, World Health Organization, 1972.
31. *Fourth General Programme of Work covering a specified period 1967–1971 inclusive. Official records of the World Health Organization*, No. 143, Annex 3. Geneva, World Health Organization, 1965.
32. *Approaches to national health planning* (WHO Public Health Report No. 46). Geneva, World Health Organization, 1972.
33. *Modern management methods and the organization of health services* (WHO Public Health Report No. 55). Geneva, World Health Organization, 1974.
34. *Health economics. Report of a WHO interregional seminar* (WHO Public Health Report No. 64). Geneva, World Health Organization, 1975.
35. *Delivery of health services in developing countries. Fourth International Conference on Social Science and Medicine, Elsinore, Denmark, 12–18 August 1978* (SHS/74.2). Geneva, World Health Organization, 1974.

36. *Application of systems analysis to health management. Report of a WHO expert committee* (WHO Technical Report Series, No. 596). Geneva, World Health Organization, 1976.

37. *Study group of experts on methods of financing health activities, Geneva, 21–25 November 1977* (SHS/RGR/77.1). Geneva, World Health Organization, 1977.

38. *Role of hospitals in programmes of community health protection.. First report of the WHO Expert Committee on Organization of Medical Care* (WHO Technical Report Series, No. 122). Geneva, World Health Organization, 1957.

39. *Hospital administration. Report of a WHO expert committee* (WHO Technical Report Series, No. 395). Geneva, World Health Organization, 1968.

40. *Hospital legislation and hospital systems* (WHO Public Health Paper No. 50). Geneva, World Health Organization, 1973.

41. Kleczkowski BM. *Approaches to planning and design of health care facilities in developing countries.* Geneva, World Health Organization, 1976.

42. *Health care: an international study.* Oxford: Oxford University Press, 1977.

43. *Health services: concepts and information for national planning and management* (WHO Public Health Paper No. 67). Geneva, World Health Organization, 1977.

CHAPTER 7

Family health

The Family Health Programme was established in 1970 to focus on the health needs of the family as a whole. At that time, the programme covered maternal and child health, human reproduction and human genetics. The last component was moved to the control of non-communicable diseases in 1972, while nutrition was added in 1971 and health education in 1973.

The motivation to create a family health programme derived largely from the growing priority given to family planning, as seen in the establishment of UNFPA in late 1969. It was also consistent with WHO's policy to "approach health in terms of the family as the basic social unit in the community" (*1*). WHO's advocacy of full integration of family planning activities into other aspects of maternal and child health was part of a holistic view of human development:

> Human development embraces every aspect of the maturation process, including its physical, biological, psychological, and social aspects. To bring about healthy development and to realize human potential, it is necessary to draw upon many areas of scientific knowledge and many components of the health service. Such areas as nutrition, communicable diseases, human reproduction, mental health, handicaps, and many others, together with the corresponding services, are related to human development. Many of these services have their greatest impact on development when they are employed early in the individual's life. (*2*)

Operationally, the concept of human development called for an integrated approach to all aspects of family health, including family planning. This was not a universally accepted policy; many nongovernmental organizations and governments supported the delivery of family planning services in a vertical, independent manner. WHO, by insisting on the health aspects of family planning, often found itself at odds with important nongovernmental organizations and bilateral agencies.

In a consultation on family health, held in late 1973, it was recommended that WHO promote family health care, to secure better understanding of the concept and of its implications for services to meet the most urgent health needs of underserved families. It could also play an important role in assisting governments to strengthen self-help in matters of family health. For this purpose, it was considered that "family health education should be a priority" (*3*).

Each component of family health was at a different stage in different Member States. Weak coverage and inadequate numbers and qualifications of human resources prevailed in most of the developing world. Also lacking was the scientific knowledge on which to base the design of services. Operational research and systems analysis were widely used to identify better methods for integrating the various components of family health into general health services.

The decade can be viewed as an effort to overcome the weaknesses of each component by evolving an integrated approach. The decade is also characterized by increasing emphasis on interagency consultations, especially with the United Nations, its four regional economic commissions, ILO, FAO, UNESCO and the International Bank for Reconstruction and Development, nongovernmental organizations such as the International Planned Parenthood Federation and the Population Council, and with sources of bilateral aid.

The World Population Conference in Bucharest, Romania, in 1974 provided an opportunity for promoting the health aspects of families. WHO worked through the Administrative Committee on Coordination subcommittee on population to harmonize the activities of the United Nations agencies in this field. Six background papers were prepared for this Conference: health and family planning, the health aspects of population trends and prospects, health trends and prospects for 1950–2000, research on biomedical aspects of fertility regulation and on the operational aspects of family planning, deterioration of the environment and population and health and human rights. The last paper was presented by WHO at the fourth United Nations symposium held in preparation for the Conference, on 'Population and human rights', in Amsterdam, The Netherlands.

The Twenty-eighth World Health Assembly, in 1975, adopted resolution WHA28.44, which welcomed the emphasis given in the World Population Conference plan of action to the interrelations between population and socioeconomic development and in turn to the national and international actions in regard to health and nutrition required to enhance the quality of life, particularly in rural and underserved areas. It requested the Director-General to intensify activities related to family health care as part of strengthening health services.

As the Organization moved to adoption of the primary health care approach, the family health programme emphasized greater involvement of the community and other sectors in promoting family health. By the end of the decade, the programme's objectives were to:

- reduce morbidity and mortality resulting from the closely related factors malnutrition, infection and unregulated fertility;
- develop and strengthen the family health component of health services, particularly as a part of primary health care and rural development;
- provide knowledge and appropriate techniques for promoting healthy reproduction, sound physical growth and psychological development of the young, and the well-being of the family as a whole; and
- promote a coordinated, intersectoral approach to improving the health and social welfare of the family as a unit.

MATERNAL AND CHILD HEALTH, INCLUDING FAMILY PLANNING

The WHO expert committee that met at the end of 1968 to discuss maternal and child health reaffirmed the statement of an earlier expert committee that the ideal to which such services should aim was to ensure that "every child, wherever possible, lives and grows up in a family unit, with love and security in healthy surroundings, receives adequate nourishment, health supervision, and efficient medical attention, and is taught the elements of healthy living" (4, 5). The meeting discussed trends in means of improving mother and child health services, such as an integrated approach to the health problems of mothers and children from conception through adolescence, the concept of continuity of care and the inclusion of family planning activities in these services. It addressed ways of reaching the entire population and of programme evaluation and operational research. Its recommendations stressed the importance of integrating related activities, while maintaining mother and child health as a "separate entity at policy and planning level so that training and services can be organized to meet the special needs of mothers and children".

The greater part of WHO's assistance to governments in improving services for children was provided jointly with UNICEF. The two organizations cooperated in assisting governments in training personnel. For instance, senior teachers of child health development received fellowships to attend a course supported by UNICEF and WHO at the Institute of Child Health, London, England; UNICEF collaborated in promoting training in paediatrics, both by providing professors for medical schools and by collaborating with other institutions in organizing postgraduate courses; WHO continued to cooperate in courses organized by the International Children's Centre, Paris, France. Training of auxiliaries and indigenous midwives was organized in a number of countries, including Algeria, Laos, Liberia, Libya and Mongolia.

UNICEF, which, until the mid-1960s, had been used primarily as a 'supply agency', began making its activities in health more operational, as seen in the late 1960s, when it attempted to bring together, in a single project, activities related to health, agriculture, education and social welfare. These were precursors of the basic services approach adopted in the early 1970s, as discussed in Chapter 1.

As UNICEF considered that its mandate gave it the right to negotiate and implement country projects independently of other agencies, it began recruiting its own health experts. Their Executive Board strongly recommended that UNICEF should concentrate on providing elementary services for children in neglected and peripheral areas, and it became even more imperative for WHO and UNICEF to coordinate their activities well, in order to avoid conflict and confusion at country level. Also, whereas both Dr Chisholm and Dr Candau considered that it would be "confusing" if UNICEF recruited doctors, Dr Mahler, when approached in 1977, had no objection, with the proviso that they would not seek to give advice contrary to WHO policy, a condition fully acceptable to UNICEF (internal UNICEF memo from E.J.R. Heyward to H.R. Labouisse, 8 April 1977).

The rapid expansion of family health programmes increased the need for systematic human resources planning and evaluation of training activities. A large proportion of WHO-assisted projects were devoted to the preparation and in-service training of health personnel in subjects related to family health. Stress was laid on use of responsive teaching methods and adaptation to local situations of materials for self-instruction designed according to new techniques (see Chapter 8). In Indonesia, for example, a 'package' for maternal and child health was put together, which consisted of interventions for improving health care under specific socioeconomic conditions. Beforehand, detailed consideration was given to exactly what auxiliary and paramedical staff could do to care for children; then, a list of behaviourally defined educational objectives was drawn up, and a problem-oriented manual on child care was written in simple language (6).

Research on child growth and development, including the WHO study on low birth weight, was assessed at a consultation held in Geneva in October 1969. Following this meeting, preliminary plans were made for a WHO-supported trial of nutritional supplementation in pregnancy, research in this area having been recommended by the Advisory Committee on Medical Research.

An investigation of mortality in childhood in several Latin American countries sharpened understanding of three interrelated problems affecting the health of mothers and children: malnutrition, infection and reproductive problems (7). While nutritional deficiency stood out as the most serious problem, the health risk to children was found to increase considerably when malnutrition was accompanied by infection, malnutrition of mothers, low birth weight and many offspring. The study further confirmed the importance of both prenatal care of mothers and perinatal care and demonstrated that breastfeeding, the educational level of mothers and the availability of water in the home have a clear effect on the incidences of various diseases.

Growth charts, used to monitor the development of children under 5 years of age, began to be used in various parts of the world. Examples were collected from 54 countries for a review in 1972, and a consultation held in November of that year agreed on and proposed a relatively simple chart that could be used internationally, with a comparable reference value. A model growth chart was finalized in 1973 for testing by auxiliaries in various settings.

Low birth weight remained a priority throughout the decade. Its etiology, prevention and social implications were discussed by a group of experts in September 1975, who concluded that the prevention of low birth weight is one of the most important challenges to public health in most countries. Stress was laid on the need for practical measures for timely interventions and for the prevention of factors that lead to low birth weight. The subject was reviewed at a workshop organized jointly by the Swedish Agency for Research and Cooperation with Developing Countries and WHO in June 1977. Birth weight distribution and percentage of low birth weight were considered to be yardsticks of development. WHO set up a task force in 1977 to study the extent and nature of low birth weight, the contributing factors before and during pregnancy and practical interventions for prevention.

The changing pattern of types of malnutrition and the distribution of malnourished children by age noted in the early 1970s (see below) was believed to be linked to changes in breastfeeding patterns, which seemed to be decreasing in various parts of the world, with serious consequences. Concerned with this trend, the Health Assembly passed a resolution in 1974 (WHA27.43) on infant nutrition, calling on governments to facilitate the promotion of breastfeeding. Furthermore, countries were urged to "review sales promotion activities on baby foods and to introduce appropriate remedial measures, including advertisement codes and legislation where necessary". By 1981, this had led to adoption by the Health Assembly of the International Code on the Marketing of Breast Milk Substitutes.

WHO initiated two studies in response to resolution WHA27.43. One was conducted in collaboration with the International Children's Centre in Paris, with financial support from UNFPA and the Swedish International Development Agency. This research project, which began in 1975 and was carried out in 10 countries, explored how factors such as the frequency and duration of breastfeeding, the quality and quantity of human milk and the interrelation of lactation and reproduction affected the health of the mother and the growth and development of the child. The second stage of the project addressed the factors that affect infant-feeding practices (e.g. social policy, legislation on maternity and working mothers, organization of medical care for mothers and children and the availability of milk substitutes) and biological studies (for instance, on the interrelations between lactation, reproduction, nutrition and the quality and quantity of breast milk). On the basis of data collected, a series of measures were implemented during the 1976–1977 biennium.

The second study, carried out in a number of developing countries, comprised a physiological and biochemical analysis of breastfeeding in various environmental and nutritional backgrounds, its relation to child growth and development and the relation between lactation, return to menstruation and ovulation.

In 1975, an interregional workshop on country projects for family health was held for members of WHO intercountry teams, to help them in adopting the 'project systems analysis' method for use at country level (see Chapter 3). As part of this managerial approach, the concept of risk was introduced, as advances in previous years had made it possible to identify individuals and groups whose characteristics or circumstances were associated with an increased risk of having, developing or being especially affected by morbid processes. This knowledge allowed for better use of the available resources, including unconventional community resources, such as teachers, traditional birth attendants and women's groups (8).

The sixth session of the expert committee on mother and child health, in late 1975, entitled its report *New trends and approaches in the delivery of maternal and child care in health services* (9). It outlined the content of mother and child health care and the priorities, including the need for manpower development. It addressed the service aspects of delivering mother and child care within the health system and outlined research needs. The main problem was not so much lack of basic knowledge as the difficulty of applying existing knowledge and giving care to all mothers and children. The committee stressed the need for applied research into appropriate, more effective methods and pointed out the importance of relevant teaching and motivation of personnel at every level of the health care system. They also described the need for appropriate, adapted technology in mother and child health care, particularly as part of primary health care, and for practical approaches to collecting and using accurate, basic health statistics at all levels.

The committee recommended that WHO encourage the regions to undertake epidemiological studies on the extent and causes of health problems occurring or originating during the perinatal period and on infant and childhood mortality and morbidity, citing the 'Inter-American Investigation' (7) as a guide for such studies. It also noted that local operational research was essential for planning, developing, testing and evaluating effective, acceptable, feasible methods for delivering mother and child health care, including family planning, which could then be gradually extended to the whole country. It was noted that these programmes also provided field training for personnel of all types and all levels of training for professionals and auxiliaries, both undergraduate and postgraduate.

Research was also needed on specific problems, such as toxaemia of pregnancy, low birth weight, psychosocial development of the child and adolescent, child-rearing practices, maternal competence in relation to mental development and productivity, long-term effects of pathological events in the perinatal stage and early childhood, the status of women and the health of the mother and child. Finally, major research efforts were required to improve the content and structure of education and training at all levels, with emphasis on primary caregivers.

During 1976–1977, the joint agency reviews and annual programme reviews that formed part of the project monitoring system were addressed. In addition, WHO was involved in 11 national programme evaluations, some of which led to concrete change. Thus, in Chile and Haiti, the evaluations pinpointed areas in which services were deficient, and changes were made to ensure wider coverage. In Malaysia, the evaluation led to a revision of the information system, with emphasis on maternal mortality, which was found to be relatively high in comparison with that among infants and children.

A WHO expert committee on the health needs of adolescents met in 1976. The meeting highlighted the need for a deeper understanding of adolescents in today's rapidly changing societies and the need for greater compassion and insight during this transitional period (10).

Resolution WHA21.43, adopted in 1968, addressed the work on health aspects of population dynamics accomplished during 1967 and requested that the programme continue along the principles set out in earlier resolutions (WHA18.49, WHA19.43 and WHA20.41), including encouraging research on psychological factors related to human reproduction. Earlier principles included recognition that demographic problems require consideration of economic, social, cultural, psychological and health factors; that the changes in the size and structure of the population have repercussions on health conditions; that human reproduction involves the family unit as well as society as a whole and that the size of a family should be the free choice of each individual family; that national administrations should decide whether and to what extent they will provide information and services to their people on the health aspects of human reproduction; that it is important to include information on population health problems in the curricula of medical students, nurses, midwives and other health workers; and that abortions and high maternal and child mortality rates are serious public health problems in many countries.

Family planning activities began in earnest in 1969, when some 20 countries decided to introduce or expand these activities, with WHO assistance and the cooperation of the United Nations and other specialized agencies. In the years that followed, with substantial support from UNFPA, WHO was able to meet the increasing demand for assistance in setting up national family planning activities as part of maternal and child care or other parts of the health services.

A WHO scientific group met in June 1969 to consider the health aspects of family planning, concentrating on its impact on the health of the mother, father, child and family and the place of family planning care in different health activities. The group stressed the importance of improving the quality and broadening the geographical coverage of studies on the effect of family planning on health, listing seven subjects for research, which included the causes of infertility and the reasons for which women resort to abortion (11). With respect to the provision of family planning in health services, the group identified various forms of 'action research', including combining family planning with domiciliary maternity care, nutrition activities and child health services, and comparing the effectiveness and efficiency of such combinations in health services at various levels of development.

Another scientific group met in November 1969 to address the subject of spontaneous and induced abortions by reviewing the epidemiology of abortion, considering the consequences in terms of maternal morbidity and mortality and fetal deaths and recommending research areas of high priority (*12*).

The logic of including family planning in mother and child health services was reinforced by the results from projects in India. Reviewed in 1970, these demonstrated that the survival of children is a strong motivation for limiting family size.

A meeting convened by WHO in 1970 brought together representatives from the United States Agency for International Development, UNDP, the International Institute for the Study of Human Reproduction, the Population Council, the University of the Philippines and the University of Novi Sad (Yugoslavia), to formulate guidelines for projects on family planning aspects of mother and child health. They emphasized the 'post partum' or 'maternity-centred' approach, as it had been found that women were highly motivated to avoid subsequent conception soon after pregnancy, childbirth or abortion. One such project, in Tunisia, was highly successful. Implemented with the International Planned Parenthood Federation, the Population Council and others, the project was part of a wider effort, supported by the country's President, that included making primary education available to all girls. Three main areas were outlined for the maternity-centred approach:

- an operational programme to improve the obstetrical, gynaecological and paediatric services of major hospitals in urban areas, where hospital-based family planning services would also be provided;
- field studies and pilot projects to test of the extension of maternity-centred family planning activities to small units and rural areas; and
- education, training and collection of data on the health benefits of family planning.

An expert committee met in 1970 to give shape to the principles and processes of planning, administering, organizing, operating and evaluating family planning programmes within overall health care systems (*13*). It considered the implications for health services of various objectives of family planning and the related legislation and assessed the prerequisites for establishing objectives, determining priorities and setting overall strategies. It also examined the use of services, health education of the public and education and training of health personnel in family planning. It endorsed the recommendations for studies made by the WHO Scientific Group on Health Aspects of Family Planning (*12*) and identified topics suitable for epidemiological and operational research, field experiments and pilot projects.

A paper on teaching of human sexuality to health professionals was prepared on the basis of a review (*14*) and served as a background document for an expert committee that met in early 1974 on the subject (*15*).

Task forces were established in the context of the Expanded Programme of Research, Development and Research Training in Human Reproduction (see Chapter 5) to discuss the acceptability of family planning and of specific methods of fertility regulation and on provision of family planning in health services. They discussed, for example, how to provide intrauterine devices or sterilization in places without medically qualified staff.

In 1974, an expert committee on the evaluation of family planning in health services discussed concepts and definitions in family planning and evaluation and reviewed experience with various techniques for evaluating the need for family planning services from the point of view of health, operational aspects and the health effects of these services, and the interaction of family planning and other health services (16). The priorities for research were considered to be: establishing and strengthening maternal and child health services within basic health services; meeting the needs in childbearing, growth and development and fertility regulation; and assuring manpower for maternal and child health care.

In many developing countries, combining family planning and family health required considerable modification of their health structures. As noted above and in chapters 4 and 6, WHO stressed operational research and systems analysis to find better methods of organization and administration. The Government of Iran, for example, initiated in 1972 a pilot project on comprehensive mother and child health and family planning in a model *sharestan* (county) of about 160 000 persons in a mainly rural setting, with WHO assistance. Similar projects were set up in Morocco, Sri Lanka and Thailand. In other countries, Colombia, India and Tunisia, for example, emphasis was placed on the mother and child health and family planning component of wider health service research programmes assisted by WHO. In Nigeria, the management techniques and project design derived by 'project systems analysis' in the states of Sokoto and Niger in 1973 were used as examples for programme development in the rest of the country during 1976–1977. The systems approach was also used in Algeria to improve the selection of appropriate techniques, by analysing the actions that were possible at each level of service and on the basis of the programme objectives.

By the 1976–1977 biennium, WHO was the executing agency, with the financial support of UNFPA, for family health and family planning projects in 18 countries in the African Region, 13 in the Region of Americas, 6 in the South-East Asia Region, 3 in the European Region, 10 in the Eastern Mediterranean Region and 12 in the Western Pacific Region. The Organization collaborated in other ways with an even greater number of countries.

NUTRITION

The assistance provided by WHO in the field of nutrition had increased rapidly and significantly during the 1960s. Protein–calorie malnutrition, nutritional anaemia, endemic goitre and avitaminosis A were common in all the WHO regions, while diseases like seasonal scurvy, rickets, osteomalacia and favism were problems of public health importance in only certain regions. The number of professional posts increased from 13 in 1956 to about 90 in 1970, the increase mostly being in field staff. The number of fellowships awarded had jumped threefold, from 75 in 1965 to 220 in 1969. In 1970, it was foreseen that the Organization would need to strengthen its efforts in this field, "not only because of its bearing on public health, but also because of the growing interest of other United Nations agencies and the member governments in this subject" (17). It was judged important that the Organization "assumes leadership in the various programmes whenever there is a health component involved".

As the nutritional status of any community is related to the quality and quantity of food available, the work of WHO was closely tied with that of FAO. UNICEF, too, was deeply involved, not only because of its concern for the health of children, but also because it provided most of the funds for field activities, especially those related to applied nutrition. These programmes consisted of field surveys to determine baseline conditions, training health personnel in food and nutrition, setting up food production and nutrition education activities and establishing supplementary feeding programmes. Such programmes were in operation in more than 60 developing countries at the beginning of the decade.

Despite the increase in the number of field staff, the percentage of WHO's budget dedicated to nutrition had declined between 1956 and 1970, from 3.4% to 1.8%. Similarly, UNICEF funding of nutrition programmes had dropped by 1969 to only US$ 2.9 million, just 8.5% of all UNICEF programme commitments. The falloff in UNICEF funding reflected disappointment in the applied nutrition programmes, which were judged to be unsustainable and not closely related to national development plans. Similar criticism was voiced by WHO staff, some of whom also found that the programmes were too dependent on ideas from abroad and on foreign aid. New approaches were needed, with a better understanding of nutrition through research.

The Director-General, in his presentation to the eleventh session of the Advisory Committee on Medical Research in 1969, said that greater emphasis should be laid on the production of protein-rich foods. The Committee agreed that the WHO research programme on nutrition should be expanded, noting that special attention should be given to the adverse effects of prenatal and postnatal malnutrition on intellectual and emotional development. WHO's nutrition research programme was addressing some of these questions, e.g. measuring the protein requirements for maintenance and growth of 1-year-old infants, testing protein-rich food mixtures and studying the relation between nutrition and infection.

Finding 'protein foods' was in keeping with the dominant paradigm at the time, which was that protein deficiency was the most important nutritional problem of childhood. It was with this paradigm in mind that the Protein Advisory Group had been established in 1955 by WHO and later (1965) expanded into a tripartite group involving FAO and UNICEF. Its terms of reference included advising on the technical and related aspects of the joint programme for improving protein nutrition and new activities, disseminating new information on the protein problem and advising on improving procedures for project evaluation and feasibility studies.

As the decade progressed, the central place of protein gave way to a more balanced view of the problem, one that addressed the total energy needs and the web of socioeconomic factors that contributed to hunger and malnutrition. Already, in 1971, the Joint FAO/WHO Expert Committee on Nutrition indicated that the protein supply must be judged in relation to other aspects of the diet, "notably, the caloric intake" (*18*). When protein intake was found to be low, it was likely that the calorie intake was equally low, "if not more so". In such circumstances, it might be better to increase the food supply rather than concentrate on providing extra protein. The Committee also noted that the main obstacles to the effective control and prevention of protein–calorie malnutrition was failure to apply preventive measures on a community basis. Ultimately, protein–calorie malnutrition can be controlled "only by general economic and social development and a coordinated approach in the fields of agriculture, education, the social services, and public health".

The relation between the nutritional status of children and infection had been demonstrated in the 1950s. The Joint FAO/WHO Expert Committee on Nutrition, at its seventh session in 1966, called for greater attention "to the prevention and control of infectious diseases which are known to have a definitive influence on nutritional status, particularly in children" (*19*). They also observed that "the single most important health problem in most developing countries is control of diarrhoeal diseases". A report on the subject prepared in 1968 indicated that "an appreciable part of the excess morbidity and mortality in children" in three-quarters of the world's population was attributable to the synergy between nutritional status and infection (*20*). The findings highlighted in this report included the fact that a child with an inadequate diet who became infected and had just one episode of diarrhoea or an acute respiratory infection could develop kwashiorkor. Shortly thereafter, the benefits of oral rehydration fluid were recognized (see Chapter 9).

In addition to the Protein Advisory Group and the Joint FAO/WHO Expert Committee on Nutrition, the Joint FAO/WHO Expert Group on Nutritional Requirements met periodically to define human requirements for major essential nutrients and for energy. In 1969, for example, it reviewed ascorbic acid, vitamin D, vitamin 12, folate and iron, while in 1971 energy and protein were reviewed.

The nutrition programme was reviewed by the Executive Board at its forty-ninth session, in January 1972. Disturbing trends were noted. The world's food production was growing at a slower rate than its population, and it was estimated that severe and moderate malnutrition affected some 11 million and 76 million children, respectively. While nearly all countries had established a nutrition unit within their ministries of health, many lacked a clear formulation or biological orientation of their national food and nutrition policies, and coordination was lacking in all phases of the programmes.

The Director-General's report outlined a number of possible areas for action. After noting that nutrition had now passed from being "just a welfare activity" to "part of the socioeconomic development plans of countries", "complementary approaches" were needed (*21*). Nutrition programmes were becoming more complex and coordination more difficult "but essential". In the future, more "mathematical instruments" would be used, such as models, systems analysis and operational research. Past and present activities should be evaluated, including the orientation of research activities. Studies on the effect of malnutrition on human development should be intensified. New conventional and unconventional protein foods were called for.

The Director-General's report also stated that WHO should continue to define the responsibilities of the health sector in determining food and nutrition policies. The global economic crisis that had further exacerbated the nutritional status of the world's children, as noted in Chapter 1, increased the pressure on international organizations to develop more effective approaches. The Director of the Family Health Division, addressing the third meeting of WHO regional advisers in nutrition, in March 1974, observed that "why there was no palpable impact" of nutrition activities was a "valid question ... in the minds of administrators" (*22*).

The deteriorating world food situation called for "deliberate and well-planned efforts of medium and long-range duration, if the present mortality was to be reduced, the suffering minimized and the quality of life improved in terms of full exploitation of inherited potentialities". Few countries had adequate machinery for planning and formulating a national food and nutrition policy. In the Region of the Americas, however, subsequent to a technical group meeting in 1969 and specific recommendations approved by all ministers of health and agriculture, the specialized agencies, WHO/PAHO, FAO and UNICEF, had, in 1971, set up an interagency project for formulating and implementing such a policy. The project also involved the Institute of Nutrition of Central America and Panama and the Caribbean Food and Nutrition Institute. The interagency working group established preliminary guidelines for food and nutrition planning, which laid down three basic policies: food supply, which included all aspects of food production, international trade in foodstuffs, food processing and food marketing; food demand, which included aspects such as income, food prices, supplementary feeding, nutrition education and consumer orientation, and the population policy; and biological use of food, including strengthening health services and expanding their coverage (in particular mother and child health programmes), the prevention and control of other communicable diseases and environmental sanitation.

The critical worldwide food situation led to convening of the World Food Conference. Held in Rome, Italy, in November 1974, it called on all governments and the international community as a whole to formulate and integrate "concerted food and nutrition policies in their socioeconomic and agricultural planning". The ninth session of the Joint FAO/WHO Expert Committee on Nutrition, held shortly thereafter, chose as its topic "food and nutrition strategies in national development" (*23*). The Expert Committee recognized that it was dealing with "difficult matters", upon which complete agreement was not always obtained. Nevertheless, the areas of consensus "were substantial". Much too little was known about the state of malnutrition. FAO and WHO would perform an "invaluable service" if they were to issue a regular review that highlighted the most significant causal factors. The heart of such work would be a demographic classification of 'at risk' groups and a report on key indicators, such as food supply, demand and prices, employment and infant mortality, and the implications for changes in nutrition status.

The Committee outlined a new approach to food and nutrition planning, following a lengthy consideration of health strategies and direct measures of nutritional improvement. The research needs identified ranged from the identification and analysis of nutrition problems in populations to political and organizational aspects of the problem. The direct measures reviewed included: food fortification, supplementary foods and feeding programmes, control of infections, maternal and child health and nutrition education. The Committee strongly endorsed the recommendation of the World Food Conference that an international mechanism be established within the United Nations system to aid in coordination of such research.

At its fifty-fifth session, in 1975, the Executive Board considered the report of the World Food Conference and, in resolution EB55.R69, requested the Director-General to "strengthen, expand, and if necessary, reorient nutrition programmes in order that WHO can better undertake its responsibilities, taking into account the relevant resolutions of the World Health Assembly and the World Food Conference" and "to seek additional financial assistance to enable WHO to undertake such responsibilities on a global scale".

A joint FAO/UNICEF/WHO expert committee met in October 1975 to consider methods of nutritional surveillance. The committee reviewed indicators that could be used for this purpose, addressed their planning and implementation and strongly recommended that nutritional surveillance systems be established as a priority. The committee also strongly recommended that international agencies coordinate their work in setting up a global nutritional surveillance system, as called for by the World Food Conference (*24*).

A series of consultations was held in 1976 to increase understanding of how to improve the nutritional status of high-risk and vulnerable populations. The subject was discussed in technical discussions organized by the regional offices and at two interregional consultations, one on the integration of nutrition and family planning programmes (New Delhi, India, October 1976) and the other on strategies for nutrition through local health services (Teheran, Iran, early November 1976). A meeting of directors of nutrition training programmes was held in Geneva in late November 1976.

The consultation in New Delhi reviewed examples of integrated projects or programmes in Bangladesh, Egypt, India, Nepal, Sri Lanka and Thailand. Noting that an effective family planning programme will result in significant improvement in the health and nutrition status of mothers and children because of proper birth spacing and a reduction in the number or pregnancies, the group recommended that there should be "an urgent move towards the operational integration of family planning programmes and nutrition-promotion measures with mutually reinforcing functional and logistic advantages" (*25*).

The consultation in Teheran reviewed both the West Azerbaijan primary health care project (see Chapter 4) and the Indian programme. A background paper (*26*) introduced the guidelines that WHO, in collaboration with UNICEF, had prepared in 1974 for nutrition activities through local health services, in which two principles were stressed. First, promotion of nutrition in vulnerable populations can be effective only if a 'package' of activities in four related areas—nutrition, mother and child care, birth spacing and health education—is delivered. Secondly, the contents of this integrated 'package' will differ according to the professional level of the worker who delivers it and according to the problems in the area in which the target population lives. The consultation agreed that, while "the health sector has neither the capacity nor the responsibility to effect the eradication of the root causes of malnutrition", health workers "are in a unique position in being able to diagnose the extent and degree of malnutrition and to moderate its consequences". They suggested the following activities as suitable for primary health care services. in most situations:

- surveillance of the nutrition of children under the age of 6 years (especially those aged 0–3), with growth charts;
- education on breastfeeding, weaning practices and improving the basic diet;
- distribution of specific nutrients in areas of high disease endemicity; and
- control of communicable diseases by immunization, prevention of gastroenteritis by health education and prevention of dehydration by oral rehydration.

Evidence from a number of small projects around the world had shown that these measures could make an impact. The challenge was to convert small-scale demonstrations into larger operations.

The consultation highlighted the need for more effective nutrition training programmes in field operations and for stronger financial and technical support from international agencies. Various obstacles were identified. As United Nations fellowships were offered through governments, the staff of many autonomous training centres were not eligible. Publications sent to governments from WHO, FAO and UNICEF often did not make their way to training centres. Even in the Americas, where nutrition activities were the best developed, deficiencies were noted; for example, there was no regional training programme for nutrition education, clinical nutrition or diet therapy, or institutional food service administration. The meeting called for a more thorough review of international nutrition training centres.

The role of the health sector in formulating national and international food and nutrition policies and plans was the subject of technical discussions held during the Thirtieth World Health Assembly, in May 1977. These led to the adoption of resolution WHA30.51, which expressed concern about "inadequate attention and commitments being given by the health and other sectors in a great number of countries to improve this critical situation". It called on the Director-General to strengthen the WHO nutrition programme, specifically by:

- strengthening research capacity, education and training in nutrition programmes;
- identifying problem areas, such as interactions between malnutrition and infection and productive capacity, and integrating relevant programmes;
- determining the most vulnerable population groups (groups at risk);
- designing systems for nutrition surveillance; and
- assisting ministries of health to introduce nutrition objectives into national development plans and to design and implement multisectoral food and nutrition policies and programmes.

A report prepared for the sixty-first session of the Executive Board, in January 1978 (27), noted that, while many international agencies, including WHO, were collaborating at country level in food and nutrition activities, "unfortunately in recent years there has been a significant amount of duplication or, even worse, of uncoordinated effort that has often resulted in confusion at country level, and in wasted or inefficient utilization of very scarce resources". To resolve these problems, the agencies of the United Nations system had agreed to establish a subcommittee on nutrition of the Administrative Committee on Coordination, which included the United Nations, UNICEF, UNDP, FAO, the International Fund for Agricultural Development, the World Food Council, the World Food Programme, UNESCO, the World Bank and WHO. At its first meeting, in September 1977, it agreed on a programme of work, which included evaluation of nutrition intervention programmes, nutrition surveillance, nutrition in national planning, action-oriented research and analysis of external resources for improving nutrition in developing countries. A permanent secretariat and an advisory group were established, which replaced the Protein Advisory Group.

The report on nutrition in the health services for the Board (27) noted that such activities were frequently based on strategies and techniques "designed from the knowledge and experiences of other countries", which, in many instances, "were not applicable to local conditions". Recommendations for dietary changes, for instance, frequently emphasized foods that were not readily available or were not acceptable to the local population. The report concluded that WHO could make a significant contribution by mobilizing and co-ordinating international resources for action at field level in countries of different areas of the world. Such action would include testing the feasibility of meeting the needs of communities, particularly the most vulnerable groups, with locally available foods; and ensuring national competence for analysing and solving national nutrition problems, due consideration being given to the economic situation of the population. The Organization was setting up an action-oriented research and training programme, and this activity was endorsed by the sixty-first Executive Board, in January 1978 (resolution EB61.R33). The direction outlined was in keeping with the primary health care approach, in which the promotion of food supplies and proper nutrition was one of the eight basic components.

HEALTH EDUCATION

In the 1960s, WHO published an annual list of references to health education in the WHO Technical Report Series. That of 1968 (*28*) was 74 pages long. Although all WHO programmes had a health education component, with increased priority for family planning and family health at the end of that decade, the programme on health education stood out in advocating its importance and searching for more effective means of achieving it.

A WHO expert committee on planning and evaluation of health education services stated that the focus of health education was on people and action. In general, its aims were to encourage people to adopt and sustain healthy life practices, to use the health services available to them judiciously and wisely and to make their own decisions, both individually and collectively, to improve their health status and their environment (*29*). Dr Dorolle, WHO's Deputy Director-General, who opened the meeting, stressed the need and scope for "far more systematic appraisal of the precise nature of the part that could be played by the general public" in making plans for various health and related technical services, a position that reflected his long commitment to the role of WHO in informing the public about health matters. The committee judged that "considerable value could be derived from even modest field studies planned to take advantage of the various practical opportunities that local health workers, teachers and other local leaders may have for making more effective use of the educational approach in their direct contacts with the people".

The report of a WHO scientific group on research in health education (*30*) suggested that an underlying objective of health education is

> the development in people of (1) a sense of responsibility for their own health and for that of the community, and (2) the ability to participate in community life in a constructive and purposeful way. The possibility of such responsible participation being carried over into other spheres of life is great. Health education thus helps to promote on the one hand a sense of individual identity, dignity and responsibility, and on the other hand community solidarity and responsibility.

Practical opportunities could be taken advantage of only where the requisite health education services existed, a realization that led the WHO regional advisers, meeting in December 1970, to call for the involvement of health education staff in the planning, implementation, strengthening and evaluation of plans and programmes that required personal, family and community involvement and action (*31*). The meeting noted that most countries still had unmet needs and potential for strengthening health education in school and teacher education programmes. The increasing number of functional literacy and vocational education programmes, which reached youth as well as adults, should include preparation in health and health education. Such programmes should be planned and implemented in close collaboration with the United Nations, UNICEF, ILO, FAO, UNESCO and other interested agencies and organizations. The same recommendation applied to programmes and projects that affected school-age children and youth.

Research that would be particularly useful included:

- studies to ascertain the practices, mores, customs and activities of indigenous health workers and their educational role and influence in health aspects of family planning;
- case studies to identify the nature, scope and impact of health education, especially in family health, in order to establish, as far as possible, cause-and-effect relations for use in similar projects or situations; and
- studies to identify indicators and tools for assessing and evaluating health education, including the time spent and the quantity and quality of effort and training performed by local health workers in different sociocultural and economic circumstances.

In a background paper prepared by the WHO secretariat for a study group meeting that took place the following week (*32*), the absence of a "well-developed scientific base on which to build health education services for important health concerns" was noted. Educational and behavioural research on family planning was judged to be in a weak state. Because of the "unique characteristics of family planning", research findings in other areas were not likely to be relevant. Of the studies that had been conducted, the largest number dealt with knowledge, attitude and practice. These studies showed a fairly high level of knowledge and favourable attitudes but much less reported practice. Validation of such results was difficult.

Some problem areas in which research was "badly needed" included the influence of education about family planning on behaviour that reduced the risk for child-bearing; when such education should begin and what should be the intended attitude and behaviour; and identification of specific educational messages that made family planning a more meaningful, real concept. A further question was how much information and understanding about the reproductive process, contraception and male and female physiology was essential to ensure consistent practice of family planning.

The study group concentrated on building up an organized health education service that incorporated the input of the WHO secretariat. It added that many findings were not readily available, thus limiting their use, and suggested that publication of the studies in a form suitable for use in operational programmes and in relevant education and training activities should be encouraged (*33*).

Further study areas were identified, but these and the others listed were likely to be realized only if "centres for health education research were established, particularly in association with schools of public health or equivalent institutions having established postgraduate programmes in health education and affording prospects and resources for interdisciplinary research". Implementation of this recommendation required a multidisciplinary approach by highly qualified research personnel who understood the educational problems encountered in health programmes. The group stressed the need for a worldwide review of existing facilities and resources for preparing health education specialists. This review would provide a basis for a long-range plan to help meet present and anticipated demands for professional manpower in health education. WHO should consider convening a consultative group of the major multilateral and bilateral agencies, voluntary agencies and foundations that provided assistance in the educational aspects of family planning care. Among other things, the group should address the role of communications tools and resources.

WHO began preparing a series of monographs on published studies and research on health education practices in 1971. The main areas documented were people's attitudes, beliefs and health practices; psychosocial and cultural factors related to health education practice; communications methods and materials; patient education; programme planning and evaluation; and health education in schools, colleges and universities. Particular emphasis was placed on topics not highlighted in earlier publications, namely, family health and education on drugs.

In a background paper prepared for the fifty-third session of the Executive Board, in January 1974, examples of practical applications of health education were given. The experience in Panama corroborated the importance of the role of ministries of health in organizing and guiding community involvement in health services. Beginning in 1970, some 600 health committees had been established in under 3 years. Each committee appointed working commissions to tackle specific problems, e.g. safe water supply or food production, and community health seminars were held, which were attended by all interested citizens. Discussions were encouraged and working groups formed to make recommendations on the basis of decisions about the problems that required attention.

In Nigeria, the Federal ministries of health and education collaborated on a health education programme for school-age children and youth. Many national staff were involved, including educational authorities, teachers, educational supervisors, medical officers, nutritionists, dentists, epidemiologists and health educators. Assistance was given by a UNESCO curriculum expert, a WHO epidemiologist, a UNICEF public health nutritionist and others; a WHO school health adviser had been in place since 1968. It should be noted that UNESCO and WHO collaboration in this field dated back to the early 1950s. After a pilot project in Lagos, the project was extended to the other 11 states, where school health programmes were set up that covered health instruction, a healthful school environment, school health services and health coordination between school, home and the community. Other experiences summarized were a project for health education of school-age children and youth in the Philippines, health education as part of the malaria eradication programme in Surinam and a rural latrine programme in Uttar Pradesh, India.

The report (*34*) noted that, despite some 25 years of work in health education involving people from all walks of life in helping to resolve preventable problems, health education had not yet received the "endorsement it deserves". Suggestions were made to improve this situation. To ensure the participation of the population in improving health services, health education should be central to the planning, organization and implementation of health policies and programmes. Health workers at every level should be better prepared in health education, behavioural sciences and communication. Practical studies of behaviour related to health should be better supported. The media should be induced to better serve the purposes of health education. Educational appeals and efforts to improve the health and well-being of school-age children and youth should receive a better response. Training institutions should be strengthened by approaches that were outlined in the report. Finally, the Organization should "take a more decisive lead in assuring ... that health education specialists, behavioural scientists, experts in communications media, and others are trained in sufficient numbers".

The reviews of the Executive Board and subsequently of the Health Assembly were generally favourable, although several delegates said they would have preferred a more analytical, critical report. Others noted that health education tended to be confined to the health services; in the field of the environment, for example, the Polish delegate considered that health education should concentrate on the "economist, the industrialist, the politician and the government administrator" (35).

The Twenty-seventh World Health Assembly, in May 1974, adopted two long resolutions: WHA27.27, on health education and WHA27.28 on health education of children and young people. The former reiterated that health education was "basic both for individual motivation and for community participation in the improvement of health conditions and should therefore form an integral part of all health programmes". Health education was important not only in health programmes but also in those for education and related socioeconomic development that affected health. It recommended that the Organization:

- intensify health education activities in all its programmes;
- endeavour to increase its support to Member States interested in planning, implementing and evaluating the health education components of their national programmes, including manpower development, strengthening of health services, promotion of environmental health and disease prevention and control; and
- cooperate more actively with the United Nations, the specialized agencies and appropriate international nongovernmental organizations and bilateral aid agencies in programmes in which health education played a part. It should be continuously alert to opportunities for inserting health education into all such programmes.

Resolution WHA27.28 would remind the world of past promises concerning children and young people. The basic principles of the WHO Constitution were referred to, "particularly the fact that healthy growth and development of the child are of basic importance and that ability to live harmoniously in a changing total environment is essential to such development". United Nations General Assembly resolution 2037 (XX), adopted in December 1965, was recalled, on the promotion among youth of the ideals of peace, mutual respect and understanding between peoples. "Considering that WHO possesses an authority and an exalted prestige based on the positive solutions found for many major health problems relying on the experience of national medical and health staffs", the Health Assembly:

deems it necessary:
1. to intensify within WHO's programmes concrete and effective action to ensure that children and young people receive a multidisciplinary health education, which is of particular importance for the development of future generations;

2. to explore and promote new approaches for tackling and solving in an appropriate way the problems posed by the health education of mothers, children and young people in order to take care of their health and of their protection against the harmful factors of modern life;

3. to support actively the basic right to health of the child and the adolescent and to promote by suitable means the improvement of the legislative provisions, together with other concrete actions aimed at ensuring a healthy future for the rising generations;

4. to invite other international organizations, particularly UNESCO and UNICEF, and, through the governments of the Member countries, national health agencies, voluntary organizations and parents, to participate actively in the implementation of activities for the health education of children and young people.

As has been noted elsewhere in this volume, the mid-1970s was a time of economic instability, unexpected budgetary expenses and, consequently, decreased funds available from the regular budget. One consequence was that support programmes, such as health education, tended to work more closely with programmes that were attracting extrabudgetary funds, which was the case for family planning. Not mentioned in this connection was the human environment, which, after the Stockholm Conference (1972), was also the object of new projects in which health education played an important part. WHO and UNICEF continued to explore means for furthering community participation, especially in the fields of rural water supplies and environmental health generally.

A meeting held in Geneva in early 1975 to establish better coordination with other services and programmes led, for example, to collaboration in preparing manuals on such subjects as the control of diarrhoeal diseases and health literacy. Guides for training village health workers in maternal and child health care, family planning and good nutrition were already being prepared.

At its twentieth session, in February 1975, the Joint UNICEF/WHO Committee on Health Policy recommended that health education be treated as a subject closely related to and supporting the new approach to primary health care, and that cases in which health education had been wholly or partly responsible for behavioural changes should be investigated. One source of such information were case studies collected from projects for family planning and environmental health as part of the community involvement study discussed in Chapter 6. It was concluded that increased access to education, both informal and formal, had led to greater involvement of people in community activities. The important role played by women was highlighted. Better communications (roads, radio, television, newspapers) appeared to have increased the readiness of communities to accept change.

Case studies were used in an FAO/WHO interdisciplinary workshop on the health education aspects of family health and integrated rural development, held in Morogoro, United Republic of Tanzania, in October 1975. This workshop, which lasted 10 days, resulted in an extensive report (36). The participants were from eight African countries; UNICEF and UNESCO representatives also participated. The workshop began by making a comprehensive list of the educational components that would be addressed. To the usual health activities related directly to children, adolescents, mothers, the family, environmental sanitation, communicable diseases, nutrition and basic education, they added farming practices, farm management and appropriate technology for agriculture. The educational tasks of a rural development worker were analysed, with particular attention to improving communication at community level as well as between agencies. Specific objectives were developed for each component identified. A panel discussion was organized early in the workshop, during which the agency participants introduced their respective programmes. It was suggested that governments and United Nations agencies were moving towards a 'package programme'. Initially, this was a package of resources provided in a particular field, such as farm inputs and extension advice or the services and supplies needed for improving the health and nutrition of infants and young children, Now, the package had expanded to include a variety of interrelated economic and social services, which added up to an integrated rural development programme. Within this, different disciplines contributed to the solution of different aspects of the same problem. Nevertheless, it was admitted that, while many people and agencies talked about integration, they were not yet themselves willing to accept integration into a joint programme. The most effective way of achieving integration was often through a problem-solving approach that brought people and staff together.

The Advisory Committee on Medical Research at its eighteenth session, in 1976, reviewed WHO's collaborative research in health education (*37*). It recognized the great significance of applied research for improving the effectiveness of health education activities. Such research should be an integral part of health services research and should continue to be the task of Member States, with WHO headquarters and regional offices advising on suitable research methods, initiating and coordinating intercountry projects, providing technical expertise and assistance for those projects, disseminating information and encouraging collaboration among Member States.

References

1. *The integration of women in development. Statement by the World Health Organization prepared for the Inter-regional Meeting of Experts on the Participation of Women in Development* (MCH/72.3). Geneva, World Health Organization, 1972.
2. *Human development and public health. Report of a WHO scientific group* (WHO Technical Report Series, No. 485). Geneva, World Health Organization, 1972.
3. *Report of consultation on family health, 5–12 November 1973* (FHE/75.4). Geneva, World Health Organization, 1975.
4. *The organization and administration of maternal and child health services. Fifth report of the WHO Expert Committee on Maternal and Child Health* (WHO Technical Report Series, No. 428). Geneva, World Health Organization, 1969.
5. *Administration of maternal and child health services. Second report of the WHO Expert Committee on Maternal and Child Health* (WHO Technical Report Series, No. 115). Geneva, World Health Organization, 1957.
6. King M, King F. *Primary child care: a manual for health workers*. Oxford, Oxford University Press, 1978.
7. Puffer RR, Serrano CV. *Patterns of mortality in childhood* (Scientific Publication No. 262). Washington DC, Pan American Health Organization, 1973.
8. *Risk approach for maternal and child health care* (WHO Offset Publication, No. 39). Geneva, World Health Organization, 1978.

9. *New trends and approaches in the delivery of maternal and child care in health services. Sixth report of the WHO Expert Committee on Maternal and Child Health* (WHO Technical Report Series, No. 600). Geneva, World Health Organization, 1976.

10. *Health needs of adolescents. Report of a WHO expert committee* (WHO Technical Report Series, No. 609). Geneva, World Health Organization, 1977.

11. *Health aspects of family planning. Report of a WHO scientific group* (WHO Technical Report Series, No. 442). Geneva, World Health Organization, 1970.

12. *Spontaneous and induced abortion. Report of a WHO scientific group* (WHO Technical Report Series, No. 461). Geneva, World Health Organization, 1970.

13. *Family planning in health services. Report of a WHO expert committee* (WHO Technical Report Series, No. 476). Geneva, World Health Organization, 1971.

14. *The teaching of human sexuality in schools for health professionals* (WHO Public Health Paper No. 57). Geneva, World Health Organization, 1974.

15. *Education and treatment in human sexuality: the training of health professionals. Report of a WHO meeting* (WHO Technical Report Series, No. 572). Geneva, World Health Organization, 1975.

16. *Evaluation of family planning in health services. Report of a WHO expert committee* (WHO Technical Report Series, No. 569). Geneva, World Health Organization, 1975.

17. *Meeting of regional advisers in nutrition, Geneva, 9–19 June 1970* (NUTR/70.8). Geneva, World Health Organization, 1970.-

18. *Food fortification, protein–calorie malnutrition. Joint FAO/WHO Expert Committee on Nutrition. Eighth report* (WHO Technical Report Series, No. 477). Geneva, World Health Organization, 1971.

19. *Joint FAO/WHO Expert Committee on Nutrition. Seventh report* (WHO Technical Report Series, No. 377). Geneva, World Health Organization, 1967.

20. *Interaction of nutrition and infection* (WHO Monograph Series, No. 57). Geneva, World Health Organization, 1968.

21. *Programme review: nutrition* (EB49/30), Geneva, World Health Organization, 1971.

22. *Report of the meeting of WHO regional advisers in nutrition, Geneva, 25–29 March 1974* (NUT/74.1). Geneva, World Health Organization, 1974.

23. *Food and nutrition strategies in national development. Ninth report of the Joint FAO/WHO Expert Committee on Nutrition* (WHO Technical Report Series, No. 584). Geneva, World Health Organization, 1976.

24. *Methodology of nutritional surveillance. Report of a joint FAO/UNICEF/WHO expert committee* (WHO Technical Report Series, No. 593). Geneva, World Health Organization, 1976.

25. *Interregional consultation on the integration of nutrition and family planning programmes. New Delhi, 5–9 October 1976* (NUT/77.3). Geneva, World Health Organization, 1977.

26. *A guideline for nutrition activities through local health services for joint WHO/UNICEF strategy.* September 1974 (NUT/74.3). Geneva, World Health Organization, 1974.

27. *The role of the health sector in the development of national and international food and nutrition policies and plans. Report by the Director-General* (EB61/24). Geneva, World Health Organization, 1978.

28. *References to health education in WHO Technical Report Series, 1968* (HE/68.2). Geneva, World Health Organization, 1968.

29. *Planning and evaluation of health education services. Report of a WHO expert committee* (WHO Technical Report Series, No. 409). Geneva, World Health Organization, 1969.

30. *Research in health education. Report of a WHO scientific group* (WHO Technical Report Series, No. 432). Geneva, World Health Organization, 1969.

31. *Report of a meeting of WHO regional advisers in health education, Geneva, 7–14 December 1970* (HE/72.2). Geneva, World Health Organization, 1972.

32. *Study group on health education in health aspects of family planning. Background notes prepared by WHO secretariat* (HE/WP/70.1). Geneva, World Health Organization, 1970.

33. *Health education in health aspects of family planning. Report of a WHO study group* (WHO Technical Report Series, No. 483). Geneva, World Health Organization, 1971.

34. *Health education: a programme review. A report by the Director-General to the fifty-third session of the Executive Board* (WHO Offset Publication No. 7). Geneva, World Health Organization, 1974.

35. *Executive Board, 53rd session* (EB53/SR/14). Geneva, World Health Organization, 1974.

36. *Educational aspects of family health and integrated rural development. Report on a FAO/WHO workshop. Mzumbe, Morogoro, 6–16 October 1975* (HED/76.1). Geneva, World Health Organization, 1976.

37. *Advisory Committee on Medical Research, eighteenth session* (ACMR18/76.13). Geneva, World Health Organization, 1976.

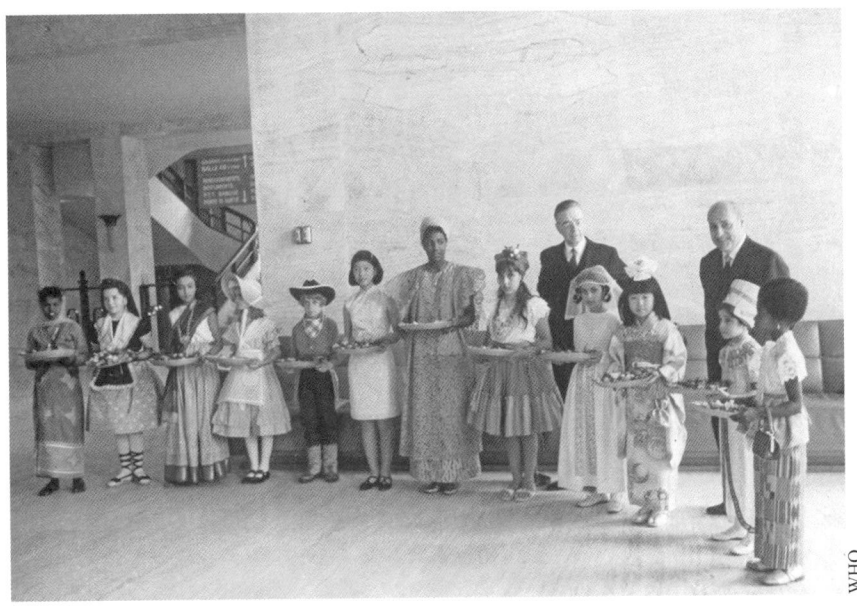

Director-General Dr Marcolino Candau (right) with Deputy Director-General
Pierre Dorolle and children in national costume at the
Twentieth World Health Assembly

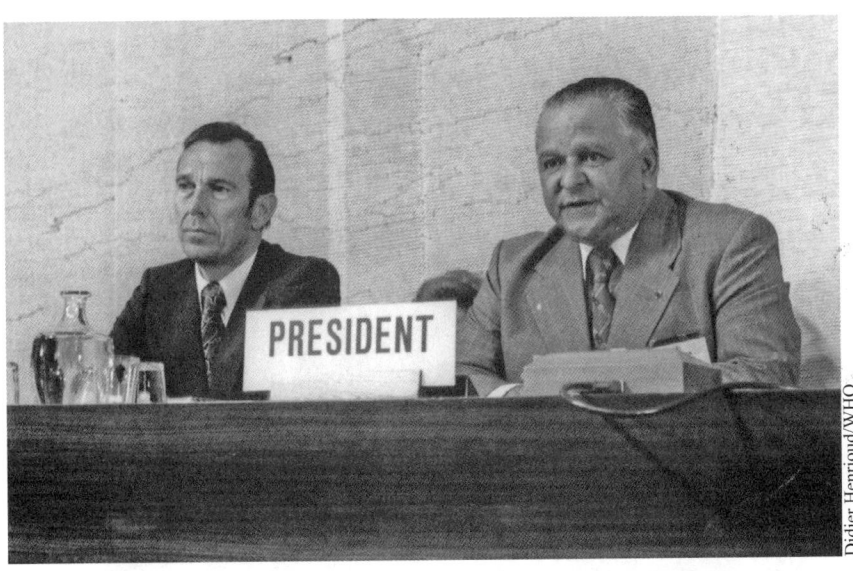

PRESIDENT

Director-General Halfdan Mahler with Sir Harold Walter, President of the
Twenty-ninth World Health Assembly

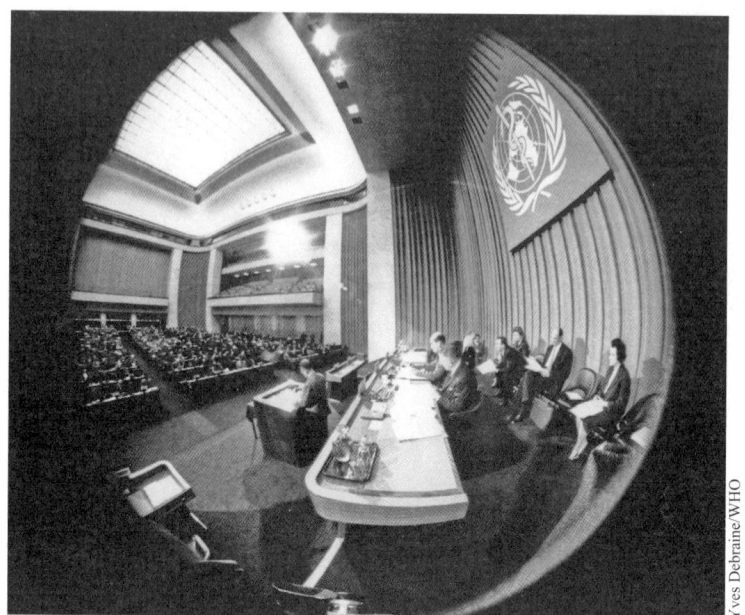

A World Health Assembly plenary session

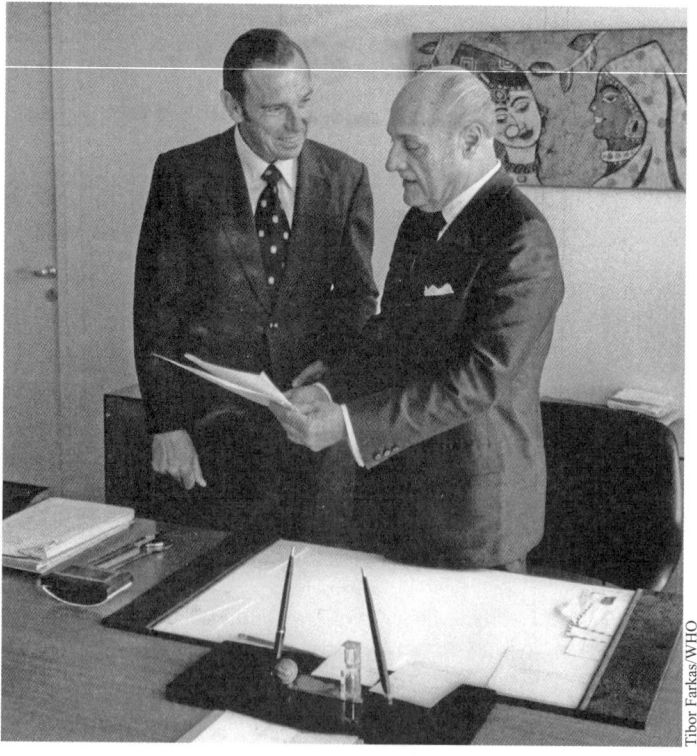

Handing over: Dr Marcolino Candau in discussion with Dr Halfdan Mahler, his successor as
Director-General, in 1973

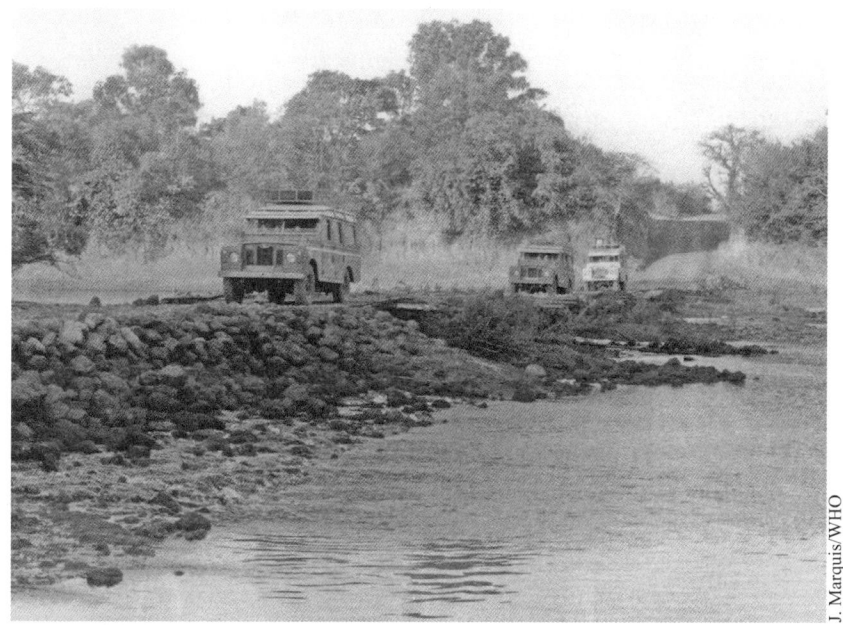

WHO Epidemiological Survey in Senegal traces disease patterns in the country.

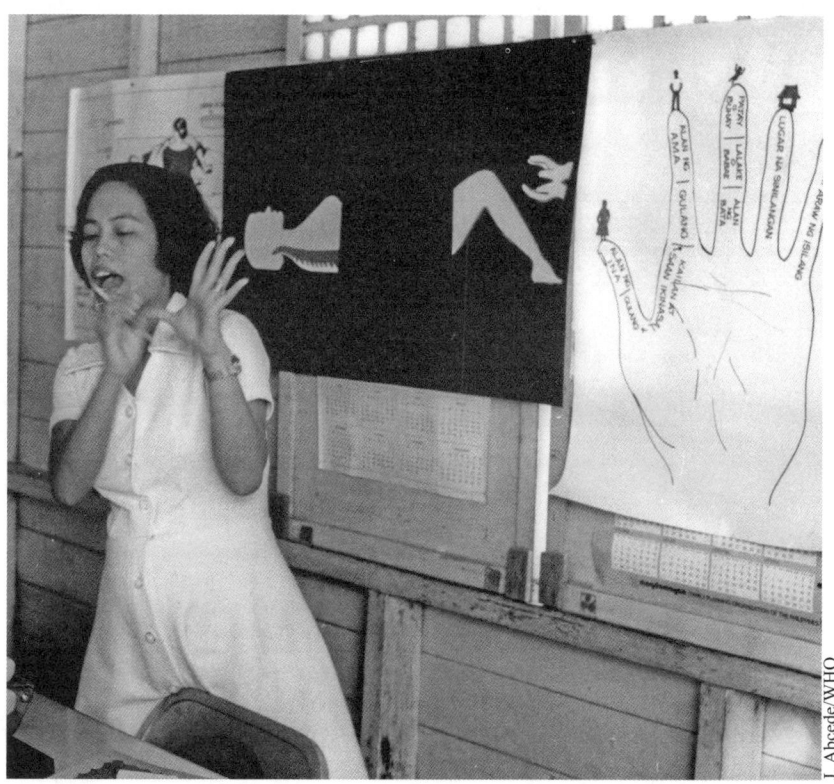

A nurse explains basic steps in child delivery to students in the Philippines.

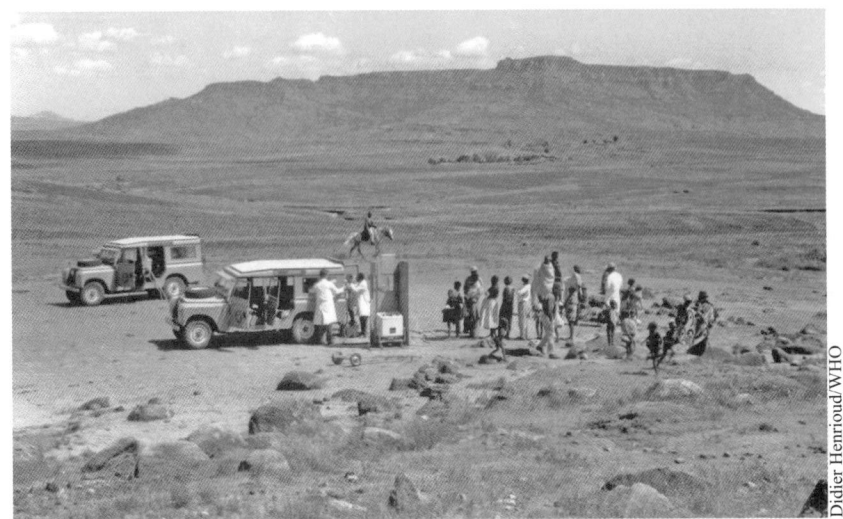

Isolated villagers in Kenya greet mobile teams bringing vaccine against tuberculosis.

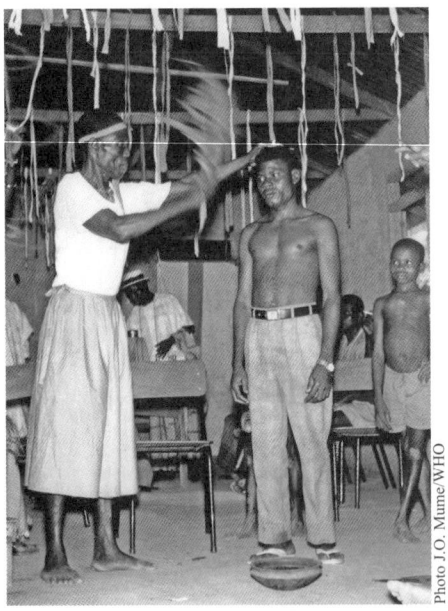

A traditional healer in Nigeria treating a patient.

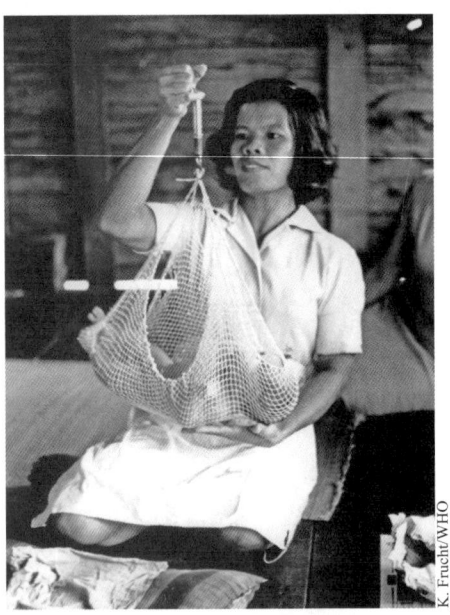

A newborn baby is weighed by a midwife in Thailand.

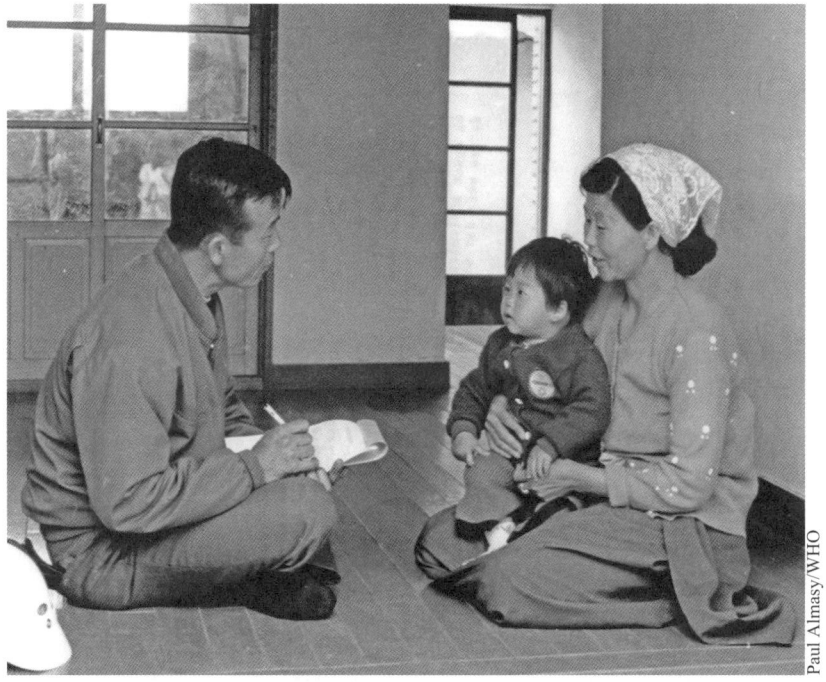

Paul Almasy/WHO

A Chinese mother discusses family planning with a health visitor.

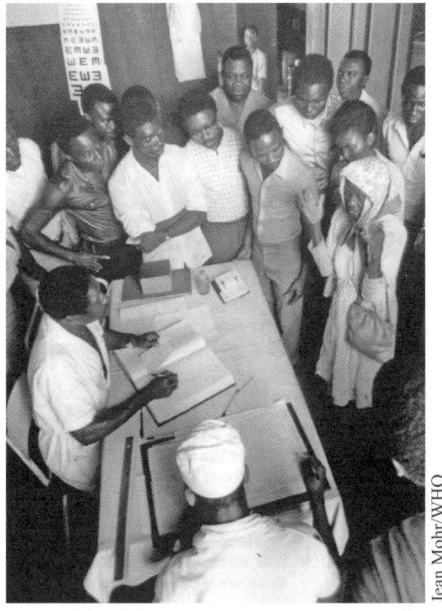

Jean Mohr/WHO

Locally trained medical students gather in a hospital in Cameroon.

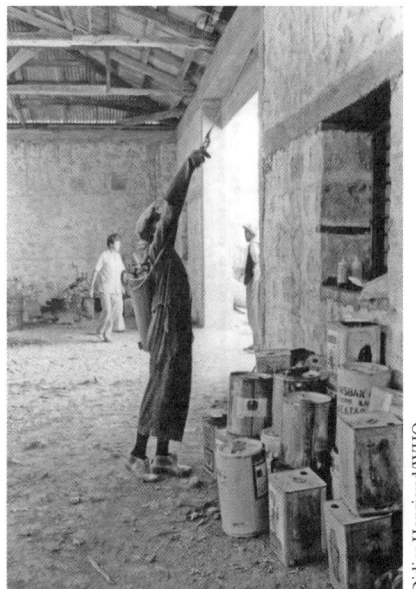

Didier Henrioud/WHO

Malaria eradication: A workman sprays factory walls with DDT in Turkey.

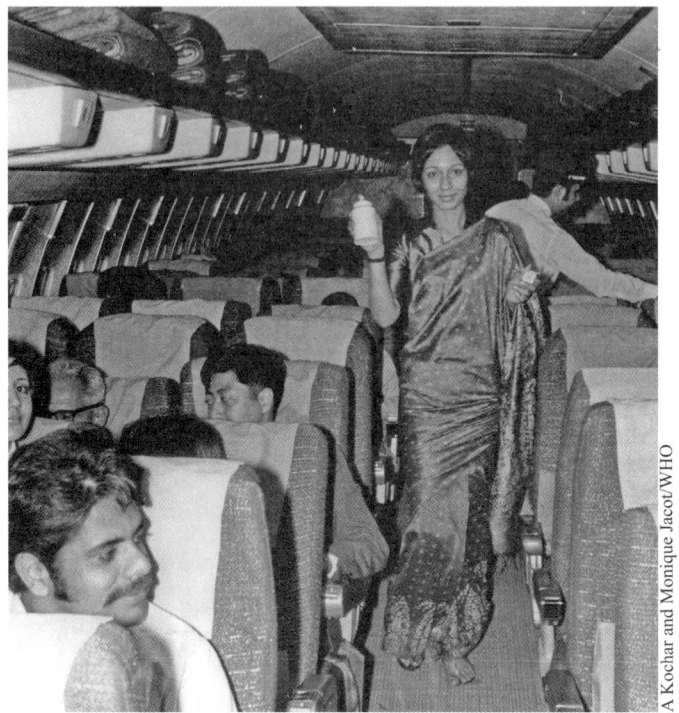

A Kochar and Monique Jacot/WHO

An air stewardess disinfects a plane leaving New Delhi in a test of insecticides on flights.

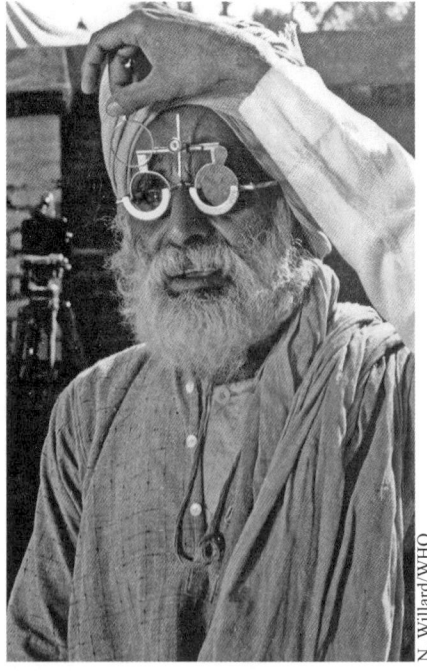

N. Willard/WHO

A patient is fitted with new glasses following an eye operation in India.

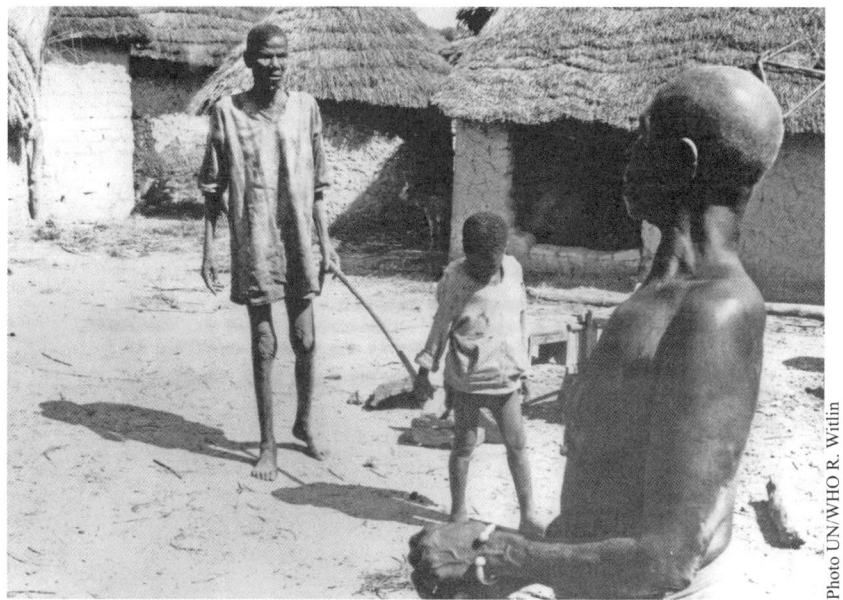

Photo UN/WHO R. Witlin

Using a stick, a child leads a man blinded by onchocerciasis - river blindness - in Upper Volta.

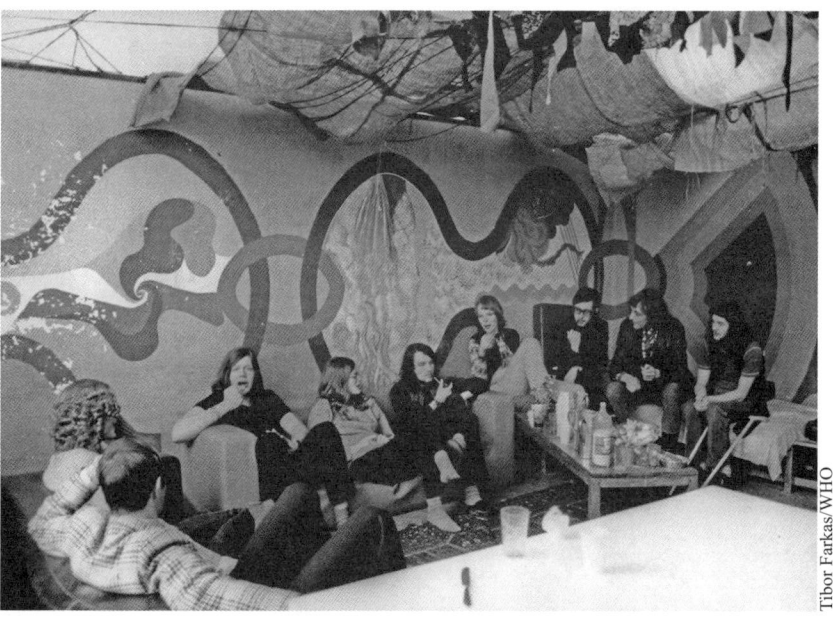

Tibor Farkas/WHO

A psychiatric clinic in The Netherlands for the treatment of depressed adolescents and young adults

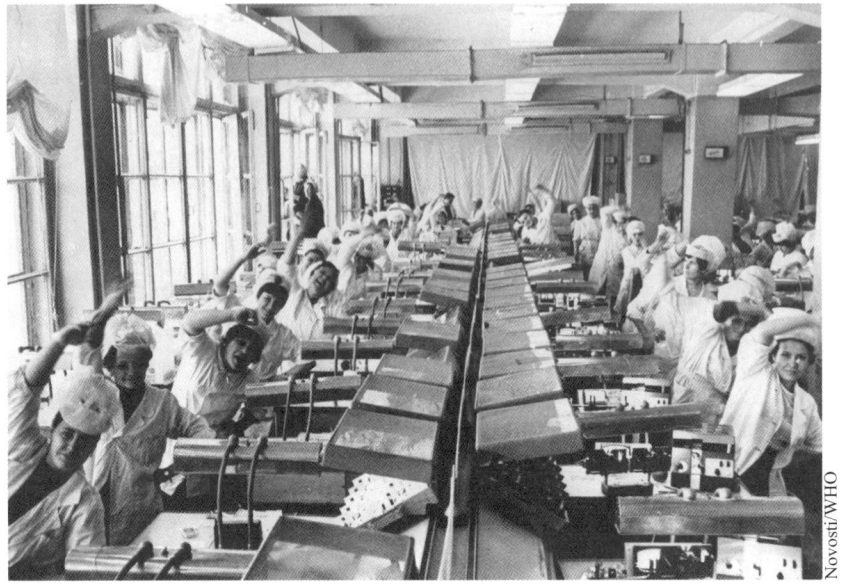

Women working in a factory pause for a session of physical exercises in the USSR

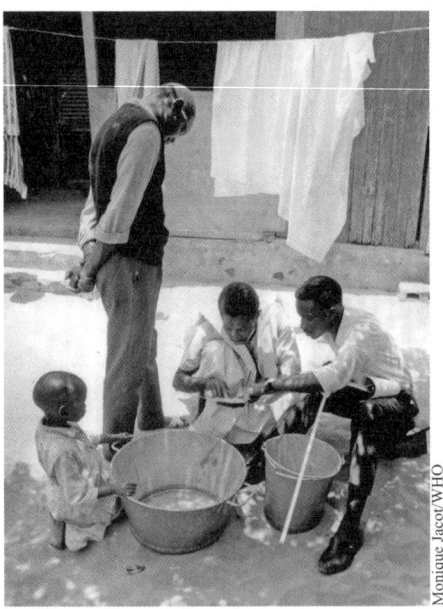

A health visitor in a village near Dakar, Senegal, asks a family about their requirements for fresh water.

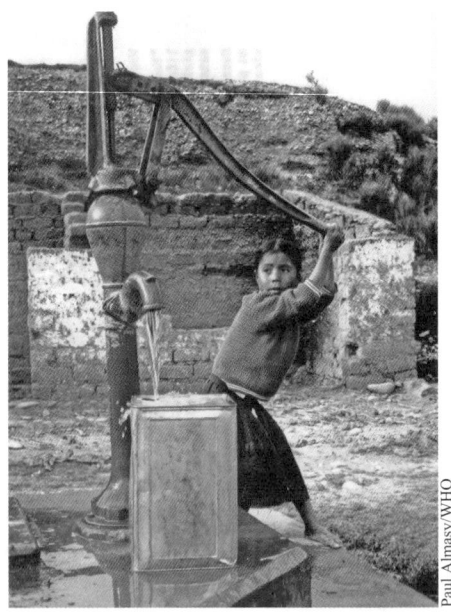

A young Peruvian girl pumps water from a well, in which the water is monitored for its quality.

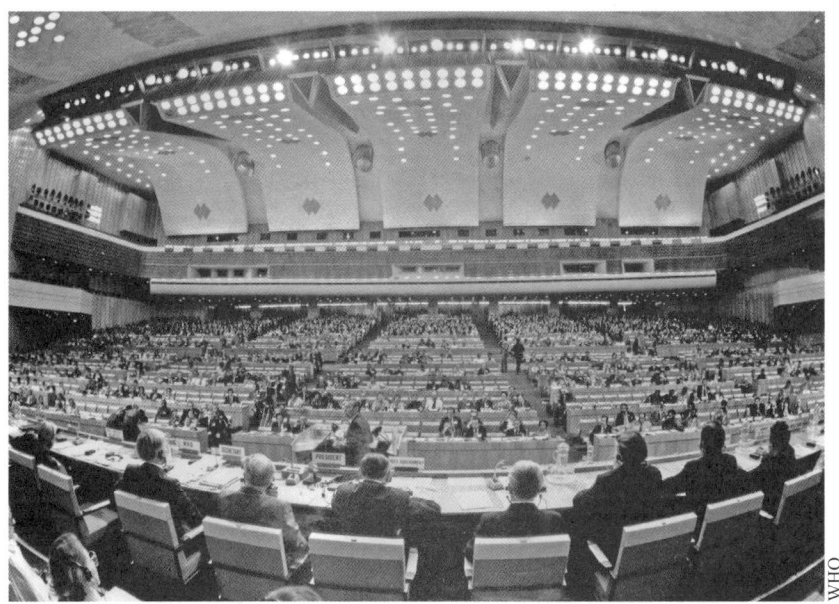

The site of the International Conference on Primary Health Care in Alma-Ata

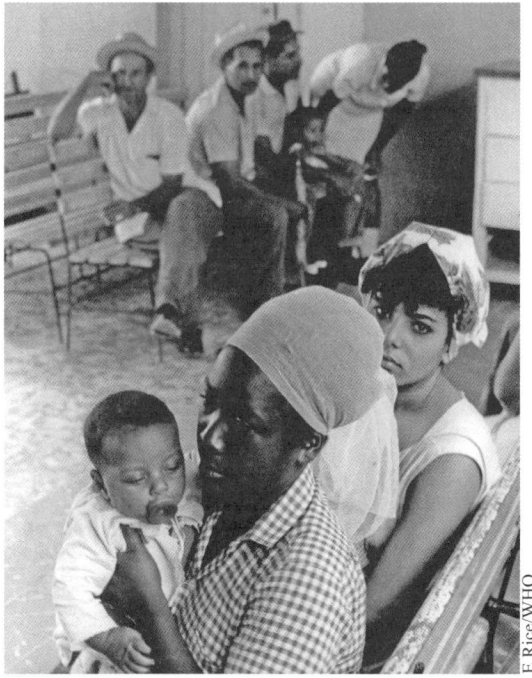

Mothers and children in a health centre in Cuba

CHAPTER 8

Health manpower development

At the beginning of the decade, the programme on health manpower development followed lines that had been well established in the early years of WHO's history: basic education in medicine, postgraduate education in medicine and public health, training of auxiliaries for the health professions and offering fellowships for training abroad. As many countries still did not have medical schools, fellowships were the only way of obtaining training. The establishment of new medical schools and strengthening existing ones continued to claim much attention.

The third decade is marked by a greater emphasis on improving the quality of teaching and on incorporating auxiliaries into the health team. Also, health manpower development, from mid-decade onwards, was placed within the wider context of national health planning. Correspondingly, greater attention was given to innovative schemes to devise national plans for both health services and human resources. The shift in emphasis grew out of the recognition that education and training on their own were no guarantee that national health services would be able to incorporate new workers in a productive manner and hold on to them. While elements of health manpower 'systems' are to be found in the first half of the decade, this chapter begins with WHO activities for improving educational programmes for all kinds of health workers, before turning to activities related to human health resources planning.

THE CHALLENGE

In 1969–1971, WHO and UNICEF jointly undertook a comprehensive assessment of their assistance to education and training programmes. Five consultants visited nine countries, several UNICEF offices and all the WHO regions to gather information on the present status and trends of education and training programmes in the light of health manpower needs and, on the basis of an assessment of the projects visited, to present conclusions and general recommendations for future action (1).

In all the countries visited, there were serious shortages of health personnel, which in one country was described as "catastrophic". In six of the nine countries, there were more doctors than nurses, and, as the need for both was great, all the countries relied heavily on auxiliary workers of one kind or another. The shortage of health workers in some instances was exacerbated by an outflow of physicians and nurses to more highly developed countries. This 'brain drain' was even encouraged in one country visited, as it promoted a "reverse flow of foreign currency".

The training received by all categories of staff was judged to be inadequate. Much of the education of health personnel was still based on western models, in some instances models that were 50 (now 80) years old. Training was not related to the needs of communities; tropical medicine was often an optional subject, even where it was most needed.

Much of the training was hospital-oriented with no attention to what was going on outside the hospital walls. Such training was seen as encouraging the 'brain drain'. Furthermore, teaching equipment was poor, especially accommodation and equipment for laboratories and practical work. There was a lack of textbooks and simple texts for teaching in national languages.

Few countries had any health development plans, and those that did tended to plan towards hypothetical norms rather than realistic solutions. Inadequate planning contributed to a host of deficiencies: no established posts for newly trained staff, inadequate provision for refresher training, lack of supervision and little attention to establishing a satisfactory career structure, especially for auxiliary workers.

Innovation was called for in: educational planning, teacher training, curriculum revision, teaching methods, the establishment of new courses to meet local needs, supervision and continuing education and review and evaluation of all aspects of educational programmes. This list was presented as a sequential one, planning leading the way for the other aspects. Planning, however, presupposes the availability of suitably trained planners. The question therefore was "Where to begin?", especially given the fact that planning was recognized at the time as a "new discipline". In 1972, the Director-General created a post in educational planning as a first step in moving the Organization in this direction.

WHO and UNICEF were called upon to help train a few educational planners for each country, and to train teachers in paedagogical methods and practices. Interdisciplinary conferences and seminars on educational subjects were also suggested. These recommendations were soon taken up by each region, as discussed in Chapter 4.

With doctors seen as playing the leading role in the health team, it was of paramount importance that medical students be given an education that was consonant with the needs of their country. In the past, WHO, with UNICEF support, had provided aid to schools to establish or strengthen departments of preventive and social medicine. The object of such aid was "to promote preventive activities in the practice of medicine" (2). The difficulty in moving in this direction is illustrated by an observation made by Dr Mahler just before he took over the post of Director-General. On that occasion, he told his audience that, despite the fact that for 25 years the concept of community-oriented physicians had been promoted, he knew of no country in which such physicians functioned as heads of health teams operating within a programme with a plan of work. One problem was the failure of medical schools to adapt medical curricula in that direction. He even advised the president of one country to close the medical schools in his country for 2 years, as they were the main focus of resistance to change. During that period, they could discuss what they were supposed to do (3).

Dr Mahler's predecessor, Dr Candau, while not inclined to using such dramatic language, nevertheless reached similar conclusions. In his review of the work of WHO in 1972, he wrote: "It would be fruitless at the present stage for developing nations to follow too closely in the footsteps of the most advanced countries. More profit can be derived from the resourceful use of existing means and a readiness to experiment imaginatively." He went further in his review of WHO's first 25 years, writing that "much of the developing world has had imposed upon it a manpower pattern that is foreign to it and that is unlikely to function properly in the conditions obtaining there" (4).

FIRST RESPONSE TO THE CHALLENGE

The USSR delegate to the Twenty-fourth World Health Assembly, in 1971, introduced a long draft resolution on the subject of training national health personnel. The draft covered the importance of current and long-term planning of the training of national health personnel in accordance with each country's objective needs and existing social and economic resources, strengthening educational institutions as an integral part of public health and education systems, and establishing a flexible system for training health personnel that took into account contemporary achievements in science and technology, together with the most recent methods for organizing teaching.

The Director-General was invited to study criteria for assessing the equivalence of medical degrees and diplomas and to suggest a definition of the term 'physician'. He was also invited to summarize and publish existing information on the curricula and syllabuses of medical schools, faculties and institutes in different countries, with a view to drawing up basic models of curricula. The draft resolution also asked him to study the phenomenon of the outflow of trained professional and technical personnel from developing to developed countries (the 'brain drain') and to address the problems of continuing education of such personnel and of training teachers for the medical education institutions of developing countries. None of these were new subjects; they were brought together to highlight their importance. The draft resolution was adopted as resolution WHA24.59.

The question of defining the term 'physician' led to adoption of resolution WHA25.42, which included the definition of the Board:

> A physician is a person who, having been regularly admitted to a medical school, duly recognized in the country in which it is located, has successfully completed the prescribed course of studies in medicine and has acquired the requisite qualifications to be legally licensed to practise medicine (comprising prevention, diagnosis, treatment and rehabilitation), using independent judgement, to promote community and individual health. (5)

Other outcomes of this resolution were more substantial, beginning with the study of the international migration of physicians and nurses.

MULTINATIONAL STUDY OF THE INTERNATIONAL MIGRATION OF PHYSICIANS AND NURSES

The delegate from Ceylon to the Twenty-fourth World Health Assembly described the problem of "outflow of health personnel" in dramatic terms. Ceylon, he said, belonged to a group of countries that he preferred to describe as "over-exploited" rather than "developing", the exploitation in his country having lasted for "nearly five centuries". Medical schools that had been built in the past were producing some 200 physicians a year, which was just enough for a nation of 12 million people. In the previous year, however, "101 young doctors had resigned from the government health services to go abroad". Ceylon expended a considerable percentage of its national budget on health and education "but would not be happy to see other more prosperous countries benefit from that".

Numerous resolutions had called on WHO to study international migration of health workers. WHA25.42, adopted in 1972, requested the Director-General to intensify efforts in this regard and to seek, if necessary, additional resources outside the regular budget to finance a study. A protocol for the study was designed in 1973, with the objectives of determining the magnitude and defining the patterns of migration; drawing up profiles of migrant physicians and nurses in terms of their demographic and social characteristics, level of education, specialty and employment history to ascertain which were most likely to migrate; identifying the factors associated with migration; identifying, in each country, the consequences of and the population groups affected by the migration of physicians and nurses; and proposing intervention strategies for each pattern of migration.

Following the first contribution, made by the Federal Republic of Germany, a group of experts was convened to review the protocol. Further funding pledges were received, and the first phase, consisting of the collection of available information, was begun at the end of 1974. The study was completed in 1977 (6). It showed that there had been a significant increase in the migration of physicians and nurses from developing countries to developed countries with free-market economies and that this trend was likely to increase. Unattractive working, service and living conditions for health workers, particularly in rural areas, poor career prospects and job satisfaction, irrelevant training programmes and lack of health manpower planning were among the reasons for this increase.

EXPANDING TRAINING PROGRAMMES

Promoting the training of national health personnel is a constitutional function of WHO. Promotion includes active participation in the educational programmes of countries. Thus, during this decade, more than 250 teachers were provided in some 70 countries. Around one-third taught nursing, and half were distributed among clinical and related fields, public health and preventive medicine (including hospital administration and statistics), and basic medical sciences. Environmental health and paediatrics and maternal and child health made up the rest.

In 1973, three main subjects were addressed by expert committees. The first (in April) was postgraduate education and training in public health; the second (in June) was continuing education for physicians, and the third (in September) was planning of medical education programmes.

The subject of postgraduate education and training in public health had not been addressed by an expert committee since 1960. On the basis of a study of the situation of public health schools carried out in 1971, the committee reviewed training programmes, institutions and associations of schools of public health. They concluded (7) that the role of WHO included providing assistance to existing institutions and promoting the establishment of new ones "committed to innovation and bold approaches, that might serve as true national and/or regional centres for health development". They suggested that WHO encourage the four existing associations of schools of public health to identify areas of common concern that could form the basis of a world federation. A number of subjects were identified that would be suitable for discussion by meetings of experts.

The task given to the expert committee that met to discuss continuing education of physicians was to review the present situation, draw up general guidelines for the organization and administration of continuing education, make recommendations for the application of educational planning and modernization of teaching methods in this field and to suggest ways of motivating physicians to pursue their studies throughout their professional career (8).

The expert committee on planning medical education programmes drew up guidelines for medical education (9), on the premise that the education of physicians and other health workers should be directed specifically towards meeting the main health needs of the society to be served. A number of planning steps were outlined, including the importance of basing policy on consultations with appropriate representatives of universities, medical schools, the practising professions, ministries of health, education, finance and planning, and the society to be served. The committee also stressed that all medical schools, especially those preparing physicians to give primary care, "should provide learning experiences in settings that approximate closely to those in which the physicians will ultimately practise: e.g., community health centres, rural health centres, maternal and child health centres". Other issues considered were the relative value of an 'open' admission policy, the need to provide data for evaluating any new policy, appropriate in-service training and continuing education of physicians.

A study group on planning schools of medicine that met in 1974 outlined methods for organizing and administering new schools and stressed that the number of physicians that were trained must be related to the total health manpower requirements of a country if a balanced 'mix' of health personnel was to be achieved (10). It discussed institutional objectives and recorded its preference for integrated teaching centres in health sciences rather than separate schools, e.g. for medicine and nursing. By this time, all the regional offices had programmes consistent with this principle, as discussed in Chapter 4.

Resolution WHA27.31, adopted in 1974, requested that the Director-General "pursue vigorously measures for the continuing education of health personnel" by assisting Member States in planning and organizing such programmes; setting, with specialists in various disciplines, specific objectives and methods of continuing education for the health professions; setting up and evaluating pilot projects in continuing education; training health professionals in communications sciences, providing leadership for programmes in this field; and encouraging and promoting research into and collecting, exchanging and evaluating information on continuing education.

A global study was initiated in 1975 on integrated, multiprofessional and community-oriented training for health personnel, with a view to determining more effective methods of preparing health workers to solve the health problems of the populations they serve.

In addition to the numerous activities regarding the training of nurses and nurse–midwives, discussed in Chapter 4, other developments were reported to the Executive Board meeting in January 1976. One was preparation of a report on behavioural sciences in nursing education, and another was the preparation of guidelines on the design and use of modular curricula and modules in teacher training and midwifery education. A design for evaluating educational programmes in nursing was tested in the field, and the training of nurses in a community setting instead of in hospitals was being tested in Indonesia.

WHO continued to collaborate with Member States in training environmental health workers, mostly sanitary engineers and sanitarians. Most of this work was carried out in the context of health services development projects. New impetus was given to this activity after adoption of Recommendation No. 7 of the United Nations Conference on the Human Environment, which stressed the need to initiate specialized training programmes in regard to environmental health. The Twenty-sixth World Health Assembly, meeting in 1973, passed resolution WHA26.59, which requested the Director-General to contribute to those training programmes

> in so far as budgetary resources permit, by providing fellowships and qualified teaching staff, by organizing long-term and short-term courses, seminars and other meetings in order to promote the acquisition of skills and the exchange of knowledge and information, on the basis of a systematic approach to the planning of training, and by studying the possibility of designating international and regional centres for the training of environmental manpower.

TEACHER TRAINING

Since 1969, a comprehensive, long-term programme had been under way to train teachers of medicine and other health sciences. This programme grew out of a consultation, held in October 1969, which recognized the importance of extending the worldwide effort to improve the preparation of health professions teachers, making the most economic use of scarce resources (11). The programme they proposed, which was designed to be comprehensive, coordinated, sequential and with a multiplier effect, comprised the identification of interregional centre(s) and fostering and supporting the establishment of other centres to serve regionally.

The first step was to designate two institutions in this field as WHO collaborating centres: the Central Institute for Advanced Medical Studies, Moscow, USSR, and the Center for the Study of Medical Education at the College of Medicine, University of Illinois, Chicago, United States. The Illinois centre functioned as a WHO interregional teaching training centre to train educational leaders and specialists for the regional teacher training centres that WHO helped to establish.

Plans were drawn up in 1971 for regional centres for training teachers of health personnel in the African, South-East Asia, Eastern Mediterranean and Western Pacific regions. The future directors of the regional centres took a 1-year course at the centre in Illinois: four in 1971 and four in 1972. A group of 27 teachers who were to work in the centres attended two 4-week seminars at the interregional teaching training centre during 1972. A 2-week seminar—conducted in French—was held in Yaoundé, United Republic of Cameroon, for deans and other high-level staff of schools of medicine in countries where regional and national teacher training centres were to be established.

By 1974, regional teacher-training centres had been established in all the regions except the European Region, as described in Chapter 4. Having fulfilled its responsibility, the Illinois centre ceased its activity as a WHO interregional teacher-training centre but continued to prepare reports and provide consultants on teacher training.

The regional teacher training centres held workshops, seminars and courses to prepare high-level staff for national centres in all Member States that wished to host one. By the end of 1977, several national centres had started to train teachers in their own settings and languages, using a variety of approaches: short intensive courses, workshops and 'internships', in which interested teachers spent a period of intensive study on subjects such as instruction strategies, selection and organization of educational experiences, audiovisual techniques and evaluation. In addition, many seminar–workshops on this subject were organized by WHO staff in support of the worldwide programme.

Three centres (two French- and one English-speaking) were set up in Africa exclusively for the training of nursing teachers; courses for future teachers of nursing were also provided in the Americas, in most countries of the South-East Asia Region and by the University Hospital of Malaysia, which offered its services to neighbouring countries.

IMPROVED TEACHING METHODS

Three collaborating centres cooperated in the Organization's programme for research in educational planning, in Shiraz (Iran), Beersheba (Israel) and Berne (Switzerland). Comparable efforts were promoted in all regions. The measures explored, suitably adapted to the needs of countries, consisted of revising curricula to be community-oriented, teacher training, formulation of procedures for objective testing and evaluation and progressive introduction of efficient educational techniques, including self-instruction.

The evaluation of teaching aids and programmed courses began in 1970. Also envisaged at the time was establishment of a media centre and the production and reproduction of simple visual aids. Within a year, this suggestion developed into a programme with the long-term objectives of evaluation of audiovisual materials by collaborating institutes and field teams; provision of an information service on evaluated audiovisual aids and the methods and equipment necessary for effective performance; encouragement and support of research on improved teaching methods; and application of newer communications media to the training of health workers. A media centre was established at WHO headquarters where teachers could obtain information on the sources and availability of audiovisual aids, see and try out examples of tested equipment and study various new approaches to education selected from faculties and institutes in different parts of the world.

A project was initiated in 1972 to meet the need for comprehensive reference materials, in the form of handbooks and manuals for various categories of health auxiliaries in training and in service, as well as material and guides for use by teachers in preparing courses. By 1974, the objectives of the programme had evolved to comprise the design, testing and dissemination of teaching and learning materials, evaluation of educational methods, material and related information services and communications techniques. The programme was reviewed by a study group in 1975, which stressed the need to apply a systems approach in solving educational problems.

Reference materials for health auxiliaries and their teachers (a health team library 'package') were distributed to hundreds of training centres. At regional level, centres in the health sciences in Cairo, Mexico City and Rio de Janeiro organized courses for teachers on the objectives, methods and evaluation of learning.

In keeping with the move towards a more holistic view of health manpower, it was decided that a long-term aim of the programme should be to encourage the gradual conversion of educational technology centres, regional teacher-training centres and other single-function educational units into multipurpose health manpower centres. Each such centre should have facilities for teacher training, for designing and producing materials and for evaluation and educational research, and should provide advice and information to institutions and individuals on programme planning and curricula. The first steps were taken to set up such a centre in Shiraz, Iran, as described in Chapter 4.

THE HEALTH TEAM

In its report of work carried out during 1974, the section dealing with auxiliary health personnel conceived the health team in the following terms:

> The team responsible for the delivery of health care to a given sector of the population may be considered as forming a pyramid, consisting of various levels of health personnel. At the base are health workers who have had short training to enable them to deliver primary health services under the supervision of staff in the two higher levels. At the intermediate step of this pyramid there is the medical assistant (*feldsher*) or community health nurse who is responsible for a rural health centre where he or she looks after patients, including those referred by auxiliaries working in villages; the person at this level is also responsible for organizing and supervising the work of the village health workers and for their training and continuing education. At the apex are the physician, the specialist and other highly qualified health personnel; they are also responsible for the district hospital to which cases are referred. Health workers at this level are also responsible for the work performed at all levels of the pyramid, and for the continuing education of intermediate level health workers.

The importance of the health team concept was stressed in WHO's approach to health manpower planning in the context of health services development. New educational approaches also contributed to this goal. For example, the Organization adopted a little-used approach in educational planning arising from the concept of the integration of teaching and service. Applied to the different levels of health care, this approach allows the student to be part of the community health service from the beginning of his or her professional training. This approach was practised most frequently in the Region of the Americas. Other regions also emphasized the importance of joint training for members of the health team.

In keeping with the community orientation of the primary health care approach, the concept of the health team had evolved by 1977:

> The 'health team' is a group of persons who share a common health goal and common objectives, determined by community needs, towards achievement of which each member of the team contributes, in a coordinated manner, in accordance with his/her competence and skills, and respecting the functions of the others. The manner and degree of such cooperation will, of course, vary and has to be solved by each society according to its own needs and resources. There can be no universally accepted composition of the health team. (*12*)

TRAINING AND USE OF HEALTH AUXILIARIES

The study carried out by the Joint UNICEF/WHO Committee on Health Policy in 1969–1971, referred to at the beginning of this chapter, found that, despite the central role seen for medical assistants and auxiliary personnel, only four of the countries visited were training them. Opposition from both the medical profession and politicians was cited as the leading cause of this anomaly. It strongly recommended that international agencies continue and expand their assistance for the training of medical assistants, health officers and auxiliaries.

In the early years of the decade, various approaches to training medical assistants were compared. Guidelines were prepared in 1970 for collecting information on the training of several groups of auxiliary personnel: medical assistants, dental auxiliaries, veterinary auxiliaries, pharmacy assistants and X-ray auxiliaries. Investigations of certain national experiences were organized, for example, that of the 'feldshers' in the USSR, which was undertaken as part of a travelling seminar in 1971 (*13*). An earlier visit of this kind had been organized in 1967 (*14*).

A study of the use of health auxiliary personnel, started in 1969 in the United Arab Republic, was extended in 1970 to include Brazil and Hungary. The principal investigators met in 1971 to assess the work done and the difficulties encountered. Three approaches to research methods in job analysis and training had been used. The approach used in Brazil was an epidemiological one, mainly in the form of a morbidity survey and a case record analysis. In Hungary, an operational research technique, a time and action study, had been used. The approach in the United Arab Republic was mainly a sociological one, with measurement of health authorities' requirements, jobs and tasks as perceived at the three administrative levels.

The role of health auxiliaries was featured in the Board's 1972 organizational study on methods of promoting the development of basic health services, the report of which indicated that the "only realistic solution which would enable coverage to be provided for the entire population, while maintaining an acceptable standard of care and hygiene in relation to local conditions, is to utilize auxiliary personnel wherever it is not possible to use professional staff" (*15*). Resolution WHA25.42, adopted in May 1972, requested the Organization to invite and assist Member States to intensify their efforts to promote the training and use of health auxiliaries as far as their present facilities permitted, with a view to improving the efficacy of the health services and extending the health coverage of the population. Two WHO consultations on the subject were held later in the year. The first proposed a descriptive formula for classifying health personnel, based on criteria of performance rather than of education. The second outlined measures that might be taken by WHO to encourage the use of medical assistants. Although the work of the 'barefoot doctors' in China had become widely known by this time, it was only in 1978 that the first WHO study tour on their training and use was organized (*16*).

WHO prepared guidelines on planning, implementing and evaluating programmes to train medical assistants and on their optimum use (*17*). Lest countries be tempted to imagine that this route would be an easy one to follow, Dr Mahler indicated in 1973 that training large numbers of health assistants was not the solution. Unless they were employed in an adequate delivery system, they constituted only a tactical or political excuse. Radical educational reforms were needed throughout the system, from elementary schools up through the university. The false notion that medical assistants and other auxiliaries were there to deliver second-rate medical care had to be dispelled. With the successful introduction of such health workers, however, one could hope that pressures for change would start a chain reaction that no one would be able to stop.

In 1973, WHO sought to collaborate in improving the situation of rural populations deprived of health care because they lived in peripheral and often remote areas. Use of 'front-line' health workers was proposed, and a working document on the training and use of village health workers was prepared in 1974 in English, French and Spanish. It dealt mainly with the training and supervision of these primary health-care workers and their role in health promotion, prevention, cure and rehabilitation, the distribution of drugs and referral, all in the context of the health team. The working document was tested in Iran and the Lao People's Democratic Republic and by many individual public health workers, and a new publication was issued in 1976 under the title *The primary health care worker: working guide, guidelines for training; guidelines for adaptation* (*18*).

In 1972, WHO participated in a study on traditional birth attendants and in 1973 organized a consultation on the role that such personnel could play in maternal and child health and family planning. Following upon this study, two interregional meetings were held, with participants from 19 countries. A guide for training and using indigenous midwives was prepared, used on a trial basis, revised and published (*19*). Regional seminars were held in the Western Pacific and Eastern Mediterranean regions in 1974, promoting the use of medical assistants.

An expert committee on the training and use of auxiliary personnel for rural health teams in developing countries was convened in late 1977. The committee confined its attention to front-line health personnel, i.e. "those who make the first contact with the population at the peripheral delivery point" (*20*). They were the first to see the sick and wounded and to bring care to pregnant women; they provided primary health care, consisting of first aid, basic curative care (simple diagnosis and treatment, referral of complex cases to a higher level), preventive care and essential educational measures. Such workers were members of (and lived in) the community they served. Their task was to help the local people find their own solutions to problems and organize themselves in such ways as to become the most active agents in their own development. The committee made recommendations on the promotion of rural health, health services, manpower and rural health teams and on national strategies for setting up rural health teams. An extensive bibliography was prepared, which included 16 films on the subject.

TOWARDS THE CONCEPT OF INTEGRATED HEALTH SERVICES AND MANPOWER DEVELOPMENT

The WHO scientific group that met in November 1970 to address the "development of studies in health manpower" first addressed the "approach to the total health system", since a "holistic approach" to health and a comprehensive analysis of the health system was needed to "provide the basis for determining health needs and future goals and for estimating the health manpower requirements" (*21*). The group reviewed past and ongoing studies in the context of national health planning. It endorsed the principles established by a WHO expert committee on national health planning in developing countries (*22*) and highlighted the principles for establishing national health services, as expressed in resolution WHA23.61, a World Health Assembly resolution that had been passed earlier in the year (see Chapter 6).

The group stressed the need for full participation of local administrators in research. Various levels of decision-making were identified, including educational institutions and the public, whose participation was imperative. The committee concluded that health manpower planning "should be given more recognition by governments as part of health planning and hence in the preparation of their economic and social policies. WHO could assist in achieving this." The group recommended promotion of studies in health planning in countries, establishment of separate study units for health manpower planning, encouraging application of the results of research on health manpower to education for the health professions, and promotion of research on methods for health manpower planning. A list of supporting activities was drawn up for WHO to carry out in conjunction with national units for the study of health manpower planning, beginning with setting up a central register of national studies under way, a bibliography, a classification of health occupations, a review of methods, an evaluation of outcomes and a better understanding of decision-making in health manpower planning. Long-term priorities included drawing up research guidelines, methods for projecting requirements for services and for estimating health needs and demands and preparation of staffing and productivity standards.

A national study of manpower that resulted directly from the work of the study group was conducted in Ceylon, which became Sri Lanka in 1972, in which WHO provided technical assistance, and UNFPA and UNDP gave financial support. Undertaken in 1971–1973, the study sought to determine the current pattern of health manpower use in the health-care system, in order to identify interventions to improve productivity and redefine the roles of the basic health occupations. It also sought to determine the needs and demands for health services in order to project future health manpower requirements, and to redefine the goals of education for the health professions. The results of the study were written up in 1975 (*23*). In a section entitled 'Aftermath', the reader learns that the urge for change in the health system had "slackened" owing to the emergence of more pressing needs in the socioeconomic life of the country, to personnel changes in decision-making at national level and to a "failure to clearly and aggressively communicate the findings and recommendations to the policy makers". Recognizing that any change of this kind could only result from a "long-lasting process", the report outlined findings for future use by Sri Lanka and other developing countries facing similar problems.

Sri Lanka was one of only a few countries that had attempted to answer or had even given thought to the question of how to rationalize the production and use of health manpower in the light of national health needs. Other countries that had undertaken manpower studies included Chile (*24*) and Colombia (*25*). In most countries, even where such studies had been undertaken, only fragmented health care was offered; highly sophisticated, centrally located medical care was provided that unduly emphasized the curative element; the number of health personnel was inadequate; and a policy on the health team concept was lacking and, consequently, health coverage was inadequate, with limited or no access of large population groups to health services.

The reasons given for this state of affairs varied. Problems specific to health manpower development included: the inadequacy or lack of national manpower policies; undue emphasis on traditional training of certain 'classical' categories of health personnel, particularly physicians, at the expense of other categories; shortage of training facilities and teachers; and a hostile attitude on the part of certain influential professional groups towards radical changes in health personnel education that would orient it more to the community or teamwork. In a more sweeping assessment, presented to the Executive Board at its fifty-seventh session, in January 1976, it was acknowledged that the sought-after breakthrough to the manpower problems of the developing world had not yet been achieved (26). Programmes were found to be "still too oriented towards the classical types of health workers, primarily physicians and nurses, and even in their training changes have been all too slow. The acceptance and development of new categories of health personnel and the retraining of existing categories also advances at a slow pace".

In response, WHO outlined a "coherent, integrated and systematic programme of collaboration with Member States in all relevant areas of health manpower development" (12). The central aim of such collaboration was to set up national programmes that integrated health manpower planning, manpower resources development and health manpower management into a single process geared to the improvement of health services. Realization of this concept, integrated development of health services and health manpower, was seen as a precondition for success in satisfying the health needs of a country's entire population.

The concept of the integrated development of health services and health manpower represented a radical change. The training of all categories of health personnel would have to be oriented towards satisfying the health needs and demands of people and not for professional interest. Priority would have to be given to meeting the health needs of the most deprived, particularly rural, communities by use of personnel with the appropriate levels of skills, first of all primary health care workers and those who provided effective support and guidance in the framework of comprehensive national health systems and services, as called for by resolution WHA28.88 (see Chapter 6). As a consequence, "a new, strong emphasis will be laid on the training and utilization of auxiliary and community health workers and their supervisors". The number of physicians, nurses and other 'classical' categories of health workers would also have to be increased, but their education would have to be made relevant to community health needs and demands without reducing its basic quality.

The report also indicated the need for a permanent country-specific mechanism for functional integration of health services and manpower development that would foster continuous dialogue, ensure efficient collaboration and coordination between various governmental and nongovernmental departments, institutions and other bodies responsible for health services and health manpower, and bring them together for the purposes of planning, decision-making and integrated development of health services and health manpower.

Other progress reports were written. One outlined the evolution of the multinational study on international migration of physicians and nurses, and another addressed the training and use of traditional healers and their collaboration with health-care delivery systems. All the reports were discussed at length by the Executive Board in January 1976 and subsequently by the Health Assembly in May of that year.

The report on the training and use of traditional healers contained proposals for collecting information, setting up appropriate training programmes and studies and research, in order "to improve the services of healers and to facilitate their collaboration with the primary health care systems" (*27*).

There was widespread agreement with the concept of integrated development of health services and health manpower within both the Executive Board and the Health Assembly. The documentation was judged to be "valuable", "useful and relevant", "extremely informative", "excellent" and a "stimulus to the discussion of the health manpower problem in Member States". The reports "showed much hard work, dedication to the cause, and a full grasp of the subject".

Additional matters raised concerned why it was so difficult to rationalize the training of health manpower, as called for by the concept. One Executive Board Member from an African country suggested that it had been a "mistake in the past to give autonomy to medical schools, since it had become a difficult matter for governments to exert influence over their curricula, with the result that these schools went on providing doctors whose training and knowledge were international in character". A Member from Latin America suggested that a "radical solution would be for medical schools to be included in, or be associated with, ministries of health, something that would not be feasible for some time to come in his region". Nevertheless, it was hoped that a meeting of the Pan American Federation of Associations of Medical Schools, held in Caracas, Venezuela, in January 1976 under the auspices of WHO, would provide a "first step in closing the gap between ministries of health and education". The representative of the World Federation for Medical Education, speaking before the Twenty-ninth World Health Assembly, indicated that "his organization strongly endorsed the proposals for health manpower development contained in the Director-General's report".

There was less unanimity on the proposals concerning traditional healers. As one Executive Board Member put it, "the use of traditional healers was a serious problem which called for thorough reflection. Countries should adopt a cautious attitude towards incorporating them into primary health services. A clear distinction should be drawn between healers using traditional therapeutic methods and other healers who indulged in little more than magic and superstitious practices." This and other, similar reservations led to use of the term 'traditional medicine' in the resolution adopted (see below), rather than 'traditional healers and birth attendants' as originally proposed. As noted in Chapter 6, resolution WHA30.49, adopted in 1977, specifically touched on the issue of training and research in traditional medicine and called on WHO to assist Member States in organizing education and research in this field.

Resolution WHA29.72 endorsed the integrated approach and requested the Director-General:

- to assist Member States in formulating national health manpower policies that were responsive to health service requirements and consistent with policy in other sectors;
- to promote the concept of integrated health services and manpower development in order to have manpower systems that were responsive to health needs, and to collaborate with Member States in introducing a permanent mechanism for application of the concept and in adapting it to the requirements of their country;
- to collaborate with Member States in strengthening health manpower planning as an integral part of overall health planning in their socioeconomic context;
- to encourage the training of health teams to meet the health needs of populations, including health workers for primary health care, and to take into account, where appropriate, the manpower reserve constituted by those practising traditional medicine;
- to collaborate with Member States in formulating and adapting effective health manpower management policies, in establishing continuous evaluation to ensure the necessary changes in a dynamic, integrated system of health services and manpower development and in devising measures to control undesirable migration of health manpower;
- to establish a long-term programme of health manpower development on the basis of these proposals in all the regions, taking into account the specific needs and possibilities of the countries in each region, and, on the basis of this long-term programme, to build medium-term health manpower development programmes with concrete aims and target indices for evaluation of the results attained, these programmes to be discussed at the regional committee meetings in 1977; and
- to study the actions taken by governments to modify their health manpower training programmes and to assist Member States in restructuring the curricula of all the members of the health team, especially for physicians at both undergraduate and postgraduate levels, to make them more relevant to the needs of their societies.

Exploratory missions had already been organized to apply the integrated development of health services and health manpower in Iran, Sri Lanka, Thailand and the United Republic of Cameroon. Many countries were assisted in setting up health manpower planning programmes, particularly in the regions of Africa, the Americas and the Eastern Mediterranean. During the discussions at the regional committee meetings in 1977, countries expressed further interest in this concept, as seen in the Ministerial Consultation on Health Services and Manpower Development, originally planned for 1976 and held in Teheran in early 1978 (*28*). Three examples of approaches to coordination were presented, from Poland, the United Kingdom and Latin America.

In his address to the Consultation, Dr Mahler expressed his conviction that the "human requirements approach" would focus much greater attention on the people themselves "instead of on the health professions". It should help people to learn to take proper responsibility for their own health, "thus avoiding an ever-greater dependence on medicine". Most importantly, he added, it should lead to fuller integration of the health sector with other sectors of society concerned with satisfying these essential human requirements.

References

1. *Joint UNICEF/WHO Committee on Health Policy: report on the eighteenth session. Official records of the World Health Organization*, No. 195, Annex 2. Geneva, World Health Organization, 1971.

2. *Promotion of medical practitioners' interest in preventive medicine, twelfth report of the WHO expert committee on professional and technical education of medical and auxiliary personnel* (WHO Technical Report Series, No. 269). Geneva, World Health Organization, 1964.

3. *The medical assistant: an intermediate level of health care personnel* (WHO Public Health Paper No. 60). Geneva, World Health Organization, 1974.

4. *The work of WHO 1972. Official records of the World Health Organization*, No. 205. Geneva, World Health Organization, 1972.

5. *Training of national health personnel. Progress report by the Director-General* (A25/7). Geneva, World Health Organization, 1972.

6. Mejia A, Pizurki H, Royston E. *Physician and nurse migration: analysis and policy implications*. Geneva, World Health Organization, 1979.

7. *Postgraduate education and training in public health. Report of a WHO expert committee* (WHO Technical Report Series, No. 533). Geneva, World Health Organization, 1973.

8. *Continuing education for physicians. Report of a WHO expert committee* (WHO Technical Report Series, No. 534). Geneva, World Health Organization, 1973.

9. *The planning of medical education programmes. Report of a WHO expert committee* (WHO Technical Report Series, No. 547). Geneva, World Health Organization, 1974.

10. *The planning of schools of medicine. Report of a WHO study group* (WHO Technical Report Series, No. 566). Geneva, World Health Organization, 1975.

11. *Training and preparation of teachers for schools of medicine and of allied health sciences. Report of a WHO study group* (WHO Technical Report Series, No. 521). Geneva, World Health Organization, 1973.

12. *Health manpower development proposals for future activities* (EB57/21). Geneva, World Health Organization, 1976.

13. *The training and utilization of feldshers in the USSR: a review prepared by the Ministry of Health of the USSR for the World Health Organization* (WHO Public Health Paper No. 56). Geneva, World Health Organization, 1974.

14. *Travelling seminar on the training and utilization of medical assistants (feldshers) in the USSR* (TAP/68.1). Geneva, World Health Organization, 1967.

15. *Organizational study of the Executive Board on methods of promoting the development of basic health services. Background documentation* (EB49/WP/6), Geneva, World Health Organization, 1972.

16. *Study tour on the training and utilization of barefoot doctors in community health services in the People's Republic of China, 10–30 August 1978* (INT/78/034). Geneva, World Health Organization, 1979.

17. *The medical assistant: an intermediate level of health care personnel* (WHO Public Health Paper No. 60). Geneva, World Health Organization, 1974.

18. *The primary health care worker: working guide, guidelines for training; guidelines for adaptation* (HMD/74.5 (Rev. 1976)), experimental edition. Geneva, World Health Organization, 1977.

19. *The traditional birth attendant in maternal and child health and family planning* (WHO Offset Publication, No. 18). Geneva, World Health Organization, 1975.

20. *Training and utilization of auxiliary personnel for rural health teams in developing countries. Report of a WHO expert committee* (WHO Technical Report Series, No. 633). Geneva, World Health Organization, 1979.

21. *The development of studies in health manpower. Report of a WHO scientific group* (WHO Technical Report Series, No. 481). Geneva, World Health Organization, 1971.

22. *National health planning in developing countries. Report of a WHO expert committee* (WHO Technical Report Series, No. 350). Geneva, World Health Organization, 1967.

23. Simeonov LA. *Better health for Sri Lanka. Report on a health manpower study* (SEA/PHA/ 149). New Delhi, Regional Office for South-East Asia, 1975.

24. Ministerio de Salud Publica y Consejo Nacional Consultivo de Salud. *Recursos humanos de salud en Chile: un modelo de analysis [Human resources for health in Chile: a model for analysis]*. Santiago, 1970.

25. Badgley RF, ed. Social science and health planning: culture, disease and health services in Colombia. *Milbank Memorial Fund Quarterly*, 1968, 46(2), Part 2.

26. *Health manpower development progress report* (EB57/21, Part I). Geneva, World Health Organization, 1976.

27. *Training and utilization of traditional healers and their collaboration with health care delivery systems* (EB57/21 Add.2). Geneva, World Health Organization, 1976.

28. *An integrated approach to health services and manpower development* (WHO/EMRO Technical Publication No. 1). Alexandria, WHO Regional Office for the Eastern Mediterranean, 1978.

CHAPTER 9

Prevention and control of communicable diseases

More than 100 pages were devoted to this subject in the history of WHO's second 10 years, reflecting the central place that it occupied in WHO's earlier programmes of work, especially that for malaria eradication. So great was the concern over the collapsing programme for malaria eradication and the uncertain prospects of the smallpox eradication programme that the governing bodies concentrated largely on these two diseases during the first years of the decade. As confidence in the smallpox campaign increased, attention was given to other diseases, particularly parasitic diseases, as reflected in the creation of the UNDP–World Bank–WHO Special Programme for Research and Training in Tropical Diseases (TDR) (see Chapter 5) and to the expanded programme on immunization.

Introducing the programme to the Twenty-eighth World Health Assembly, in 1975, the responsible assistant director-general said that the programme had four main aims: (i) to adapt the knowledge gained from technological progress to the conditions prevailing in countries; (ii) to place the problem of communicable diseases in its proper social and economic perspective; (iii) to integrate the fight against communicable diseases into overall health services; and (iv) to ensure coordinated action at national level, at regional level (particularly with regard to areas that were neighbours or were comparable epidemiologically) and at global level (*1*).

EPIDEMIOLOGICAL SURVEILLANCE AND QUARANTINE

Quarantine is one of the oldest public health services to have been organized at an international level. A set of international sanitary conventions emerged from a series of international meetings held between the mid-nineteenth and the mid-twentieth centuries, which were brought together in the *International sanitary regulations*. These regulations mainly address a selected group of diseases and apply to all forms of international transport.

During the latter part of WHO's second decade, a new approach to disease control was introduced, epidemiological surveillance, which replaced the old concept of epidemiological intelligence (*2*). It was defined as "the exercise of continuous scrutiny of and watchfulness over the distribution and spread of infections and factors related thereto, of sufficient accuracy and completeness to be pertinent to effective control," and grew out of improved epidemiological methods, especially as regards the processing and analysis of data and the use of laboratory and field studies (background document for reference use at the technical discussions on national and global surveillance of communicable diseases, April 1968). As a consequence of this development, the Unit of Quarantine was merged with that of Epidemiological Surveillance in 1968, and, by the end of the decade, the programme was called only Epidemiological Surveillance.

The bringing together of surveillance and quarantine was part of a strategy designed to move away from the concept that disease prevention could be accomplished only by quarantine measures. As a first step, it was necessary to revise the *International sanitary regulations*, which dated back to 1952. Detailed revision of the *Regulations* was first carried out by legal and technical experts at two meetings of the Committee on International Quarantine in 1967. These were sent to Member States for comments and suggestions. A revised set of *Regulations* (with the word 'Health' replacing 'Sanitary') was then reviewed by a subcommittee that met during the Twenty-second World Health Assembly, in 1969. With the adoption of the *International health regulations* in 1969 (resolution WHA22.46), the Committee on International Quarantine changed its name to the Committee on International Surveillance of Communicable Diseases.

The Director of the Division for the Control of Communicable Diseases used the example of typhus during discussions at the Twenty-second World Health Assembly to explain the significance of the changes. To begin with, he said, "quarantine methodology had a very limited effect on the spread of the disease." (*3*) Elimination of typhus from quarantinable diseases would improve its control, as many countries did not report its occurrence because of possible harm to their economy. If it were not quarantinable, "but under surveillance, outbreaks were more likely to be reported and they could be effectively controlled, mainly by the use of insecticides."

Immunological surveys can provide objective information about the presence or absence of a given infection in a population and thus serve as a useful adjunct to surveillance. With this in mind, a WHO scientific group was convened in November 1969, which established the basis for international coordination of multipurpose serological surveys, including the role of serum reference banks (*4*). The meeting recognized that new serological methods were desirable to advance knowledge of diseases that were highly prevalent in certain areas, including parasitic and some bacterial diseases such as leprosy and tuberculosis. In order to coordinate serological studies throughout the world, it was considered that a programme for continuous collation of information on blood and serum collections, compilation of results and dissemination of information would be useful.

Information on all diseases covered by programme was disseminated regularly through the daily WHO epidemiological radiotelegraphic (later telex) bulletin and in the *Weekly epidemiological report*, which also contained technical guidance and epidemiological notes on a number of other diseases of international importance, and reports on the importation of cases—often fatal—of diseases into countries where doctors were unfamiliar with them.

As effective international surveillance depends on the quality and geographical coverage of national surveillance, the WHO programme emphasized assistance in strengthening national surveillance. A prerequisite was training of a cadre of epidemiologists in Member States who were also trained in surveillance methods. Another essential element of the strategy was the presence of technicians and allied health personnel to observe and report outbreaks with particular symptoms in their communities.

Training was one of the main features of the programme. Various approaches were used, including international and regional seminars on the methods and coordination of epidemiological surveillance. Intercountry centres for epidemiological surveillance were established in the African Region (Abidjan, Nairobi and Brazzaville in 1974), and a new centre was set up in the Americas in 1975, the Caribbean Epidemiological Centre in Port-of-Spain.

Technical manuals were prepared on the surveillance of nine diseases: four diseases under the *Regulations* as from 1 January 1971 (smallpox, yellow fever, cholera and plague) and five diseases under international surveillance (louse-borne typhus, louse-borne relapsing fever, influenza, paralytic poliomyelitis and malaria). In 1975, a general guide on surveillance of communicable diseases was prepared, with emphasis on operational aspects and the rational use of manpower.

During its nineteenth session, in November 1976, the Committee on International Surveillance of Communicable Diseases undertook a broad review of the basic concepts underlying the *International health regulations*. The Committee considered that the *Regulations* would continue to be of value, despite changing epidemiological circumstances. As the *Regulations* represented the maximum measures that should be taken, Member States could reduce their requirements on international travel at any time in accordance with the current epidemiological situation.

The Committee took the occasion to express its concern that the vaccination certificate requirements notified to WHO by many States were not in accordance with the practice and policies of entry to those countries; this situation often resulted in unnecessary difficulties for travellers.

ERADICATION OF SMALLPOX

It was the delegate of the USSR to the Eleventh World Health Assembly, in 1958, who proposed that WHO should undertake the global eradication of smallpox. This proposal was agreed to the next year, when the Twelfth World Health Assembly adopted resolution WHA12.54, which emphasized the "urgency of achieving world-wide eradication" and recommended that the health administrations of those countries where smallpox was still present organize and conduct eradication programmes "as soon as possible."

Progress in the first years was patchy. Although several countries initiated mass vaccination programmes, most were handicapped by factors such as insufficient supplies of potent and stable freeze-dried vaccine, inadequate transport and the lack of a suitably designed plan and strategy. The Organization was limited to providing technical assistance and guidance, with no increase in resources under the regular budget. Furthermore, not all the regional offices were ready to promote the campaign fully; only the Pan American Sanitary Organization had an established programme, which dated back to 1950. Several countries where the disease occurred were not yet Members of the Organization, e.g. China and Viet Nam. More importantly, there were four large smallpox-endemic territories in Africa that either no longer participated in WHO (South Africa) or were represented by colonial powers (Mozambique and Southern Rhodesia).

In 1966, new impetus was given to the programme by the decision of the Nineteenth World Health Assembly (resolution WHA19.16) to intensify the global effort and to increase the Organization's participation. Nevertheless, this decision was made with "grave reservations" (*5*). The Director-General did not consider that smallpox eradication was possible. Rather than risk an eradication campaign that might suffer the same fate as that for malaria (see below), the highest priority was given to "the establishment of permanent basic health services" (5). Dr Candau had previously stressed the importance of the basic health services (see Chapter 6), which might explain the slowness with which some regions initially gave their full support to the eradication campaign.

Four sources of funding were envisioned in the original plan: the WHO regular budget, which in the first year allocated US$ 2.4 million; contributions to the WHO Voluntary Fund for Health Promotion, Special Account for Smallpox Eradication; bilateral contributions; and contributions from other international agencies. It was originally estimated that US$ 48.5 million would be needed for a 10-year programme (1967–1976). Voluntary contributions were sought through mailings and visits to governments and other potential donors. Ultimately, international assistance between 1967 and 1979, when eradication was certified, amounted to some US$ 98 million, of which US$ 34 million came from the WHO regular budget.

The strategic plan for eradication was two-pronged: mass vaccination with freeze-dried vaccine of assured quality assessed by special teams, and a surveillance system for the detection and investigation of cases and the containment of outbreaks. The surveillance was to be based on a reporting system in which all existing medical and health units participated. This being a new concept, which might be difficult to implement in highly endemic countries, a three-phased programme for its development was proposed, during which reporting, field investigation, control procedures and laboratory study of cases were steadily improved.

The WHO Scientific Group on Smallpox Eradication, meeting at the end of 1967, defined smallpox eradication as "the elimination of clinical infection by variola virus" (6). Proof that smallpox had been eradicated presupposed the presence of a case detection system sufficiently effective to reveal the presence of the disease in an area before more than two or three generations of cases had occurred. When, within an arbitrary period of 2 years, no endemic case of smallpox had been detected and outbreaks due to imported infection had been promptly controlled, the country could be said to be 'smallpox-free'. The word 'eradicated' could be used only when the disease was absent from an entire continent. At this time, smallpox was no longer present in Europe, North America or Australia including Oceania.

At the beginning of 1967, an estimated 10–15 million cases were occurring annually in 31 endemic countries or territories with a total population of more than 1 billion. Despite budgetary constraints, which forced the programme initially to expand operations with consultants rather than full-time staff, activities steadily increased during the first year. In 1968, the number of endemic countries with special eradication programmes increased from 12 to 19, and agreements for the commencement of programmes was reached in eight others. In 1969, 23 countries reported transmission, eight fewer than in 1968, and in five of them transmission was interrupted. By 1970, only 18 countries recorded endemic cases, and in six of these transmission was interrupted.

Progress was reported in surveillance reports in the *Weekly epidemiological report* every 2–3 weeks; more extensive summary reports were prepared twice a year. Each year, one or two international meetings were arranged for senior smallpox eradication programme staff from regional offices and endemic countries, annual conferences were held for WHO's regional smallpox advisers, and biennial meetings were held of the research group concerned with monkeypox and related problems.

The WHO Expert Committee on Smallpox Eradication that met in November 1971 was asked to assess the present situation and to consider the strategy and method to be used in the years to come (*7*). Experience had shown that surveillance was the essential element of eradication, and WHO was called upon to intensify its efforts to support and coordinate programmes. When the incidence of smallpox decreased to zero in all countries and the absence of the disease was beyond doubt, it was hoped that the surveillance programmes could take on increasing responsibility for other communicable diseases.

By 1973, smallpox had been confined to five endemic countries: Bangladesh, Ethiopia, India, Nepal and Pakistan. A brief account of the efforts made to bring about successful conclusion of the campaign is given for India and Ethiopia.

In India, the national campaign, which had been in operation since 1962, was intensified in 1967. Progress was, however, less than had been anticipated, as outbreaks were not being detected early enough. In the summer of 1973, WHO staff and Indian national and state health personnel agreed on a strategy to detect outbreaks more quickly and to contain them promptly. The plan was for some 100 000 health staff to undertake 10-day village-by-village searches to detect cases, with containment teams following rapidly to stop outbreaks. Surprisingly, the initial search in several northern states revealed thousands of cases in areas where only a few hundred had been reported routinely. Case searches were repeated in heavily endemic areas every 1–2 months and less frequently in low-incidence areas. So great were the numbers reported that state and national health authorities were tempted to replace the surveillance and containment policy with one of mass vaccination, but this was resisted. Gradually, the searches were transformed into house-to-house searches, and the number of smallpox cases steadily decreased. With the mobilization of additional staff and the provision of emergency funds, 'Operation Smallpox Zero' was begun in January 1975.

New instructions were issued. As there were so few outbreaks, it was decided that each should be dealt with as an "*absolute* emergency, with maximum mobilization of staff and volunteers". Whereas previously the containment teams had consisted of three or four persons, they would now consist of "15 or 20 workers or more, headed by the District Medical Officer of Health assisted by a national or WHO epidemiologist" (*6*). Operation Smallpox Zero was successful. In all, only 308 outbreaks and 1436 cases were detected in India after 1 January. In April, some 115 000 health workers undertook week-long, house-to-house searches throughout India. The last case was recorded in May 1975, and India celebrated 'freedom from smallpox' in August of that year.

Field operations did not begin in Ethiopia until early 1971. The challenges were formidable: most of the population was widely scattered over this vast country, where roads were few and health services sparse; people suffering from the mild variola form of smallpox travelled and spread the disease; several ethnic groups resisted vaccination. With only 67 available staff, resources were initially concentrated in four southwestern provinces, where the health service structure was better, although one or two staff in each of the other nine provinces began surveillance. By the end of the year, more than 26 000 cases had been found, an unexpectedly high number, as Ethiopia had been reporting only a few hundred cases each year for the entire country.

Steady progress was made during 1973 and 1974, and the number of cases decreased to 17 000 in 1973 and to less than 6000 in 1974. A severe drought in late 1974, however, resulted in an estimated 200 000 deaths and extensive refugee movement. Working conditions became increasingly difficult, particularly in areas where there was armed conflict. At the end of the year, a major revolution took place, the Emperor was deposed and a new Government took charge. In some areas, smallpox eradication teams were attacked; several were kidnapped, and on one occasion two Ethiopian vaccinators were killed. Despite these obstacles, the programme continued and was strengthened by the donation of the services of three helicopters, which proved invaluable by permitting investigations in even the most remote areas. By the end of July 1975, only 131 known active outbreaks occurred in 13 clusters spread over a little more than 1% of the country's total area.

As Ethiopia was by then the only known endemic country, WHO was able to make additional resources available, and the number of personnel grew to somewhat more than 1000. The revolutionary Government declared the programme to be of the highest priority. Activity intensified, and, in July 1976, an outbreak was found in the Ogaden Desert, which proved to be the last in the country. Unfortunately, smallpox had by then spread to neighbouring Somalia; emergency control programmes were instituted there, but it was not until 26 October 1977 that the world's last case was found and isolated in the town of Merka and all his contacts were vaccinated.

From 1973, international commissions were constituted to visit previously endemic countries to determine, on the basis of reports and field visits, whether the surveillance conducted over at least the past 2 years had been adequate to detect cases of smallpox. Eradication in South America was certified in 1973 and in Indonesia in 1974. Between 1975 and 1979, 15 international commissions visited 11 countries in Asia and 34 countries in Africa. In December 1979, the Global Commission agreed that eradication had been achieved and recommended that routine vaccination throughout the world be stopped.

Applied research contributed greatly to the rapidity with which smallpox was eradicated. Initial research showed that the new bifurcated needle was effective and that the technique of multiple-puncture vaccination could be learnt easily even by persons with little education. This needle permitted the vaccination of 100 persons from a standard vaccine vial, while conventional methods permitted vaccination of only 25. Moreover, the vaccination 'take' rates were generally higher. The methods for producing and testing smallpox vaccine were perfected by collaborating laboratories.

WHO encouraged field staff to undertake epidemiological studies, the results of which were widely distributed. Of particular importance was the early finding in western and central Africa and in Madras State, India, that smallpox spread less rapidly and less easily than was thought and that prompt detection and immediate containment of outbreaks was the most cost–effective means of pursuing the goal of eradication. Studies also showed that cases seldom occurred among adults in endemic areas, and few cases occurred among people who had previously been vaccinated. Vaccination campaigns therefore focused on children and on ensuring that all individuals had a vaccination mark. New approaches were used for surveillance, in schools and markets; sampling techniques applicable to developing countries were designed for use in quality-control studies; and, in meticulous studies of smallpox transmission, it was possible to demonstrate that essentially all cases resulted from face-to-face contacts between affected and susceptible persons. No less important were the studies of monkeypox, which showed that human-to-human transmission of the disease was sufficiently difficult that it was highly unlikely that infection with the monkeypox virus could become endemic.

Intensive efforts were made to identify all laboratories that might have smallpox virus and to persuade them to destroy the virus or to transfer their specimens to the WHO collaborating laboratories in Moscow, USSR, or Atlanta, Georgia, United States. A smallpox vaccine reserve of 200 million doses was set up in Geneva in 1976, which was later reduced to 5 million doses. The two collaborating centres continued to study smallpox virology and the potential for an effective antiviral agent, should one ever be needed for therapy.

MALARIA: FROM ERADICATION TO CONTROL

The global eradication campaign was launched in 1955. The resolution adopted by the Eighth World Health Assembly, in that year (WHA8.30), called for a programme for the worldwide eradication of malaria. The Malaria Eradication Special Account, which had been established to help finance the Organization's expanded activities, proved of critical importance in financing the early years of the campaign. When this source of funding dramatically decreased in 1965, the Organization was obliged to allocate regular budget funds to meet programme operating costs. As a consequence, the Health Assembly began to scrutinize the programme more closely, which led to growing pressure on the Organization to re-examine its strategy. Furthermore, other priorities, particularly family planning and smallpox eradication, began to receive greater attention. Of even greater importance was the call (8) to integrate the malaria programme into basic health services, especially in countries where eradication was not foreseeable in the near or medium-term future.

After 2 years of study, the Twenty-second World Health Assembly, in 1969, adopted resolution WHA22.39, which continued to call for eradication of the disease but recognized the many problems that had blocked progress. Furthermore, WHO was asked to continue to provide assistance in studying the socioeconomic impact of malaria and of its eradication and to find a method for socioeconomic evaluation of the programmes under way. The review carried out during the previous 2 years had attempted to evaluate the impact but had been thwarted by lack of adequate reliable data.

For more than two decades, the malaria programme had been run as an independent, 'vertical' programme. The 1969 Health Assembly resolution now identified the role of the basic health services as "crucial" in malaria eradication and thus "increased attention to their development" was needed. WHO called upon the Expert Committee on Malaria to review the principles of malaria eradication and to recommend a strategy more suitable to the current situation. At its fifteenth meeting, in October 1970, the Committee reviewed the practices of malaria eradication, emphasizing their "time-limited" nature (9). Where eradication could not be envisaged within a predetermined time, a malaria control programme was called for, control being defined as "an organized effort to carry out those anti-malaria measures that are possible with the available resources and suitable under the prevailing epidemiological conditions, with the objective of achieving the greatest possible reduction of mortality and morbidity."

The Committee acknowledged that training had always been given high priority by WHO. More than 100 courses had been organized over the previous decade, at various training centres around the world. National training centres, assisted by WHO, had provided programmes for some 8500 staff in more than 280 courses. The new strategy of malaria eradication, however, called for more comprehensive training of malariologists.

A large international conference was organized by WHO in late 1972 on the subject *Malaria control in countries where time-limited eradication is impracticable at present* (*10*). The organization of malaria control activities was seen to require activities at three levels: central, intermediate and peripheral. At the central level, a team should be integrated into a communicable disease control unit, consisting of a malariologist and a sanitary engineer or 'sanitarian'. They would be responsible for overall policy-making, conducting feasibility studies and the overall planning and management of the programme. The intermediate level was seen as the backbone of activities, consisting of a medical officer with a solid grounding in public health administration and epidemiology, assisted by a trained, experienced senior malaria health inspector. At the peripheral level, there would be supervisors and small teams to perform activities such as the conduct and updating of geographical reconnaissance or delimitation of vector-breeding places, training and supervision of spraymen and drug administrators, collection and microscopic examination of blood slides from fever patients and suspected malaria cases, treatment of malaria, regular reporting of results, feedback of data to the intermediate level and health education of the public.

Particular attention was given to research. Many questions remained: Why are certain anophelines, or strains of them, efficient vectors whereas others are not? What is the course of the disease in semi-immune populations and its effect on their working capacity during periods when the disease is quiescent? How can different staining or concentration techniques improve the diagnosis of malaria? How is the biochemistry of malaria parasites related to their biological cycles in the body of the host?

At its sixteenth meeting, in November 1973, the Expert Committee continued to refine issues raised at its earlier sessions. The importance of integrating antimalaria programmes into the health and socioeconomic context was discussed extensively. In order to determine which socioeconomic targets were feasible, these aspects had to be an important component of the feasibility survey carried out in the early stages of programme planning. Studies of the cost–benefit type based on purely economic criteria fell short of what was needed. The interrelations between malaria and certain features of underdevelopment (e.g. primitive agricultural methods and human ecology conducive to contact between man and mosquito) were so close as to require not only a complete study of the effect of the campaigns on socioeconomic conditions but also a study of the effect of the latter on the malaria situation (*11*). Special attention was given to the impact of large-scale development projects on malaria and on the importance of including appropriate antimalaria measures in such projects from their inception.

The massive epidemics in the Indian subcontinent resulted in more than a tripling of reported cases from that area between 1972 (nearly 2 million cases) and 1976 (6.5 million cases). Particularly disturbing were the appearance of major epidemics in countries that in the 1960s were judged to be on the way to eradicating malaria. Against the background of meetings and studies to find new approaches to the problem and in light of the rapid deterioration of the malaria situation in a number of countries, WHO continued to promote, organize and coordinate antimalaria activities at national and international levels. Efforts were made to obtain international and bilateral assistance for malarious countries. WHO organized regional meetings on specific malaria problems and border meetings in several regions. New training programmes were set up, which were more comprehensive, as called for in the strategy adopted in 1969.

In an "analytic summary" of WHO's work, prepared at the end of 1973 (*12*), the "solution" to the problem of malaria was found to be "inseparable from the solution of that of socioeconomic advance in the developing countries". The use of all technical methods "must go hand in hand with the expansion of basic health services in rural areas, with the provision of more trained personnel, with better health education, and above all with an improvement in the economic conditions of underprivileged communities in tropical areas."

The deteriorating situation led the Executive Board at its fifty-fifth session, in January 1975 (resolution EB55.R37), to establish an ad hoc committee on malaria to identify all aspects of the problem that required attention, with emphasis on the formulation of regional strategies, reorientation of national programmes and the design, production and adequate supply of antimalarials and insecticides.

A paper prepared by the secretariat for consideration by the ad hoc committee (*13*) described various issues, including WHO's role as perceived by the Director-General. Reference was made to the unfavourable turn taken by the programme since 1969: while the strategy outlined in 1969 was considered to be sound, it was admitted that the Organization has been unable to implement it. This was judged to be due to the fact that no one— governments, national or international institutions or individuals—connected with the programme was psychologically prepared to admit even partial failure and to break away from the past, leading to the conclusion that "it was probably a mistake to stipulate that 'global eradication' remained the objective when it was obviously out of reach for decades to come, with the means at our disposal." The views of the ad hoc Committee were requested in the hope that it would lead the Board to make a "strong statement" that would help to promote the radical change in attitude without which no fresh impulse could be given to the programme.

The ad hoc committee limited itself to proposing a role for WHO consisting of six points:

- recognition of WHO's leadership role as mandated by the Constitution;
- WHO's role in attracting international contributions to technically and economically sound programmes;
- a greater role for the WHO regional committees and regional offices in formulating regional approaches;
- close coordination among WHO secretariat at all operational levels, with the proviso that permanent WHO malaria teams would be required only exceptionally, while WHO could remain involved in field research "particularly to develop operational models and/or test various methods (drug regimes, insecticides) in the field";
- the continuing need for an active role of WHO in antimalarial activities that involved several countries; and

- a role for WHO in initiating plans for the design, production and distribution of antimalarials and insecticides in liaison with other international institutions and with industry, while recognizing that its own resources could be used only for emergency cases and in limited amounts.

The Executive Board at its fifty-seventh session, in January 1976, endorsed the report of its ad hoc committee and outlined the role of WHO as follows:

- assist countries in taking more realistic, flexible approaches in antimalaria programmes;
- intensify coordination with other international organizations and bilateral agencies;
- emphasize and assist in the extension of training in malariology at both national and international training institutions, including formulation of training courses in this field suitable for all public health workers in malarious countries; and
- assert the Organization's leading role in making overall plans for the design, production and distribution of antimalarials and insecticides.

When the Twenty-ninth World Health Assembly addressed the same subject, it added two further lines of action for the Organization to pursue:

- assist countries in conducting operational studies and setting up research facilities for various aspects of malaria, particularly for immunizing agents, new chemotherapeutic substances and biological methods of control; and
- promote the use of bioenvironmental methods of malaria control whenever feasible.

The first point, concerning research, became an essential feature of TDR, which was launched in 1975 (see Chapter 5 and below), while the second point was incorporated in later programmes.

The TDR programme for malaria started along four lines: chemotherapy, immunology, parasite biology and cultivation in vitro, and applied research. The work of the chemotherapy group included research on the mechanism of action of antimalarial drugs, improvement of drugs in clinical use, improvement of existing and new drug screening procedures, design of new drugs and clinical studies.

Immunological research in malaria had seen a "major renaissance" in 1976–1977 owing in part to the successful establishment of continuous cultivation of *Plasmodium falciparum* in vitro (*14*). The programme was oriented mainly towards research on malaria antigens, mechanisms of immunity and immune evasion, immunodiagnostic tests, immunopathological phenomena, development of blood state, sporozoite and gamete vaccines in animal models and, eventually, vaccination against malaria in humans.

The priorities for field research emerged from regional advisory committees on medical research and included baseline assessment and monitoring of drug sensitivity in *P. falciparum*, evaluation of community participation in antimalaria activities, chemoprophylaxis for children in malaria endemic areas, approaches to malaria control in problem areas and the strain distribution of *P. falciparum*.

OTHER PARASITIC DISEASES

The Organization's work on parasitic diseases other than malaria concentrated on schistosomiasis, filariasis, onchocerciasis, trypanosomiasis and leishmaniasis. The objective of the programme was to assist governments by providing the necessary expertise for taking control measures against prevalent parasitic diseases, with the aim of reducing transmission—and hence morbidity—to a level at which the disease was no longer of public health importance.

During this period, epidemiological studies were undertaken on methods of monitoring changes in disease situations and patterns, on assessing the public health and socioeconomic importance of various parasitic diseases, and on the value of measuring morbidity patterns as an index of the impact of the disease. Two aspects of the relation between parasitic diseases and socioeconomic development were stressed: the degree to which parasitic diseases are an obstacle to economic development, and the degree to which economic development aggravates the prevalence of parasitic diseases.

Schistosomiasis

While schistosomiasis was an acute problem in some countries, proof of its public health importance was lacking in others. Furthermore, the available control methods, although beginning to show some signs of effectiveness, had not yet proven themselves on a large scale. The WHO Expert Committee on Schistosomiasis that met in 1972 to review the status of knowledge about control techniques noted that reluctance to undertake campaigns against the disease might be due, in part, to lack of confidence that the results would be favourable (*15*).

Long-term investigations on the pathology of schistosomiasis infections were carried out in Brazil and Nigeria. The research on snails addressed their ecology, physiology, biochemistry and immunochemistry. At a meeting of the directors of laboratories collaborating in molluscicide testing and evaluation, held in 1970 in Washington DC, United States, discussions centred on how to improve coordination among the laboratories involved and the role of the chemical industry in the programme. The WHO Snail Identification Centre in Copenhagen investigated differences in the susceptibility of various species of snails to different strains of schistosoma, which might account for the significant variations in the prevalence of the disease.

Work in the field of chemotherapy mainly concerned the action of chemicals on schistosomes, with clinical trials of promising compounds. The possible long-term adverse effects of drugs remained a matter of great concern. Late in 1971 and again in June 1972, WHO convened groups of experts to review information on the available antischistosomal drugs. Although the newer drugs were judged to be highly effective, it was recommended that the search for less toxic drugs should continue.

In view of its acute nature and its widespread distribution, schistosomiasis was ranked next to malaria in importance. Its association with water development schemes, especially those involving man-made lakes, was the basis for several studies to understand how the disease develops in different ecological situations and to devise appropriate control strategies. In 1968, discussions were held on the feasibility of a schistosomiasis control project in the context of man-made lakes, involving several large international organizations (*16*).

In July 1970, WHO convened an informal group of specialists in snail ecology to discuss schistosomiasis transmission in man-made lakes and to recommend an appropriate research programme. Pilot schemes for schistosomiasis control were proposed in the United Republic of Tanzania, which were linked to an FAO fisheries project in nearby Lake Victoria. Other water development schemes in Africa demanded WHO's attention as well, so that by the early 1970s the Organization found itself carrying out surveys in several project areas, including Lake Victoria. Activities related to man-made lakes were extended to South America in 1976.

Interest in the control of schistosomiasis took a sharp upswing in 1975. The Member from the United States of the fifty-fifth session of the Executive Board "in the interest of stimulating some action" with regards to the schistosomiasis programme, introduced a draft resolution, noting that there had not been a resolution on the topic since the Fifth World Health Assembly (*17*). The Board's resolution (EB55.R22) requested that the Director-General report on the matter to the Twenty-eighth World Health Assembly.

The report of the Director-General (*18*) indicated that both the prevalence and the incidence of schistosomiasis were increasing globally. While some striking successes in control had been achieved in China, Israel, Japan and Venezuela, the steady increase in the prevalence of the disease demonstrated that better control was necessary. Thus, research on all aspects of schistosomiasis occupied a primary place in the work of the Organization.

With regard to control, the Twenty-ninth World Health Assembly heard that there had been a "disproportionate reliance on a single control tool in the past, usually molluscicides" (*19*). A more "holistic philosophy" of control was required, which took into account the etiological complexity of the disease and the "vital importance of the interest, involvement and participation of the community in controlling the infection in its own area". An international conference on schistosomiasis, held in Cairo in October 1975 under the auspices of the Ministry of Health of Egypt, with the United States Government, UNEP and WHO, further stressed the need for a combination of measures to control schistosomiasis.

A scientific working group on schistosomiasis was established in 1977 within TDR (see Chapter 5 and below). Initial attention was given to carrying out multicentre trials on the drug Praziquantel. The group also recommended that major clinical pharmacological testing centres be set up and supported in countries affected by the disease.

Filariasis

In a review of filariasis by an expert committee that met in 1973 (*20*), it was concluded that more attention should be paid to the public health importance of filarial infections and the efficacy of control methods. Epidemiological studies should be extended, standardized study protocols should be designed, longitudinal studies should be conducted to compare the effects of vector control and mass chemotherapy alone and in combination against the natural variations in endemicity, and further studies were needed on vector bionomics in different parts of the world. The committee found particularly alarming the steadily spreading risk resulting from rapid urbanization in many endemic countries of Africa and Asia. The main urban vector of filariasis, *Culex pipiens fatigans*, thrives in foul water, which is one of the major results of overcrowding and lack of sanitary facilities.

The ideal filariasis control programme would combine application of insecticides against the vector with a mass chemotherapy campaign and planned improvement of sanitary facilities to eliminate the vector's breeding sites. In practice, control programmes tended to emphasize either the first or the second of these three methods. Where vector control was considered too difficult or ineffective, diethylcarbamazine, the only drug then available that could be safely used for mass treatment, was administered. Early experience with the drug, however, indicated primary treatment failure, as seen by persistent microfilaraemia, some secondary failure, in which microfilaraemia recurred, and some new infections. More sensitive techniques were needed to obtain greater accuracy in evaluating the effects of mass chemotherapy.

Use of more sensitive measuring devices showed that the presence of ultra-low-level microfilaraemia, undetectable by most commonly used techniques, can result in infection of a significant proportion of mosquitoes. This and other findings shed light on why mass treatment with the drug had not so far succeeded in eliminating the disease in any population.

Within the Organization's interregional programme of field investigation on filariasis, the epidemiological dynamics of the disease in India were studied in 1973, and trials were initiated with diethylcarbamazine salt.

A consultation in 1975 advised on the planning of laboratory and field studies for better understanding of the epidemiology of filarial infections and for designing the most effective, economic means of control.

Experimental drug development was handicapped by the fact that most human filarial parasites do not infect laboratory animals. One avenue explored in a WHO-supported laboratory in Paris was to use a filaria of marsupials that is transmitted by *Aedes* and *Culex* as a laboratory model.

By the end of 1977, control of filariasis was continuing in all endemic countries. The newly established TDR programme initiated a number of research projects: to search for new drugs, to study the feasibility of designing a vaccine, to study the mechanism and prevention of immunopathological lesions in infected persons and to identify maintenance and culture methods for filarial parasites. A programme of epidemiological research was set up to find methods for detecting persons at high risk and to improve methods for controlling transmission, particularly by use of relatively simple measures, such as 'self-help'.

Onchocerciasis

The most important development in the control of onchocerciasis (river blindness) during this decade was the launch of a programme in the Volta River Basin, involving seven countries: Dahomey, Ghana, Ivory Coast, Mali, Niger, Togo and Upper Volta. The feasibility of control was agreed upon at a technical meeting held in 1968, involving WHO, the United States Agency for International Development and the Organisation de Coordination et de Coopération pour la Lutte contre les Grandes Endémies (*21*). The main method chosen was aerial larviciding of breeding sites. It was thought at the time that the chances of success would be greatest if the operations were carried out in ecological zones sufficiently large to obviate the need for continuous control of the whole area in order to protect it against re-invasion by the onchocerciasis vectors.

Studies were undertaken to estimate the probable economic effects of eradication of the disease in the countries involved. Several years were needed to gain accurate knowledge of the flight range and longevity of the principal vector, *Simulium damnosum*, and the best means for controlling its breeding during the dry season. Morbidity surveys were carried out, with special attention to the relation between infection and blindness, one of the consequences of heavy infestation of humans by the microfilariae.

The control area covered about 700 000 km², with some 10 million inhabitants. More than 1 million were estimated to have onchocerciasis, of whom at least 70 000 were considered 'economically blind'; many more suffered serious visual impairment. Because no drugs were available that would clear existing infection, it was foreseen that the programme would last as long as any infection persisted. As this could be as long as 15 years, a 20-year control programme was envisaged.

A steering committee was set up in 1972, comprising representatives of each of the sponsoring agencies (WHO, FAO, the International Bank for Reconstruction and Development and UNDP). As the executing agency, WHO was assigned the task of implementing the programme, which was formally established on 1 January 1974 with its headquarters in Ouagadougou, Upper Volta. The first year of activity was devoted to setting up structures, recruitment and training of staff, setting up infrastructure, purchasing equipment and supplies, complementary surveys and intensification of research. Actual control operations began in February 1975.

A scientific advisory panel was formed, made up of nearly 200 technical and scientific workers, providing a pool of expertise that could be called upon, as necessary, for advice on all aspects of the disease and its control. An ecological panel, comprising a small group of specialists with wide experience in river-basin ecology, the epidemiology of diseases in river basins and the ecological effects of pesticides, was set up by the steering committee to guarantee protection of the environment.

Meeting in Paris in June 1974, the sponsoring agencies, the participating countries and the donors agreed to simplify the management of the programme. A joint coordinating committee was established, headed by an independent chairman and with representatives of the donors, the seven participating governments and the four sponsoring agencies, which was responsible for overseeing the planning and implementation of the programme.

To provide the joint coordinating committee with continuous, independent evaluation of the technical aspects of the programme, WHO formed a scientific and technical advisory committee, composed of 12 members of the scientific advisory panel. The steering committee established an economic development advisory panel to assure continuous review of information on the effect of the programme on economic development.

During 1976 and 1977, phases II and III of the control programme were conducted according to schedule; operations now covered the full project area. The overall administrative responsibility of the programme was transferred from WHO headquarters to the Regional Office for Africa at the beginning of 1977. With the institution of larvicide operations, chemotherapy research was intensified in collaboration with TDR.

A WHO expert committee on the epidemiology of onchocerciasis, which met in 1975, recommended inter alia that better systems be devised and applied for gathering information on the disease and, in view of the importance of both onchocerciasis and other causes of blindness in tropical Africa, that special attention be given to tropical eye diseases in the training of physicians and auxiliaries (*22*).

A consultation held in 1975 selected films, photographs and slides available from WHO, the International Bank for Reconstruction and Development and private collections for use in preparing a film intended for physicians and medical auxiliaries on the epidemiological, entomological and clinical aspects of onchocerciasis.

Trypanosomiasis

African trypanosomiasis (sleeping sickness), estimated at the time to threaten the health of some 35 million people in Africa, was seen as a serious obstacle to the development of 6 million km^2 of fertile land. In the early years of the decade, operational research on the control of human and animal trypanosomiasis was conducted in Kenya within a project financed by the UNDP, with WHO as the executing agency. The use of helicopters for spraying insecticide (dieldrin) in a water-in-oil emulsion was tested. A notable scientific advance made in the course of this project was a simple laboratory test for distinguishing between *Trypanosoma rhodesiense* and *T. brucei* isolated from animals or from members of the Glossina genus without requiring a direct test of infectivity in a human volunteer. Use of this test demonstrated for the first time that not only cattle but also sheep and reedbuck were reservoir hosts of trypanosomes dangerous to man.

The use of aerial spraying continued, with satisfactory results, even in dense thicket. Studies of environmental contamination resulting from the spraying operations showed that there was little danger associated with spraying, as long as the dosages of the active ingredient of dieldrin were kept low.

Efforts to control the disease foundered on the difficulty of maintaining adequate follow-up to operations that were often initiated with overly ambitious targets. With regular medical surveillance, the human reservoir of infection, which is particularly important in the case of *T. gambiense*, can be maintained at a low level; however, early diagnosis is important, as successful treatment at late stages of the disease is difficult. To improve surveillance methods, the Organization supported research on simple diagnostic tests, suitable for field use in rural populations.

By mid-decade, several diagnostic methods were available. In 1975, a parallel evaluation of serological tests was made by seven laboratories on identical samples of sera collected at four African centres. The joint FAO/WHO Expert Committee on African Trypanosomiasis, which met in 1976, concluded that the average cost of surveillance (US$ 0.44 per inhabitant per year) was too high for many countries where the disease was endemic, and the search for cheaper methods remained a priority.

The drugs that were then available for treatment lost much of their effectiveness in the face of a growing number of drug-resistant strains. Research on the chemotherapy of trypanosomiasis addressed the possibility of exploiting the fact that several trypanosomicidal drugs have a particular affinity for the DNA in trypanosome kinetoplasts.

In 1975, as part of the TDR programme, a task force on trypanosomiasis chemotherapy met to define research priorities in order to plan a collaborative programme comprising research on biochemistry, the design of new trypanocides, experimental screening methods for use in vitro and in vivo and clinical trials. By 1977, trials had begun on four therapeutic compounds.

American trypanosomiasis (Chagas disease) was at the time widespread in Central and South America, disabling thousands of people, including young adults, and necessitating hospitalization. Assistance in setting up Chagas disease control programmes was provided to a number of Member States in the Americas, as was support for a comprehensive programme of research on its ecology and epidemiology.

A TDR scientific working group on Chagas disease met in 1977 in collaboration with PAHO to agree on a programme of research on new control methods, including longitudinal epidemiological studies, new chemotherapeutic agents and immunology and vector control.

Leishmaniasis

As the health service infrastructure necessary for detecting leishmaniasis was lacking in most endemic areas, it was almost impossible to assess its importance as a world health problem with any accuracy. *Kala-azar* (visceral leishmaniasis) and mucocutaneous leishmaniasis are killing diseases, often after long periods of disablement and hospitalization. The cutaneous form usually has less severe health effects, although it affects individual well-being, particularly of women in traditional societies for whom it can represent a devaluation of life of the same order as crippling or blindness. It was believed that lack of data on the prevalence of the cutaneous form and its less obvious threat to health explained why, in some countries with a considerable leishmaniasis problem, the efforts made for its control were disappointing and why even drugs for its treatment were often lacking in endemic areas.

During the early years of this decade, research was aimed principally at the immunological aspects of the disease. Strains of human and animal *Leishmania* were identified, maintained and distributed as a service to research laboratories by the International Reference Centre for Leishmaniasis, in Jerusalem, and institutes in Belo Horizonte, Brazil, and Moscow, USSR. In time, the Jerusalem centre took over responsibility for collecting *Leishmania* species. By 1974, improved methods of preservation had been designed and a method for identifying strains on the basis of antigenic characterization of excretion factors had been further refined. By 1975, this centre was able to produce an inoculate that was identical in virulence and free from contamination, allowing preparation of a reference strain for vaccine production. The WHO International Reference Centre for Immunoglobulins, in Lausanne, Switzerland, studied the fundamental aspects of cell-mediated immunity in leishmaniasis.

For studies on pathogenesis, therapy and immunity in leishmaniasis in vitro, WHO provided assistance for finding a reliable experimental model with tissue culture techniques. By 1973, the Liverpool School of Tropical Medicine in England had screened some 180 known and potential antileishmania compounds, and it was expected that this work would provide a stimulus to the development of suitable drugs by pharmaceutical research institutes.

The leishmaniasis research programme was reviewed by a TDR-administered scientific working group in late 1977, which concluded that the public health importance of leishmaniasis had been underestimated and decided to initiate programmes to obtain better information on its distribution and prevalence. Moreover, leishmaniasis was considered to be a valuable model for studying the principles of host defence mechanisms, particularly macrophage action.

EXPANDED PROGRAMME ON IMMUNIZATION

The Director-General, in his introduction to *The work of WHO* for 1971, noted that the success of the global smallpox eradication programme was a striking example of what can be done. Similar results could be obtained in the control of measles, whooping cough, diphtheria and poliomyelitis (*23*). The idea of building on the success of the smallpox eradication campaign had been discussed informally during the International Conference on the Application of Vaccines against Viral, Rickettsial, and Bacterial Diseases of Man, sponsored by PAHO in December 1970, which was attended by leading vaccine specialists, epidemiologists, public health officials and immunization managers from around the world (*24*).

WHO initiated the Expanded Programme on Immunization (EPI) in 1973. The programme and budget statement for 1975 (*25*) mentioned that "Immunization is the most effective and rapidly applicable measure of preventive medicine available to health authorities". Resolution WHA27.57, adopted in 1974, called on Member States to "develop or maintain immunization and surveillance programmes against some or all of the following diseases: diphtheria, pertussis, tetanus, measles, poliomyelitis, tuberculosis, smallpox and others, where applicable" and requested WHO to collaborate closely with governments in setting up their programmes, in mobilizing efforts to make quality vaccines and other equipment and supplies available to meet country needs, to support educational and research activities and to establish a special account under the Voluntary Fund for Health Promotion.

The Joint UNICEF/WHO Committee on Health Policy discussed the EPI in 1975 and agreed that both WHO and UNICEF should renew their interest and double their efforts in assisting countries in extending immunization to their children (*26*).

Discussions during the Twenty-ninth World Health Assembly, while supporting the idea of building the EPI on the success of the smallpox eradication campaign, brought to light some of the constraints and problems that the new programme would face. To begin with, as stressed by the delegate of the United States, national plans "must include measures for the acceptance of full financial responsibility by the countries themselves as quickly as possible", a position supported by the USSR delegate, who also noted that the discussion had shown that there was a "whole series of unsolved problems" (*27*). These included the need for vaccines suitable for use in tropical countries, the difficulty of ensuring timely transport, dependence on other countries to make needed supplies and equipment available, and the difficulty of maintaining a continuous programme for an indeterminate time.

At the conclusion of the Health Assembly discussion, the representative of the Executive Board reported that the Board

> considered that it was the responsibility of WHO to stimulate the interest of Member States in the immunization programme …. It was for the countries concerned to decide on their own national programmes …. It was for the government concerned, as well as for the public health administration, to decide on a programme and to afford it a high priority. A detailed plan should be drawn up for the immunization of all children, starting with the most vulnerable groups, and it should be based on existing health services, taking into account particularly the development of maternal and child health and primary health services. (*27*)

The Health Assembly went on to adopt resolution WHA29.63, which commended the Director-General's intention to merge the smallpox eradication programme and EPI, recommended that research be conducted to evaluate the effectiveness of vaccination in countries with different climatic and socioeconomic conditions, and to find qualitatively new, more effective, heat-stable vaccines.

The Director-General, reporting on the outcome of the Twenty-ninth World Health Assembly to the Executive Director of UNICEF, said that "without your active cooperation we cannot promote the Programme with the success that it requires since your experience constitutes a major asset in the planning and management of operations, as well as in the supply and distribution of vaccines and other equipment." (letter dated 19 August 1976). Shortly thereafter, the Director-General proposed that "UNICEF take full responsibility for the provision of vaccine for the Programme ... EPI should preferably be part of UNICEF's 'social package' or of primary health care activities but only exceptionally develop as a programme per se." (note for the record of the Director General's discussion with Mr Heyward and Mr Egger, UNICEF, New York, 20 October 1976).

As approved in resolution WHA30.53, adopted in 1977, the programme objectives were to immunize all children of the world by 1990, particularly against diphtheria, pertussis, tetanus, measles, poliomyelitis and tuberculosis, and to reduce morbidity and mortality from other selected diseases of public health importance for which safe and effective vaccines currently exist or become available.

The initial activities, supported by UNICEF, UNDP and several bilateral funding sources, included establishing a focus for programme activities in each regional office, running training seminars and assisting national programmes in planning, implementation and evaluation.

In 1977, priority was given to regional and global plans to serve as the foundation for activities under the Sixth General Programme of Work. The plans included promotion of research to improve the quality and stability of vaccines and to improve cold chains and the logistics of supplies, equipment and vaccines.

BACTERIAL AND VIRAL DISEASES

Cholera control and emergence of the Diarrhoeal Diseases Control Programme

In 1970–1971, the seventh pandemic of cholera occurred, which affected some 40 countries, mainly in Africa and the Middle East, many of which had not been touched for decades.

Some governments chose not to notify the presence of cholera, which probably contributed significantly to its spread in the latter part of 1970. WHO was inundated with requests for supplies for cholera control, particularly for intravenous fluid, which was the mainstay of treatment at the time.

WHO hurriedly put together a paper entitled *Principles and practice of cholera control* (*28*), which had chapters on various aspects of cholera as well as a concise review intended "especially for those areas where cholera has been unknown for many decades and where the approach or the appearance of the disease would confront the health authorities with unfamiliar problems". Knowledge about cholera had expanded to a remarkable degree during the pandemic that had started in Indonesia in 1961. The paper highlighted the search for more effective therapy, fuller understanding of the pathogenesis and pathophysiology of the disease, the use of animal models for studying immunity, a critical assessment of the vaccines presently available, and the prevalence and importance of the carrier state.

The most dramatic development described in this publication was the use of oral rehydration therapy. Oral hydration had been studied in the 1960s, and, while some of the results were promising, there was still uncertainty about its safety; some paediatricians actively resisted its use on these grounds. As evidence mounted of its effectiveness and acceptance, WHO promoted its use more widely and encouraged countries to produce packets of oral rehydration salts locally and ensure expertise in their safe use. In effect, oral rehydration therapy was taken out of the research wards of hospitals and made a household remedy. 'Crash' training courses were organized and special guidelines prepared on its use.

A pharmaceutical firm in Geneva was engaged to produce packets of oral rehydration salts, which WHO then purchased in bulk and sent to countries. Recognizing that the cost of producing oral rehydration salts in Switzerland was too high, WHO sought the assistance of UNICEF to procure packets of salts of good quality at a reasonable price. UNICEF responded with enthusiasm. The availability of cheap packets of salts made it easier for national health workers to use and gain experience and confidence. A field trial in the Philippines demonstrated that peripheral health workers could (after a brief training) treat acute diarrhoea in children under 5 years of age. The results of this and other experiences were incorporated in guidelines that emerged in 1976 as a booklet entitled *Treatment and prevention of dehydration in diarrhoeal diseases* (*29*).

The Thirty-first World Health Assembly, in resolution WHA31.44, endorsed the priority accorded to this problem in WHO's Sixth General Programme of Work and noted the action already taken by the Organization to launch a major attack on diarrhoeal diseases. Later in 1978, WHO launched a global diarrhoeal diseases control programme in collaboration with UNICEF, UNDP and the World Bank.

Throughout this period, WHO continued to promote the search for improved cholera vaccines, by supporting research on cholera immunology in laboratories in various countries, including controlled vaccine field trials in the Philippines, with support from Japan. A consultation held in 1971 concluded that there was no immediate prospect of improving upon the then available vaccine, which was of limited efficacy. Various cost–benefit analyses had shown that improved sanitation was more effective than immunization in preventing diarrhoeal diseases. Emphasis continued to be laid on long-term planning for cholera control through improved sanitation, a message that was widely promoted in inter-regional seminars and training courses.

In 1973, after extensive visits to gather information on the efficacy of various cholera control measures, a consultation was held to help the Organization set up an expanded programme, with the ultimate aim of wider surveillance and more effective control of cholera and other acute diarrhoeal diseases. The basis of the programme was the early detection of outbreaks in rural areas, particularly by persons such as village headmen, religious and community leaders and teachers, so that medical staff and auxiliaries could institute treatment promptly and apply appropriate control measures. In the following year, to provide a firm basis for appropriate diagnostic services, WHO published a brief volume entitled *Guidelines for the laboratory diagnosis of cholera* (*30*).

In 1977, interdisciplinary working groups on diarrhoeal diseases were created at head-quarters and in the regional offices, which promoted oral rehydration as part of primary health care in the management of dehydration associated with diarrhoea. This was the fore-runner of the global programme described above.

Other acute bacterial diseases

Technical cooperation with developing countries for the diagnosis and control of other acute bacterial diseases with high morbidity and mortality (pertussis, tetanus, diphtheria, cerebrospinal meningitis, other coccal infections and plague) gradually improved during the decade. WHO collaborating centres continued to assist in the preparation of simplified guidelines for the diagnosis and treatment of these diseases, as well as in field research and reference work.

The control of tetanus, pertussis and diphtheria was strengthened by the promotion of immunization programmes, while research to improve the vaccines used continued. WHO collaborating centres assisted in the quality control of diphtheria and tetanus toxoids and other combined vaccines by testing national products. These diseases were included in the expanded programme on immunization (see above).

Support was provided for the development and testing of live oral vaccine against *typhoid fever* and to immunological studies on local intestinal immunity. A controlled field trial of killed oral typhoid vaccine in India was completed in 1969, and vaccine trials in the following years showed promising results. Killed oral typhoid vaccines were tested in field trials in India and Chile later in the decade but were not found to be effective.

Growing concern with resistance of enterobacteria and related organisms to antibiotics led to a WHO meeting on the subject in October 1977. The participants reviewed methods for surveying resistance and recommended simple methods, the use of which would generate internationally comparable data (*31*).

An international study of live and killed *plague* vaccines was initiated in 1969, with participating laboratories in India, the United States and the USSR. At its meeting in October 1969, the expert committee on plague reviewed its position regarding natural foci of plague, control and research. It emphasized the importance of surveillance of plague foci, which are spread throughout the world. Concerning the control of plague, the committee noted that rodent and insect control was by far the most effective measure, vaccination being of secondary importance. WHO provided assistance for studies of plague and its control in Burma, Indonesia and Viet Nam. In the Americas, assistance was provided for investigating the epidemiological and ecological factors that contribute to the maintenance of plague foci and to the occurrence of epizootics.

A controlled field trial of two *meningococcal meningitis* vaccines was initiated in 1967 in Upper Volta. Further laboratory and field studies of vaccines were sponsored by WHO in Nigeria and Senegal. The initial results, reported in 1971, indicated that the vaccine had not prevented the spread of infection in the trial population. Encouraging results were reported, however, after large-scale controlled trails coordinated by the Organization and carried out in Egypt (1972) and Sudan (1973). The results of these and other vaccine trials were reviewed by a study group that met in 1975, which also discussed other aspects of the disease and its control. The need for further research became evident; for instance, disagreement among laboratories indicated that improved strain testing was needed, and better understanding was required about which strains were particularly virulent. The possibility of developing other types of immunizing agent and live attenuated vaccines should be explored. Although field trials had been conducted, the efficacy of vaccines in infants and young children had still not been proven (*32*).

An international cooperative study to compare the incidence and epidemiological patterns of *streptococcal* and *staphylococcal* infections was carried out in areas with different ecological situations. A further aim was to establish effective control systems for these infections. A study was conducted in Nigeria of the prevalence of streptococcal infections and their sequelae, particularly rheumatic fever and rheumatic heart disease.

Leprosy

The priorities of the WHO leprosy control programme reflected the recommendations made in 1965 by the expert committee on leprosy: treatment of infectious cases, surveillance of their contacts and release from control of tuberculoid and indeterminate patients who had already completed the required period of disease inactivity and treatment. Training of national personnel in these methods continued to be an important part of WHO's work throughout this period. Some 24 countries were assisted.

The expert committee met again in June 1970 and recommended that regular treatment of lepromatous and borderline patients should be continued for at least 10 years after inactivity of the disease had been achieved, before they were released from control. It also stressed the importance of integrating leprosy control into national general health services.

To make leprosy control more effective, plans were drawn up in 1974 to permit joint leprosy and tuberculosis control programmes. By late 1976, when the expert committee on leprosy met again, it had become clear that the strategy had major shortcomings, including the difficulty of determining when infectious cases had been cured. Research was proposed, in the hope that it would yield improved methods for controlling leprosy (*33*).

WHO had started to intensify its leprosy research programme in the late 1960s, emphasizing those fields in which rapid improvement in leprosy control could be expected, such as the possibility of preventing leprosy by means of vaccination with BCG, trials of new chemotherapeutic agents, improved means for cultivation of *Mycobacterium lepra* in vitro

and improving the diagnostic value of lepromin, an extract of human tissue infected with
M. leprae. The possibility of preventing leprosy by means of BCG vaccination was suggested in a research project in Burma in 1964. By 1973, however, it had become clear that
the slight benefit that had been realized did not justify general use of this vaccine.

Diaphenylsulfone (Dapsone®) continued to be the drug of choice during the early
years of this decade. Studies were nevertheless undertaken with other drugs, including
rifampicin, clofazimine and thalidomide, and studies of the skin reaction induced by lepromin continued.

In several WHO collaborative research projects, *M. leprae* was transmitted to animals
(mostly mice) to assess their suitability as experimental models. In 1972, a major development occurred: the finding that the nine-banded armadillo offered considerable promise as
an animal model for leprosy transmission. Furthermore, use of this animal would allow
production of *M. leprae* in large quantities. Leprosy was therefore included in the TDR (see
Chapter 5), and, for the first time, a WHO-coordinated research strategy was formulated,
with three main objectives: designing a skin test for detecting subclinical infection, making
a specific antileprosy vaccine and devising immunotherapy methods.

In 1977, TDR funded 24 immunology projects in 11 countries and 21 chemotherapy
projects in 9 countries.

Tuberculosis and other respiratory infections

The WHO tuberculosis programme began as a vertical, stand-alone programme, with
control approaches used in industrialized countries. By the late 1950s, it had become clear
that this approach was not working in developing countries, and new directions were sought.
A series of studies supported by the Indian Government, WHO and the British Medical
Research Council in two Indian institutions (the Tuberculosis Chemotherapy Centre in
Madras and the National Tuberculosis Institute in Bangalore) provided the basis for integrating tuberculosis programmes into general health services. The results indicated the
efficacy of home treatment with intermittent regimens and showed that most cases of
tuberculosis could be diagnosed by bacteriological examination of patients with respiratory
symptoms attending general health services.

These findings provided the basis for a new strategy, which was presented at the eighth
session of the Expert Committee on Tuberculosis that met in 1964. The Committee reported
that "specific tools now available for preventing and curing tuberculosis make it possible
to plan and execute effective antituberculosis programmes under practically any epidemiological or socioeconomic conditions." (*34*) To this end, WHO provided assistance to nearly
60 countries, covering all aspects of tuberculosis control, including vaccination with BCG,
case finding and treatment.

At its ninth session, in December 1973, the Expert Committee reaffirmed the direction
set out. The national programme "must be country-wide", "permanent", "adapted to the
expressed demands of the population" and "integrated in the community health structure" (*35*). WHO continued to give priority to direct BCG vaccination, ambulatory treatment
of bacteriologically confirmed cases and the promotion of standardized, operationally simplified methods and techniques.

In a two-page review of WHO's efforts to promote research (*36*), which was part of a larger report prepared for the fifty-third meeting of the Executive Board on the subject 'Interrelationships between the central technical services of WHO and programmes of direct assistance to Member States', the Indian experience was categorized as "the cornerstone of an entirely renewed tuberculosis control policy of worldwide relevance", which called for "central direction and the concentration at the central level of a core of scientists with the required degree of knowledge and experience, able to effectuate under the guidance of high-level advisory groups, the synthesis of multiple contemporary research endeavours and trends in biology, medicine and public health practice." This positive review of the project in India was followed by a less favourable assessment of subsequent research, which, as discussed in Chapter 5, was contributing to isolation of research stimulated at headquarters from the regional programmes of direct assistance to governments. The tuberculosis projects were characterized as "a vast array of individual 'research projects'".

The results of two WHO-assisted 5-year prospective studies revealed that there was no scientific basis for the common practice of giving BCG-vaccinated children regular tuberculin tests to decide on the need for revaccination. The tuberculin test itself reinforces sensitivity to a further test, and therefore regular testing cannot reveal whether sensitivity has really waned. A major concern during this period remained the perfection of BCG production techniques to ensure that sufficient vaccine of adequate quality was available when needed.

WHO-assisted studies showed that microscopic examination of sputum samples from persons seeking help for persistent symptoms yielded a high proportion of positive results, and that auxiliary personnel in peripheral health units could reasonably be expected to undertake sputum microscopy in addition to their routine work, thus making reliable diagnosis of tuberculosis available to the population covered by basic health services.

WHO also provided assistance for investigations of the efficacy and applicability of various chemotherapeutic regimens at a number of institutions in developing and developed countries. To identify regimens that provided maximum benefits for minimum expenditure in personnel, time and money, studies were undertaken to determine to what extent the duration of treatment and the initial intensive phase could be shortened and whether interim treatment could be provided with a longer interval between doses.

Regional teaching and training programmes were used to demonstrate methods of tuberculosis control under socioeconomic, cultural and administrative conditions similar to those in the trainees' countries.

Sexually transmitted diseases and endemic treponematoses

Once the prevalence of clinically active *yaws*, *pinta* and endemic *syphilis* had been decreased dramatically as a result of mass campaigns supported by UNICEF and WHO and community-wide application of long-acting penicillin, WHO initiated studies on the extent of continued low-level transmission of infection and the potential recrudescence of endemic *treponematoses*. These studies confirmed that the incidence had dropped abruptly in areas where the campaign had been conducted, with evidence of continued low-level transmission of infection in a number of areas. Projects were prepared during 1968 to establish whether both the disease and infection could be controlled by intensive environmental measures.

WHO-supported studies brought to light increasing spread of *gonococcal* infection by infected asymptomatic women and evidence that gynaecological complications and sterility resulting from gonorrhoea were becoming more frequent. In the European Region, a pilot surveillance project for all venereal diseases was established in 1969 with the health administrations of France and Sweden with the aim of improving and accelerating epidemiological work, contact- and case-finding and reporting and statistical exploitation of information by modern data processing at national and international levels.

At a meeting held in November 1974 on the role of health education in the control of sexually transmitted diseases, the consequences for the individual and the community of the global increase in gonorrhoea, syphilis and other sexually transmitted diseases was stressed. The seriousness of the problem of gonorrhoea was further emphasized by two groups of scientists convened by WHO in 1975. WHO-assisted research explored the question of to whom, how and where case-finding, preventive and health education activities should be directed in France, India, Nigeria and Senegal.

The aims of the WHO research programme on gonorrhoea were to standardize bacteriological and serological diagnostic methods, making them more sensitive and more reliable; to study the structural and antigenic components and the different biotypes of gonococci; to increase knowledge about host–agent relations; to monitor changes in the sensitivity of the gonococcus to therapeutic agents; and to evaluate and standardize treatment regimens.

The research supported or coordinated by WHO centred on two areas with respect to the treponematoses: the ultrastructure, biochemistry and metabolism of treponemes and the factors necessary for their survival and possible culture; and host–agent interactions, the humoral or cellular basis of immunity and the possibility for specific immunization.

Viral, chlamydial, rickettsial and related diseases

The WHO programme on viral diseases consisted of surveillance, support for laboratory methods for viral diagnosis, support for preventive and control measures and encouraging applied research. These activities were carried out in conjunction with a network of collaborating centres that served as sources of authoritative advice to national virus laboratories and as centres for training virologists in research and in diagnostics. The collaborative centres also provided prototype strains of virus, diagnostic and reference reagents, antigens and cell cultures to selected laboratories in all parts of the world.

At the beginning of the decade, almost all the reference centres were in developed countries. Each had responsibilities for providing technical support in specific areas. In 1973, the Organization extended its work on reagents by establishing a collaborative programme in which several laboratories in developed countries would assist laboratories in developing countries, first by providing small amounts of antigens so that the laboratories could obtain experience and then by helping them to prepare their own antigens.

In 1969, the WHO team for special studies in virology in Africa started working at the East African Virus Research Institute, in Entebbe, Uganda. One of their studies was a detailed investigation of poor serological responses to live *poliovirus* vaccine in children living in warm climates.

With the arrival of the *influenza* season, efforts are mobilized to identify the specific virus strain responsible as early as possible to allow time for the preparation of vaccines. Every year, WHO provided each national centre, of which there were some 80 in 55 countries in 1968, with a complete set of influenza reagents to assist them in identifying strains and to ensure the comparability of results between laboratories. In 1969, the directors of the WHO virus reference centres met to review work and plan the future programme. They agreed that WHO should continue to support the reagents programme, proposing that it be expanded to include animal influenza viruses and their antisera. They also suggested that the Organization find means of obtaining better epidemiological information on influenza and other diseases.

Work on animal strains of influenza viruses led to a rapid increase in information on the antigenic relationship between strains of animal and human origin. As the system of nomenclature used at that time was not designed to show such relations, a group of consultants met in September 1970 to prepare a revised system, which shows not only the antigenic type of ribonucleoprotein (i.e. influenza type A, B or C) but also the character of the haemagglutinin and neuraminidase antigens of A-type strains.

The role of animals in the spread of influenza was reviewed at a consultation in January 1973. By then, it had become apparent that both wild and domestic birds constitute a reservoir of the influenza A virus that circles the world. As many as 15% of sera from 500 domestic ducks in one study in the Western Pacific Region, and in chickens in the Kamchatka Peninsula in the USSR were found to have antibodies to the influenza A virus. By 1975, the prevailing opinion was that birds were the original host and main reservoir of the A type.

A scientific group was convened in September 1975 to review the WHO programme on viral diseases. Like its predecessor, it recommended continuation of the reagents programme and the network of collaborating centres as well as the virus reporting system, which had developed steadily. Furthermore, they recommended that WHO provide more direct assistance to countries, in the form of aid in epidemics, immunization, training to laboratories and support for scientific research.

The WHO scientific group on viral *hepatitis* that met in 1972 recommended that infectious or epidemic hepatitis should be called 'viral hepatitis type A', and serum hepatitis should be called 'viral hepatitis type B'. The first phase of a collaborative study to evaluate a WHO antiserum to detect hepatitis B antigen was completed in 1974 in 27 laboratories in as many countries. An expert committee met in 1976 to review advances in the field of hepatitis A and B.

Outbreaks of *yellow fever* in five West African countries in 1969 led to the establishment of a unit in Abidjan, Côte d'Ivoire, to collect and disseminate information and to assess the nature and possible risk for spread of disease as soon as the first cases occurred. The Organization also trained emergency aid teams that could move into an area immediately on receipt of a request from a government, to provide expert diagnostic services and advice on control measures as well as preliminary supplies of vaccine and insecticides. In March 1971, a WHO expert committee on yellow fever met in Entebbe to review current knowledge of the disease in Africa and the Americas and to make recommendations for future action and research. WHO assisted national laboratories in strengthening their capabilities for yellow fever surveillance. The use of viscerotomes was encouraged, and these were made available to the offices of WHO representatives and stockpiled for use in emergency situations at the centre in Abidjan.

Owing to the increasing threat of yellow fever, the programme for surveillance of *dengue haemorrhagic fever*, yellow fever and *Ae. aegypti* in the Americas was strengthened by the establishment in 1975 of a scientific advisory committee covering all three areas, which replaced the former committee concerned with dengue only. To coordinate surveillance and control measures, a technical advisory committee on dengue in the South-East Asia and Western Pacific regions was created in 1974, which prepared guidelines for the diagnosis, treatment and control of the disease and outlined the fields in which applied research was required.

WHO assisted the Republic of Korea in planning and organizing a trial of inactivated *Japanese encephalitis* virus vaccine.

Lassa fever virus was first isolated in north-eastern Nigeria in 1969, and outbreaks of the disease continued in subsequent years. Its rapid spread led WHO in 1972 to initiate a serological survey in West Africa to ascertain its geographical extent and real prevalence, including subclinical cases. A new virus, *Ebola* virus, resembling Marburg virus, was characterized in high-security laboratories after dramatic outbreaks in Sudan and northern Zaire. WHO staff members and consultants were sent to the sites of the outbreaks as part of WHO emergency aid in epidemics.

One approach to the control of disease-carrying insect vectors is to use viruses that are pathogenic for them. In order to ascertain the safety of insect viruses, the Organization prepared the antigens necessary for conducting serological surveys in populations that had been or might be exposed heavily to such viruses, in order to determine the degree of human and animal infection they might cause.

Chlamydiae were increasingly recognized as agents of sexually transmitted diseases. An outline of recommended criteria for their laboratory diagnosis was published in 1976.

Louse-borne typhus remained endemic in parts of the highlands of Africa and South America. Continued support was given to strengthening facilities for epidemiological and laboratory surveillance of louse-borne typhus and other rickettsial infections in the Andean region. In Bolivia, a trial of attenuated typhus E strain vaccine was completed during 1975.

VETERINARY PUBLIC HEALTH

The work of WHO in veterinary public health started with a few major zoonoses, and food hygiene, rabies and brucellosis were discussed first by the Health Assembly in 1948. In the late 1950s, comparative medicine was added when the WHO programme on chronic degenerative diseases was expanded and the programme of medical research enlarged. Although more than 150 infections were recognized as zoonoses in the 1970s, the WHO programme focused on a few that were important hazards to human health, some also being of major economic importance. These were: rabies, brucellosis, animal tuberculosis, leptospirosis, echinococcosis (hydatidosis), taeniasis–cysticercosis, toxoplasmosis, viral encephalitides and psittacosis–ornithosis. Emerging zoonoses, such as animal influenzas and Marburg disease, were also studied for their scientific and potential epidemiological interest.

The Twenty-second World Health Assembly, in 1969, asked the Director-General (resolution WHA22.35) to consult with the Director-General of FAO about finding a method and criteria that could be used by Member States in surveillance and evaluation of zoonoses control programmes, in which their economic importance would be evaluated. WHO and FAO therefore convened a small group of consultants to plan pilot studies in selected areas. They concluded that the substantial expense involved (for example, US$ 250 000–300 000 for a study restricted to the economic consequences of trichinosis in swine alone) could be justified only when the results were to be used to select the most suitable methods for effective control of the disease. The Executive Board, in resolution EB49.R11 on the subject in January 1972, recognized that such studies "would entail substantial expense, unless carried out in countries or institutions already engaged in related work on zoonoses". The Director-General was asked to maintain an "active interest" in the studies and to provide assistance "within the available financial resources".

Most requests for assistance in the field of veterinary public health came from countries in the Americas, because of the long-established interest of PAHO in this field and the important role of the animal industry in the economy of the region. Requests for assistance fell into three main categories: zoonoses control, food hygiene and veterinary public health education. The requests for assistance in controlling zoonoses mostly concerned the surveillance and control of rabies and brucellosis. Requests for assistance in food hygiene were for studies on the microbiological aspects of food control, both hygienic and technological; hygiene standards and related laboratory methods; natural toxicants in food, especially fish; food legislation and administration; and the strengthening of food hygiene services, especially laboratory services. Education and training received high priority in WHO, the main aim being to provide training in veterinary public health and its component subjects at the postgraduate level. Attention was also paid to training auxiliary personnel.

In the WHO programme on rabies, considerable attention was given to solving difficulties in diagnosis and field control, but emphasis was also laid on the immunization of humans and animals and post-exposure treatment. At its sixth meeting, in December 1972, the expert committee on rabies summarized what was known about rabies and recommended that research be undertaken or intensified on a vaccine, on pathogenesis and immunity, on diagnosis and on the ecology and control of rabies in wildlife (*37*). In 1975, the results of field trials with the human diploid cell rabies vaccine were reviewed at a WHO consultation held at the Pasteur Institute of Iran, Teheran.

One of the most important problems in brucellosis is controlling infection in sheep and goats and preventing virulent *B. melitensis* infection in man. As the test-and-slaughter method is not applicable in countries where sheep and goats are the main asset of rural or nomadic people, the coordinated research programme devoted much attention to immunization of these animals and of humans. Attempts were also made to use the available diagnostic and vaccination procedures to reduce the rate of animal infection in highly endemic areas to a level at which the more radical test-and-slaughter policy would become feasible. Efforts were made to standardize antigens for humans and animals and the procedures for skin tests.

The epidemiology of leptospirosis was improved through WHO-coordinated research and a network of WHO/FAO reference centres that provided standardized reagents and provided assistance in identifying serotypes, carrying out epidemiological investigations, preparing vaccines and training personnel. Considerable improvements were made in diagnostic methods, such as the demonstration of leptospirosis by immunofluorescence, isolation by direct culture in suitable media and application of sensitive serological techniques. Other zoonoses dealt with in the WHO programme included hydatidosis, trichinosis, toxoplasmosis and animal tuberculosis.

The programme was reviewed by the Executive Board in January 1973. Possible lines for future development included increasing field activities in regions other than the Americas, where the programme was already well developed, undertaking surveys in groups of countries with similar types of husbandry and a clear description of the steps necessary for dealing with problems, on a regional basis where possible. A joint FAO/WHO expert committee on veterinary public health met in late 1974 to define the functions of public health veterinarians in the control of zoonoses, food hygiene, environmental health, comparative medicine and other, related disciplines.

Food hygiene is concerned with the conditions and methods of food production, processing, storage and distribution and aims at ensuring safe, wholesome products that are fit for human consumption. The WHO programme concentrated on foodborne infections and intoxications and hygienic standards, especially from the microbiological point of view. All measures, such as surveillance, investigation and reporting, that could be used to protect humans against foodborne diseases were included in the programme. The importance of uniform laboratory methods for food examination and simplified techniques for use in developing countries was stressed. WHO, in cooperation with the International Commission on Microbiological Specifications for Foods of the International Association of Microbiological Societies, promoted studies on standardization of methods, interpretation of the significance of microorganisms in food and plans for sampling the most important food items in international trade.

Comparative medicine remained an essential element of the Organization's general veterinary public health activities, as findings obtained in animal models can have significant applications for human disease. The WHO/FAO programme on comparative virology, for example, involved 135 laboratories organized in 16 teams, each team being responsible for a distinct group of animal viruses.

In 1976, the programme on the ecology of influenza viruses in animals and their relation to human influenza was expanded. A number of new strains of influenza virus with new properties were isolated from a large number of bird species. In some areas, up to 5% of apparently normal migrating birds were found to be carrying the virus. Some strains isolated from these birds were indistinguishable from human strains of Victoria/75 (H3N2).

VECTOR BIOLOGY AND CONTROL

The vector biology and control programme, like those for epidemiological surveillance and TDR, was considered a 'support' programme (*38*). Its objective was to provide advice and assistance to Member States on the ecology, biology and control of the arthropod vectors and mammalian reservoirs of human diseases, ensuring the safety to humans and the environment of any control measures that were recommended. The approach used involved supporting and coordinating research through a network of international reference centres and collaborating laboratories, direct studies by regional offices, direct investigations by WHO research units and establishing standard procedures, performing surveys and acting as a clearing house for information.

Resistance of vectors and pathogen reservoirs to pesticides

The Organization carried out investigations on the biochemical, physiological and genetic mechanisms of resistance, including cross-resistance and multiple resistance. By the 1970s, some 20 standard methods for determining the susceptibility or resistance of major vector species to insecticides and of rodents to rodenticides had been developed. Data collected in the field were stored in computers, and relevant information was widely distributed through a quarterly, *Information circular on insecticide resistance, insect behaviour and vector genetics*, which was reviewed by expert committees on insecticides and summarized in reports. A monograph on insecticide resistance of arthropods, issued in 1958, was reviewed and updated in 1971 (*39*).

Resistance testing by the Organization led to the conclusion, in 1968, that the number of resistant species had grown significantly in recent years. By 1973, the results of more than 8000 susceptibility tests had been accumulated, of which some 850 were computerized. They indicated that 61 species had developed resistance to DDT, of which 19 were anophelines, while 91 species (39 anophelines) had developed resistance to dieldrin.

The Expert Committee on Insecticides, meeting in 1975, confirmed that in the 7 years since it had last considered the subject, 10 new vector species and a new family, the reduviids, vectors of Chagas disease, had developed resistance. More than 100 vector species had been reported to be resistant, and this number was increasing every year. Evidence had accumulated to show that "resistance has been caused as a side effect of agricultural pesticide usage" (*40*). Despite the harmful effects of resistance, the Committee emphasized that all the evidence showed that "vector control was likely to depend on substantial, continued use of pesticides for at least a decade". The Committee recommended that WHO continue to encourage, stimulate and wherever possible support research on the fundamental aspects of resistance. These studies should include quantitative studies on factors that influence the rate of development of resistance in vector control programmes; further studies on mechanisms of resistance; and studies on resistance in field populations of important vector species.

Recognizing the serious impact of resistance on many programmes, the Committee emphasized the importance of thorough initial and reorientation training in detecting resistance for all staff engaged in vector control. The coverage by the quarterly *Information circular*

was "too complex and technical to be of benefit to those in charge of field control operations"; what was needed was a document in "simple language explaining the basic facts of
resistance, its detection, and methods for coping with it." It also suggested that WHO should
prepare another circular for nontechnical administrators and intermediate supervisory staff,
describing important developments in vector control techniques.

The Committee paid considerable attention to the role of heavy, regular application of
pesticides in inducing resistance. It recommended that the existing collaboration between
WHO and FAO be used to advise Member governments to monitor the import, manufacture,
marketing and use of all pesticides, so that warnings could be given of possible future
resistance. Whenever possible, regulations should be introduced to control the entry and
use of such pesticides.

Testing and evaluation of new pesticides

A collaborative programme for testing and evaluating insecticides for use in malaria
eradication was begun in 1960. It was later expanded to include tests of new compounds
against other vectors. By the 1970s, six WHO collaborating centres and more than 40 insecticide manufacturers were involved in screening new compounds for insecticidal activity
and their safety for humans. The 150–200 new compounds that had been evaluated each
year 10–20 years earlier had, however, been reduced to only 10–20 new candidates per year.

Each candidate compound was subjected to a series of evaluation stages, each succeeding
stage posing more stringent criteria of safety and effectiveness. Particular attention was
given to the biodegradability of the compounds, their effects on aquatic and other forms of
life and their persistence in the environment. The programme was reorganized at the end
of 1977 to allow more rapid evaluation of new pesticides. Also, compounds already in the
scheme were re-evaluated in new types of formulations for malaria control and for the
control of other vectors, especially *Simulim* and *Glossina*.

Safe use of pesticides

The topic of the safe use of pesticides grew in importance in public health and agriculture
during this decade. WHO undertook research on the inherent toxicity of compounds to
humans and animal, their mode of action and routes of absorption, methods to determine
the degree of absorption and protective measures to reduce exposure to pesticides. Close
collaboration was maintained with FAO concerning the large-scale use of pesticides in
agriculture.

The Expert Committee on Insecticides, meeting in late 1972, reviewed the use of insecticides, molluscicides and rodenticides in public health and the health aspects of pesticides
not directly associated with vector control (*41*). The Committee stressed the importance of
international organizations working together, "particularly in education and training, in
those countries where the use of pesticides for economic reasons has outstripped the present
capacity of the authorities to cover the safety aspects adequately."

Discussions were initiated in 1973 with agricultural organizations and the chemical
industry to promote studies on minimum acceptable safety measures for agricultural

application of pesticides of moderate or high mammalian toxicity. In 1973, steps were taken to expand the scope of the programme, to assess the overall environmental effects of pest control, whether for public health or other purposes. Data on pesticide poisoning began to be collected that year. Investigations on the possible effects of long-term exposure to DDT continued in both Brazil and India.

With the International Agency for Research on Cancer, WHO extended the toxicological investigation of new pesticides to include testing for possible mutagenicity and carcinogenicity.

Specifications for pesticides and equipment for vector control

Specifications for new insecticides are drawn up concurrently with their evaluation in the later stages of testing. The first edition of *Specifications for pesticides used in public health*, designed to provide both the manufacturer and the purchaser with a set of specifications for meeting the requirements of public health programmes, was published in 1956; a second edition appeared in 1961. The recommendations of the WHO Expert Committee on Pesticides, meeting in 1963, concerning the equipment used to apply and disperse pesticides, were published in 1964, with a second edition in 1974 (*42*). With FAO, a comprehensive registry of equipment suitable for use in vector control operations was established in 1975 (*43*).

Emergency operations

The most promising rapid method for control of adult mosquito populations was ultra-low-volume application of insecticide by aircraft. Early field trials carried out by the Aedes Research Unit in Bangkok, Thailand, with malathion gave positive results and led to larger trials in other areas.

Given the difficulty of finding pilots specially trained in making ultra-low-volume applications or suitably equipped aircraft at short notice, trials were undertaken with ground equipment for applying non-thermal ultra-low-volume fogs of insecticides. The outbreak of yellow fever in West Africa and the demonstration that insecticidal fogs were applicable against epidemics in towns and villages led to the purchase and storage of equipment and insecticides where they were rapidly accessible.

The WHO Vector and Rodent Control Research Unit in Jakarta, Indonesia, initiated and supervised ultra-low-volume aerial application of insecticides for the control of mosquito vectors in a severe outbreak of dengue haemorrhagic fever in Java in 1973.

Emergency assistance was also provided in cases of foodstuffs contaminated by insecticides.

Applied ecology

Field investigations of various vectors in a range of climatic zones were pursued to determine the population dynamics and ecological features important for their chemical, biological and genetic control. Thus, studies were conducted on *Ae. aegypti* in West Africa, India and Indonesia, on *C. tritaeniorhynchus* in Indonesia and the Republic of Korea, on *C.p. fatigans* in India and Indonesia, on *An. gambiae* and *An. funestus* in tropical Africa, on *An. stephensi* in India and on *An. aconitus* in Indonesia.

The scientific group on vector ecology that met in 1971 stressed the importance of understanding the basic mechanisms that underlie the abundance of vectors in relation to the development of resistance and the "disturbing accumulation of chemicals in the environment" (*44*). It reviewed existing approaches for collecting data and outlined surveillance techniques for the major vectors of disease.

During 1973, ecological study of vertebrate (especially mammalian) reservoirs of disease was intensified. Methods were found to analyse the population structures and densities of vertebrates, their role in disease transmission and the appropriate means for their control.

A scientific group on the ecology and control of rodents of public health importance, which met in late 1973, summarized current knowledge in the field. They found that effective use had not been made of various improvements in rodent control achieved during the previous two decades. Also, information about the effectiveness of various control techniques was deficient. The recommendations covered information needs, studies to be undertaken, pilot schemes for control and continued collaboration with FAO in this area (*45*).

The WHO Arbovirus Vector Research Unit in Enugu, Nigeria, carried out ecological studies on several *Aedes* species known to be vectors of yellow fever and other important arboviruses. Research was extended in 1975 to other parts of Nigeria to obtain information on the distribution of mosquitos in different ecological areas. These studies were coordinated with similar work by the Office de la Recherche scientific et technique outre-mer (ORSTOM) in Côte d'Ivoire and Upper Volta, the Pasteur Institute, Bangui, Central African Republic, and other research groups to ensure that the findings were comparable and to paint a comprehensive picture of the ecology of virus vectors in this part of Africa. In 1976, dengue virus was isolated at the University of Ibadan, Nigeria, from material provided by the Vector Research Unit.

Other investigations still under way at the end of the decade included a study of the vectors of filariasis in Indonesia, Samoa and the United Republic of Tanzania; a study of the ecology of potential reservoirs and vectors of plague in western Java; and a study of possible rodent reservoirs of the newly described Ebola virus following the 1976 epidemic in Sudan and Zaire.

Biological, genetic and environmental control

The placing of severe restrictions on the use of DDT by the United States and other developed countries in 1969 handicapped many programmes in which it was relied upon for disease vector control. Continued use of highly persistent organochlorine insecticides, such as DDT and dieldrin, were recognized threats to the environment. Although the United States delegate to the Twenty-fourth World Health Assembly said that his Government "would limit the availability of DDT to countries where it was used in malaria control",

WHO recognized that substitutes were needed, leading the Organization to search for alternative control methods, chemical or otherwise (*46*).

After the adoption of resolution WHA22.40 in 1969, which requested the Director-General to "stimulate and intensify research on the development of alternative methods of vector control," a report was prepared for consideration by the Twenty-third World Health Assembly, in 1970 (*47*). Noting that the increased resilience of many vectors, due to the development of resistance to insecticides and the destruction of natural enemies, had increased the need for more insecticides in the environment, the report went on to suggest that it had now become "self-evident that the study of the basic ecology of the vectors should have been first undertaken as the essential background for an enlightened choice of the methods for control." Against that background, the report suggested that alternative methods of control, "while they might prove to be more economical in the long run, will certainly be more arduous." It was estimated that an adequate assessment of possible methods would take 5 years.

Five categories of control method were outlined: biological control, involving the use of fish and arthropod predators, insect and helminth parasites and fungal, bacterial or viral diseases of vectors; genetic control, involving the release of males that have been radiosterilized, chemosterilized, are of cytoplasmically incompatible strains, are sterile hybrids, carry genetic translocations or have deleterious genes; traps and attractants; hormones and natural toxins; and environmental sanitation, which more than all the other methods is closely associated with the development and economic status of the country concerned. Resolution WHA23.33 recommended that the proposed plan of work be taken into account in preparing the regular budget for 1972.

A search for biological control methods was initiated during the 1960s but intensified in the early 1970s on the basis of the recommendations of the Health Assembly. A collaborating centre examined diseased or parasitized arthropods sent from the field and, through a network of collaborating laboratories, identified the parasites and pathogens involved. Subsequent studies on the microorganisms or parasites isolated and on their efficacy in controlling diseases were conducted in WHO field research units and collaborating centres. The use of larvivorous fish was explored in several projects.

A major problem encountered with biological methods of control was a lack of uniform, stable microbial cultures and a lack of adequate tests for human and environmental safety. By 1975, priority was being given to entomopathogenic fungi and spore-forming bacteria, which could be produced locally. The vectors seen to be priorities were mosquito species the larval forms of which are amenable to larviciding, as adult insects are usually resistant to insect pathogens.

A 7-year study was launched in 1969 of the feasibility of controlling mosquitos by genetic means; the study was conducted by a research unit in New Delhi, India, jointly sponsored by the Indian Council of Medical Research and WHO. The experiments included control by releasing 'sterile males'. The unit assisted in creating a nucleus of scientists fully conversant with the techniques used.

The first scientific working group on biological control of insect vectors of disease was held in 1977 within TDR. The group reviewed the scheme for isolating and characterizing biological control agents, protocols for safety tests and designs of field trials.

Vector control in international health

Pursuant to a resolution of the Twenty-first World Health Assembly, the Organization provided descriptions and assisted in the design, assembly and testing of a vapour 'disinsection' system for large aircraft. A comprehensive report on aircraft disinsecting with the dichlovos system was prepared in 1973, on the basis of extensive tests carried out in the United States. Its use was approved by the Committee on International Surveillance of Communicable Diseases in 1974, and the Twenty-seventh World Health Assembly, in 1974, approved the report of the Committee that contained a section on vector control in international health.

In 1972, the Organization published a manual entitled *Vector control in international health* (*43*), which was compiled with the help of experts in the fields covered.

Tropical disease research programme

The establishment of the TDR programme is described in Chapter 5. The period 1976–1977 saw completion of the planning phase of the Programme and transition to a preparatory phase of organization and pilot activities, leading to full operation of projects. Scientific working groups were convened for various aspects of each of the diseases included in the Programme and the biological control of disease vectors, as described above. Groups were also established for epidemiology and biomedical sciences, both being cross-disease groups, i.e. oriented towards research on problems common to more than one of the diseases covered by the Programme, such as development of surveillance systems for 'tropical diseases' (epidemiology) and parasite cultivation (biomedical sciences).

Collaboration was sought with the pharmaceutical sector in order to gain access to their expertise in drug and vaccine development and to stimulate their interest in investing in this field. Five types of involvement were foreseen: participation by industry-affiliated scientists in scientific working groups, screening of agents in research projects by laboratories in industry and non-profit institutes, contracts for technical services, clinical evaluation of new drugs and vaccines, and training of scientists and technicians.

The 'research strengthening group' met for the first time in October 1977 to establish the main policy guidelines for four programme objectives: to strengthen research and training institutions, so as to assist tropical countries in setting up the infrastructure necessary to cope with problems related to disease control; to support the training of persons from tropical countries, so that scientists and other research personnel of the highest quality were available to meet manpower needs; to encourage and assist in the diffusion, interpretation and integration of new knowledge, so as to influence health policies and their implementation favourably; and to contribute to the rapid transfer of knowledge, technology and skills to affected countries that were relevant to their health objectives and within the sphere of TDR. Under the aegis of this programme, pilot activities continued in Ndola, Zambia, and were initiated in centres in Nairobi, Kenya; Kuala Lumpur, Malaysia; and Cotonou, Benin (*48*).

A planning consultation on socioeconomic research took place in December 1977. With respect to disease prevention and control, proposals and recommendations were made on behavioural and socioeconomic feasibility; anthropogenic environmental disease and development activities; behavioural, organizational and related issues in disease control; the use of quantitative operational criteria for decision-making to ensure optimal intervention strategies; and decision-making and the economic consequences of vector-borne parasitic diseases.

PREVENTION OF BLINDNESS

A WHO programme for the prevention of blindness, as such, was established only at the end of 1976. Previously, a range of activities, some dating to the early years of WHO's creation, had dealt with various aspects of the problem, particularly trachoma, xerophthalmia, onchocerciasis and cataract. Resolution WHA22.29, adopted in 1971, asked the Director-General to collate the available information on the extent and the causes of preventable and curable blindness and to propose activities that the Organization would carry out within its programme of work. The responses received to requests for information were incomplete, and further analysis was required. A study group was convened in November 1972, which recommended caution in formulating priorities at an international level, giving as its reason the limited resources available and the concern that an international programme would lose its impact if it were too diverse (*49*). The group went on, however, to note the need for concerted international action through an acceptable, effective coordinating mechanism. As a consequence, WHO intensified its contacts with nongovernmental organizations active in the field. In particular, as a result of restructuring and strengthening of the International Agency for the Prevention of Blindness in 1974, greater collaboration between this organization and WHO allowed for considerable expansion of the programme.

WHO continued its activities in specific areas. Thus, for example, trachoma control programmes were reviewed at the nineteenth session of the Joint UNICEF/WHO Committee on Health Policy in 1972, which endorsed the strategy, while recommending that increased support be given to improving methods for the diagnosis, treatment and control of trachoma. Relatively large comparative therapeutic trials were initiated that year to better define the benefits that could result from the use of different schedules of treatment or different antibiotics known to be safe and effective.

Direct WHO support was continued to a number of countries. Advisory services and supplies were provided in the European Region, while an intercountry project on trachoma control was launched in the Eastern Mediterranean Region.

A comprehensive report (*50*) was prepared on vitamin A deficiency and xerophthalmia following a meeting held in November 1974 in collaboration with the United States Agency for International Development on the diagnosis, epidemiology, prevalence, treatment and prevention of xerophthalmia. The report included guidelines for programmes of action and indicated areas in which future research was needed.

Preliminary assessments of the problem of blindness were made in Bangladesh, Burma and India in 1973, in northern Nigeria in 1974 and in Guatemala in 1975. In all these countries, the priorities identified were trachoma, xerophthalmia and onchocerciasis.

The programme established in 1976 for the prevention of blindness was initially intended to address these priorities, as well as cataract, eye injuries and glaucoma. The long-term objective was to introduce adequate eye care and to promote eye health at the peripheral level, especially through health education, intersectoral coordination of activities, promotion of national programmes and mobilization of extrabudgetary resources, in collaboration with other organizations in the field, notably the International Agency for the Prevention of Blindness.

References

1. *Official records of the World Health Organization*, No. 227 (WHA28/SR/A/4). Geneva, World Health Organization, 1975.
2. World Health Organization. *The second ten years of the World Health Organization 1958–1967*. Geneva, 1968.
3. *Sub-Committee on International Quarantine, second meeting. Official records of the World Health Organization*, No. 177. Geneva, World Health Organization, 1969.
4. *Multipurpose serological surveys and WHO serum reference banks. Report of a WHO scientific group* (WHO Technical Report Series, No. 454). Geneva, World Health Organization, 1970.
5. *Smallpox and its eradication*. Geneva, World Health Organization.
6. *Smallpox eradication. Report of a WHO scientific group* (WHO Technical Report Series, No. 393). Geneva, World Health Organization, 1968.
7. *WHO Expert Committee on Smallpox Eradication. Second report* (WHO Technical Report Series, No. 493). Geneva, World Health Organization, 1972.
8. *Integration of mass campaigns against specific diseases into general health services. Report of a WHO study group* (WHO Technical Report Series, No. 294), Geneva, World Health Organization, 1965.
9. *WHO Expert Committee on Malaria. Fifteenth report* (WHO Technical Report Series, No. 467). Geneva, World Health Organization, 1971.
10. *Malaria control in countries where time-limited eradication is impracticable at present. Report of a WHO interregional conference* (WHO Technical Report Series, No. 537). Geneva, World Health Organization, 1974.
11. *WHO Expert Committee on Malaria. Sixteenth report* (WHO Technical Report Series, No. 549). Geneva, World Health Organization, 1974.
12. *Report of the World Health Organization in 1973: analytic summary* (PCO/74.1). New York, United Nations, Economic and Social Council, 1974.
13. *Development of the antimalaria programme: report by the Ad Hoc Committee on Malaria of the Executive Board* (EB57/19, Annex 2). Geneva, World Health Organization, 1976.
14. *Annual report 1977: Scientific working groups on malaria* (TDR/AR(1)/77.2). Geneva, World Health Organization, 1977.
15. *Schistosomiasis control. Report of a WHO expert committee* (WHO Technical Report Series, No. 515). Geneva, World Health Organization, 1973.
16. *Inter-agency consultation on man-made lakes, Geneva, 2–3 July 1968. Record of discussions* (CPD/69/2). Geneva, World Health Organization, 1969.
17. *Official records of the World Health Organization*, No. 224 (EB55/SR/9). Geneva, World Health Organization, 1975.
18. *Schistosomiasis. Report of the Director-General* (A29/18). Geneva, World Health Organization, 1976.

19. *Official records of the World Health Organization*, No. 234 (WHA29/SR/B/14). Geneva, World Health Organization, 1976.

20. *WHO Expert Committee on Filariasis. Third report* (WHO Technical Report Series, No. 542). Geneva, World Health Organization, 1974.

21. *Onchocerciasis control in the Volta River Basin area. Information paper* (OCP/74.1 Rev. 3). Geneva, World Health Organization, 1977.

22. *Epidemiology of onchocerciasis. Report of a WHO expert committee* (WHO Technical Report Series, No. 597). Geneva, World Health Organization, 1976.

23. *Work of WHO 1971. Official records of the World Health Organization*, No. 197. Geneva, World Health Organization, 1971.

24. *International conference on the application of vaccine against viral, rickettsial, and bacterial diseases of man, Washington DC, 1970* (PAHO Scientific Publications, 226). Washington DC, Pan American Health Organization, 1971.

25. *Official records of the World Health Organization*, No. 212, section 5.1. Geneva, World Health Organization, 1975.

26. *Joint UNICEF/WHO Committee on Health Policy. The expanded programme on childhood immunization* (JC20/UNICEF-WHO/75.4). Geneva, World Health Organization, 1975.

27. *Official records of the World Health Organization*, No. 234 (WHA29/SR/A/16). Geneva, World Health Organization, 1976.

28. *Principles and practice of cholera control* (WHO Public Health Paper No. 40). Geneva, World Health Organization, 1970.

29. *Treatment and prevention of dehydration in diarrhoeal diseases: a guide for use at the primary level.* Geneva, World Health Organization, 1976.

30. *Guidelines for the laboratory diagnosis of cholera.* Geneva, World Health Organization, 1974.

31. *Surveillance for the prevention and control of health hazards due to antibiotic-resistant enterobacteria. Report of a WHO meeting* (WHO Technical Report Series, No. 624). Geneva, World Health Organization, 1978.

32. *Cerebrospinal meningitis control. Report of a WHO working group* (WHO Technical Report Series No. 588). Geneva, World Health Organization, 1976.

33. *WHO Expert Committee on Leprosy. Fifth report* (WHO Technical Report Series, No. 607). Geneva, World Health Organization, 1977.

34. *WHO Expert Committee on Tuberculosis. Eighth report* (WHO Technical Report Series, No. 290). Geneva, World Health Organization, 1964.

35. *WHO Expert Committee on Tuberculosis. Ninth report* (WHO Technical Report Series, No. 552). Geneva, World Health Organization, 1974.

36. *Organizational study on the interrelationships between the central services of WHO and programmes of direct assistance to Member States. Official records of the World Health Organization*, No. 223 (EB53/WP/1), Annex 7. Geneva, World Health Organization, 1975.

37. *WHO Expert Committee on Rabies. Sixth report* (WHO Technical Report Series, No. 523). Geneva, World Health Organization, 1973.

38. *Meeting on medium-term programming for communicable disease prevention and control, Alexandria, 23–27 October, 1978* (CD/MTP/78.1). Geneva, World Health Organization, 1978.

39. *Insecticide resistance in arthropods* (WHO Monograph Series, No. 38). Geneva, World Health Organization, 1958.

40. *Resistance of vectors and reservoirs of disease to pesticides. Twenty-second report of the WHO Expert Committee on Insecticides* (WHO Technical Report Series, No. 585). Geneva, World Health Organization, 1976.

41. *Safe use of pesticides. Twentieth report of the WHO Expert Committee on Insecticides* (WHO Technical Report Series, No. 513). Geneva, World Health Organization, 1973.

42. *Equipment for vector control*, 2nd ed., Geneva, World Health Organization, 1974.

43. *Vector control in international health*. Geneva, World Health Organization, 1972.

44. *Vector ecology. Report of a WHO scientific group* (WHO Technical Report Series, No. 501). Geneva, World Health Organization, 1972.

45. *Ecology and control of rodents of public health importance. Report of a WHO scientific group* (WHO Technical Report Series, No. 553). Geneva, World Health Organization, 1974.

46. *Official records of the World Health Organization*, No. 194 (WHA24/SR/A/9). Geneva, World Health Organization, 1971.

47. *Research on alternative methods of vector control. Report by the Director-General. Official records of the World Health Organization*, No. 184, Annex 9. Geneva, World Health Organization, 1970.

48. *Annual report 1977: research capability strengthening working group programme area III* (TDR/AR(1)/77.13). Geneva, World Health Organization, 1977.

49. *The prevention of blindness. Report of a WHO scientific group* (WHO Technical Report Series, No. 518). Geneva, World Health Organization, 1973.

50. *Vitamin A deficiency and xerophthalmia. Report of a joint WHO/United States Agency for International Development meeting* (WHO Technical Report Series, No. 590). Geneva, World Health Organization, 1976.

CHAPTER 10

Prevention and control of noncommunicable diseases

The scope of the programme for the prevention and control of noncommunicable diseases grew during the third decade of WHO's existence, as elements were shifted from other programmes: radiation medicine from environmental health, human genetics and immunology from biomedical sciences, and the health of working populations from organization of health services. Furthermore, a new programme element, 'other chronic diseases', was added. The emphasis remained, however, on applied research, for better understanding of the diseases and to improve preventive and control measures.

MENTAL HEALTH

Under the guidance of Dr Brock Chisholm, WHO's first Director-General, who was a psychiatrist, WHO addressed the subject of mental health early in its history. It was in fact the first international governmental organization to encourage work in this field. In the 1960s, when new forms of therapy became available, the prospect of effective care in the community opened up. As noted in the annual report of 1968, advances in in psychopharmacology and social therapy had changed the face of mental illness, and the mental health services in many countries might require fundamental reorientation (1).

As there were insufficient trained personnel to deal with mental disorders, two approaches were proposed: preparing basic health service staff to work in mental health and promoting psychiatric training as an integral part of the medical curriculum. Field experiences with these approaches were reviewed in 1973 at a WHO seminar, followed in 1974 by a WHO expert committee meeting on the organization of mental health services in developing countries (2). These reviews showed that there were so few staff with specialized mental health skills that services could be extended only by involving others. Furthermore, a general approach to the problem would be unlikely to work, and new types of training should be considered. Specialists should provide both in-service training and supervision of front-line mental health workers. The specialists would first have to be trained in teaching and supervising methods, preferably in their own country or, failing this, in their own culture.

Various studies were undertaken to understand better the epidemiology of different mental disorders, including how they differed from one population to another. In an international study of schizophrenia, for example, initiated in 1967, it was found that internationally applicable and acceptable procedures could be used for assessing psychiatric patients and that the psychopathology of major functional psychoses such as schizophrenia is similar, in spite of vastly different cultural and socioeconomic conditions. Later follow-up revealed that the course and outcome of schizophrenia in developing countries were better than those in richer ones.

The results of this study reflected the general conclusion that the prevalence of mental disorders in developing countries was no less than that in developed ones. The prevalence was high throughout the world, at least 1% of any population being incapacitated by severe mental disorder at any given time and 10% being so affected at some period during their lives.

To give the measurement of mental illness a solid foundation, standardized approaches to psychiatric diagnosis, classification and statistics were promoted. Annual seminars were held on this subject, each devoted to one major group of disorders. The eighth such seminar, in 1972, recommended that particular attention be given to education, including publication of glossaries, reports and teaching manuals; research, which should include new models of classification and further standardization of rating procedures and diagnostic processes; and standardization of statistical reporting.

Reference networks of experts were created, one to monitor the programme, coordinate national research and collate information on advances in psychiatric epidemiology and another to follow advances in standardization of classification and psychiatric diagnosis. A project for monitoring mental health needs was launched in 1976 in seven countries, in which methods for the creation, maintenance and evaluation of a mental health component of national health information systems were devised and tested.

A comparative study of patients with depressive disorders was initiated in 1974 to identify means for assessing depressive conditions in various cultures and to explore the influence of sociocultural factors on the occurrence, course and outcome of these disorders. Similar studies were undertaken on the problems of suicide, drug dependency and alcoholism.

In resolution WHA28.84, the Twenty-eighth World Health Assembly, in 1975, recognized that mental disorders constitute a major public health problem in all parts of the world and noted that effective methods for reducing mental morbidity and its consequences were now available. It asked the Director-General to assist Member States in strengthening the mental health component of their general health services through research on the epidemiology and biology of mental disorders; finding new, effective methods of treatment and control of such disorders; improving the training of personnel in mental health services and research; and improving communication in this field by setting up information systems and standardizing classification and terminology. Although the programme had already been providing similar assistance, the recognition afforded by this resolution reinforced its commitment. One of the key features of the 'new' programme was its commitment to seeking simple, effective methods for treating conditions that were widespread and of major public health importance, such as acute psychoses and chronic psychotic states, as well as conditions the prevalence of which varied among the regions. In addition to recognized psychiatric disorders, the programme also addressed suicide, dependence on alcohol and abusive drug substances, and juvenile delinquency.

New projects were initiated to demonstrate the effectiveness of approaches that had been the subject of recent reviews. In one collaborative study, for example, four developing countries (Colombia, India, Senegal and Sudan) set up services for patients with conditions of high priority, making use of a wide range of health workers. Simple, nontechnical training programmes and manuals were designed and tested, and simple screening methods were designed. By the end of 1977, it was found in all four countries that approximately 15% of all patients seeking health care at the primary level suffered from definite mental disorders, in many cases in combination with physical disorders. It was also shown that even brief training in mental health had a strikingly beneficial effect on the attitudes of health staff towards such disorders, and they were able detect most mental health problems and provide treatment with a limited range of 'essential psychotropic drugs'. An earlier project had shown the advantages of methods for assessing acute psychotic conditions that could be used by rural health workers.

A study on the prevention of suicide was undertaken with the collaboration of experts in several countries, and the results were published in 1968 (3). An investigation was carried out in several European countries with a view to improving the reliability of suicide statistics. The initial results showed that, even in the same country, coroners or their equivalents can give different verdicts on the basis of the same case history of a reported suicide and that the divergences may be sufficiently great to invalidate comparisons of published suicide rates within and between countries. The results of an investigation in 25 countries in all the WHO regions on procedures for ascertaining suicide were published in 1974 (4).

Early in the decade, WHO drew up plans for stimulating national surveys on dependence on alcohol and other drugs. Planning for coordinated services in a number of European countries was initiated in 1970, on the basis of information from those countries, and training courses were conducted in which representatives from countries in other regions participated.

The Twenty-fifth World Health Assembly, in 1972, in its resolution WHA25.62, recognized that the abuse of dependence-producing drugs continued to be a worldwide problem, with serious adverse effects on health. It stated that the Organization had an obligation to provide medical leadership, guidance and technical assistance in the field of drug dependence in the form of education, prevention, treatment and rehabilitation, and to conduct research. The Director-General was asked to explore means of increasing financial support to an expanded programme on drug dependence. The United Nations Fund for Drug Abuse Control provided funds to initiate several projects.

Throughout this period, the Organization maintained its statutory functions with regard to dependence-producing drugs, in collaboration with the United Nations Commission on Narcotic Drugs, the Permanent Central Narcotics Board and the Drug Supervisory Board. Research on the "dependence liability" of drugs and on the neurochemical and pathophysiological consequences of short- and long-term use of these substances continued to be supported. The Organization advised governments on setting up and using integrated services for prevention, early detection, treatment and rehabilitation at the community level.

An expert committee that met in November 1972 paid particular attention to application of the epidemiological approach to studying drug dependence (5). Another expert committee, meeting in 1973, assessed various approaches to the prevention of problems associated with nonmedical use of several dependence-producing drugs, including alcohol, amphetamines, barbiturates and opiates (6). The committee emphasized the importance of evaluating the effectiveness of prevention programmes and the assumptions on which they were based. It recommended that WHO also address the prevention of alcohol-related problems. A scientific group on progress in methods for evaluating the dependence-liability of drugs, meeting in 1974, proposed that multidisciplinary research should be conducted to bring together the results of preclinical and clinical assessments of the dependence-inducing potential of drugs with those of epidemiological studies on patterns of drug use (7). An interregional study of the epidemiology of drug dependence became operational in 1975. A general method for evaluating programmes for treating drug dependence was devised in 1977, and plans were made for testing it in seven countries.

The mental health of adolescents and young persons was the subject of a WHO-sponsored regional conference held in Stockholm, Sweden, in 1969 for countries of the European Region. Various aspects of juvenile delinquency were discussed, and a report was published in 1971 (8). A pilot project on juvenile delinquency was initiated in nine countries, which resulted in a reassessment of WHO's role in this field when it was completed at the end of 1975. In the area of child mental health and psychosocial development, an expert committee met in late 1976 (9), and information was collected on mental health education programmes relating to the use and abuse of alcohol, tobacco and drugs in European countries in order to assess their short- and long-term effects.

In 1973, the programme was extended to cover the behavioural sciences and neurosciences, with greater emphasis on psychosocial factors in health. The latter development was endorsed in 1974, when the Twenty-seventh World Health Assembly adopted resolution WHA27.53, which asked the Organization to "initiate programmes concerning the role of psychosocial factors and their influence on health in general, and mental health in particular" and to organize multidisciplinary programmes to explore these factors. This resolution stemmed from technical discussions that had been held that year on the role of health services in "preserving or restoring the full effectiveness of the human environment in the promotion of health", which led to an unpublished document, *Promoting health in the human environment in 1975, a review based on the technical discussions held during the Twenty-seventh World Health Assembly, 1974*. This document focused on the social and human aspects of the human environment and is rich with ideas that touch on aspects of importance to other programmes of the Organization. For example, the conclusions and recommendations for the future role of health services include the statement that there appeared to be a growing desire on the part of health services in both developed and developing countries to provide health care that took into account the psychological, social, cultural, economic, rehabilitation and physical needs of the individual. That would, however, require a radical change in the roles and attitudes of health personnel and in the concept of team work. More emphasis should be placed on preventive and human medicine and the use of nonmedical, social solutions to health problems.

The programme of mental health was expanded in 1975 to reflect the relations between mental health and disability prevention and rehabilitation. Rehabilitation was stressed as an integral part of overall mental health care, and attention was called to the mental health needs of disabled persons whose primary impairments are physical.

At the regional level, programmes were mounted to respond to the increased awareness of mental health in Member States. In some regions, programmes were initiated to address the growing problem of drug dependence. Activities were initiated to design simple, economical, effective methods for mental health care that could be integrated fully into general health services.

The Advisory Committee on Medical Research in 1972 had recommended increased attention to research in the neurological sciences and in mental functioning in order better to understand human behaviour, both normal and abnormal. An expert advisory panel on neurosciences was therefore established in 1973, which held a series of consultations over subsequent years with the objective of facilitating work in developing countries. In 1977, a study group was convened in Addis Ababa, Ethiopia, to review the application of recent advances in neurosciences for the control of epilepsies, infections of the nervous system, nutritional neuropathies, cerebrovascular diseases and Parkinson disease (*10*).

The medium-term mental health programme for the period 1975–1982 was shaped by these directions. One new development was establishment of a coordinating group for the WHO Mental Health Programme. This broadly based group would meet every 2 years and consist of WHO staff members and representatives of a wide range of disciplines concerned with mental health, including the heads of WHO collaborating centres, representatives of United Nations agencies and governmental and nongovernmental organizations and public health administrators. At its first meeting, in 1976, the group agreed on the content of the medium-term programme, the focal points for each activity and methods for coordinating work. Shortly afterwards, coordinating mechanisms were established at regional and national levels.

CANCER

At the beginning of the decade, the Organization's activities with regard to cancer were primarily in the fields of histopathological classification and clinical cancer control. Assistance and advice to governments for the organization of cancer control services began to feature more prominently in the early 1970s, pilot studies of cancer control services having shown what could be accomplished.

The programme on histological classification was initiated in 1957 to devise a uniform system of nomenclature, deemed essential for comparative studies on cancer. By the early 1970s, the programme involved 19 international reference centres and a number of collaborating laboratories, in which more than 200 pathologists in almost 50 countries worked. The centres organized periodic meetings with their collaborators to discuss problems in the classification, nomenclature and diagnosis of a set of pathological specimens that had been circulated to all collaborating centres. Clinical histories and follow-up data were analysed to relate morphological aspects of the tumours to their biological activity. The first volume of the WHO *International histological classification of tumours* was published in 1967, dealing with lung tumours. By the end of 1977, 18 volumes had been published.

A meeting was held in 1974 to consider whether the published classifications should be modified to suit the needs of paediatric pathologists, particularly for their use in clinical trials and epidemiological studies, and the form of a publication on the classification of tumours in childhood.

An international collaborative study on breast cancer and lactation, which had begun in 1964, was completed in 1969. The study covered 4400 breast cancer patients and 13 000 controls in six countries with different incidences of breast cancer and different lactation patterns and habits. It showed that lactation patterns bear no relation to the incidence of breast cancer but that, in all the areas covered by the study, women who bear their first child when they are under 18 years of age have only about one-third the breast cancer risk of those whose first child is born after they have reached the age of 35 years. This result led to a study of hormone patterns in young women and girls in areas of high and low incidence of breast cancer.

Four international reference centres were established for the evaluation of four types of cancer: melanoma and cancers of the stomach, breast and ovary. The centre in Milan, Italy, began conducting studies of melanoma in 1971. Breast cancer was the focus of the centre in Villejuif, France, where an inquiry into the economics and cost–effectiveness of mass screening for the early detection of breast cancer was initiated in 1973.

Several pilot projects for cancer control were already under way in 1968. With the assistance of the Norwegian Agency for International Development, a project was initiated in 1970 in Madras State, India, based on the detection and treatment of cancer of the cervix uteri and oropharyngeal cancer, the two major types of cancer in that area. The aim of the project was to devise methods for adequate coverage and follow-up in the framework of the existing health services, and to train personnel in these techniques. The project ended in 1973, by which time registration and follow-up systems had been established, health education in the community carried out, and diagnostic and treatment facilities set up.

Other types of assistance programmes were established by 1974. In the African Region, for instance, assistance was given for cancer control in Zanzibar. In the Americas, support was provided to Brazil to upgrade its cytology laboratories. In the Eastern Mediterranean Region, cancer control programmes were assisted in Democratic Yemen, Iran, Iraq, Libya and Tunisia.

The International Agency for Research on Cancer (IARC), which was established in 1966, is a specialized agency of WHO. Its main focus at the time was identification of environmental carcinogens, in both epidemiological and laboratory studies carried out in collaboration with national cancer institutes. Beginning with studies of the causes of tumours of the digestive system, the IARC extended its studies to include other systems. Also, while air and water pollution received considerable emphasis, contamination of foods by natural or added substances was also studied. An example of a naturally occurring carcinogen is aflatoxin, a contaminant produced by fungal action on groundnut meal.

Nearby populations with different patterns of cancer incidence provided a starting point for studies of possible causal factors. For example, surveys showed that the prevalence of oesophageal cancer increased by more than 10-fold from west to east over a distance of less than 650 km along the southern shore of the Caspian Sea. In 1970, IARC started studies of dietary practices and personal habits in collaboration with the Institute of Public Health Research, Teheran, where an IARC Regional Centre was established.

In addition to specific studies, IARC systematically collected data on cancer incidence from cancer registries in all parts of the world to provide material for studies on the etiology of cancer. It was hoped that population-based registries would provide an early warning system to signal the introduction of new carcinogens into the environment. A feasibility study completed in 1973 showed, however, that annual variations in cancer incidence were much greater than had been anticipated. Given the long lag between cause and effect, such a system was deemed to be ineffective.

The Agency's training programme awarded fellowships and organized short courses, although rising travel costs and necessary increases in stipends limited the number of 1-year fellowships that could be offered to around 10 each year.

Following a recommendation by the Executive Board in January 1973, international cooperation in cancer research was considered by the Twenty-sixth World Health Assembly, which led to a long-term programme of international cancer research in collaboration with IARC. Three roles were envisioned for WHO: continuation of the existing programme of support, service, training and dissemination of information; establishment and maintenance of a nucleus of expert knowledge to assess and use new developments in diagnosis, therapy and causation; and coordination of research on cancer and allied fields including genetics, virology, immunology, biochemistry and comparative medicine.

The report presented to the Twenty-seventh World Health Assembly in 1974 stressed the need for international cooperation in basic, environmental and clinical research and in cancer services. It was proposed that WHO serve as an intermediary or focal point to integrate the work of national, intergovernmental and nongovernmental organizations in cancer; that WHO stimulate national efforts with technical assistance and advisory services; that the terminology, classifications and methods be standardized; that the current situation in various fields of cancer be reviewed and evaluated; that new methods, such as immunodiagnosis, and the practical application of research findings be promoted; and that skilled manpower for both cancer research and health care be made available.

In pursuance of the resolutions of the Twenty-sixth (WHA26.61) and Twenty-seventh (WHA27.63) World Health Assemblies, the WHO regional offices became more active in coordinating the efforts of Member States to control cancer. A meeting in Geneva brought together WHO and IARC staff members to consider further action, and concluded that the regional offices should furnish aid, advice and expertise to countries to enable them to formulate integrated cancer control programmes within their existing health systems; establish the facilities required for health education in cancer and for training health workers in early detection; set up referral services; evaluate the work done; and introduce modern methods of management into the organization of cancer programmes. The meeting also recommended that assistance be provided for establishing or strengthening national or regional cancer centres (*11*).

In the African Region, particular attention was paid to establishing cancer services within general national health services, and practical procedures were outlined for enlarging cancer programmes. In the Region of the Americas, WHO provided assistance for setting up cancer registry subsystems, evaluating clinical trials on different types of cancer, and establishing cervical and uterine cancer control programmes. Support to the countries of the South-East Asia Region included technical assistance in training in cytology and cytopathology and strengthening radiotherapy facilities. In the Eastern Mediterranean Region, a regional cancer control programme was elaborated as a model for national programmes, and regional reference centres were set up in existing cancer institutes to study the most effective ways of controlling the main types of cancer prevalent in the Region.

An ad hoc committee of the Executive Board was established in 1977 to make recommendations on all WHO's activities in the field of cancer, including those of IARC. Its report was reviewed by the Board in January 1978, which went on to approve the recommendations contained in the report, in particular:

- that the main function of WHO with respect to cancer should be as expressed in the Sixth General Programme of Work, namely to promote cancer prevention and control, including coordinated cancer research;
- that, whereas the range of functions of the IARC was acceptable, the activities of WHO headquarters should be strengthened to constitute an adequate and coherent plan of action;
- that the cancer programme of WHO headquarters and the programme of the IARC should retain their separate identities but should be better coordinated;
- that the interdisciplinary team for internal coordination of the WHO cancer programme should be maintained; and
- that the Director-General should establish a permanent coordinating committee to address high-level programme policy issues covering the range of problems directly or indirectly connected with cancer prevention, control and research.

A report on the importance and potential of cancer chemotherapy for developing countries was submitted to the Advisory Committee on Medical Research in 1977 (*12*). The report stressed that drug-sensitive tumours are commoner in developing than in developed countries. Another significant conclusion concerned the expertise gained in developing countries from the use of natural products in traditional medicine, which could lead to a rational approach for the isolation of biologically active substances. After a review of the subject, the Advisory Committee recommended (*13*) that WHO:

- explore means for making cancer chemotherapy drugs available at reasonable cost for patients in developing countries;
- strengthen existing cancer control services in developing countries and advise on the establishment of such services when necessary;
- update knowledge regularly, including the WHO textbook on cancer chemotherapy (*14*), and emphasize conditions in developing countries;
- assist in training medical and paramedical personnel in cancer chemotherapy; in particular the inclusion of oncology in the curricula of training programmes would be highly desirable; and
- encourage and stimulate rational screening of drugs used in traditional medicine, with a view to establishing their cytostatic and other activities. This could be linked to WHO research on tropical diseases, in which plants were being screened for their activity in other diseases.

CARDIOVASCULAR DISEASE

The Organization's main concerns in this respect were atherosclerosis, ischaemic heart disease, arterial hypertension, cerebrovascular disease, rheumatic fever and cardiomyopathy. Particular attention was given to devising preventive measures that would reach the whole community. The studies on prevention were interrelated with epidemiological, clinical and experimental investigations designed to throw light on the etiology, development and course of cardiovascular disease. A number of activities were carried out jointly or in close cooperation with the International Society of Cardiology and relevant regional and national institutions.

The programme received continuous support from WHO's governing bodies. The last resolution adopted during this decade, by the Twenty-ninth World Health Assembly, in 1976 (resolution WHA29.49), invited the Director-General to prepare a long-term programme in this field, with emphasis on promoting research on prevention, etiology, early diagnosis, treatment and rehabilitation; and coordinating international cooperation in this field.

Earlier, in 1973, a meeting convened by WHO of leading specialists in cardiology had drawn up guidelines for a worldwide cooperative effort for the control of cardiovascular disease. Up to then, most of the Organization's activities had been in developed countries. In 1975, the Organization extended its activities to the problems of developing countries and suggested that regional research and training centres in cardiovascular disease control be established within university departments of preventive medicine, with existing personnel and facilities. The main function of such centres would be the education and training of health personnel at all levels by direct involvement in field projects. Essential functions of the centres would also be to define problems, design projects and carry out surveys, pilot studies, evaluation of treatment and basic and applied research.

In most cases of *ischaemic heart disease*, advanced atherosclerosis in the coronary arteries is the predominant feature, and occlusive coronary atherosclerosis with thrombosis is a common precipitating cause of the acute stage of the disease. Acute myocardial infarct is often the first recognized clinical manifestation of ischaemic heart disease, and mortality from this cause is highest within the first few hours after onset. Consequently, a multidisciplinary approach is needed both for preventing advanced coronary atherosclerosis and thrombosis and for providing immediate treatment for all patients suspected of having acute myocardial infarct or presenting symptoms that indicate a high risk for heart failure.

In 1968, a long-term programme to study ischaemic heart disease was launched in the European Region, comprising projects for prevention, the collection of better information on the extent and impact of the disease in the community and treatment, including rehabilitation and long-term follow-up of patients. In 1971, the second phase, covering the years 1973–1977, was approved. In this phase, the programme was expanded to include the public health problems of hypertension, stroke, rheumatic fever and rheumatic health disease, congenital heart malformations and chronic chest diseases.

As part of this intensified programme, a registration system for acute myocardial infarct was established, after testing in Göteborg, Sweden, and Prague, Czechoslovakia. Eighteen registers were in operation by 1971 in 15 European countries. Most patients with acute myocardial infarct were found to have experienced symptoms such as chest pain, arrhythmia or abnormal fatigue in the days or weeks preceding the acute attack, and study of use of these symptoms for early diagnosis of imminent myocardial infarct were incorporated in the registration system. At the end of the study (1974), simplified registration and surveillance systems for patients with myocardial infarct were drawn up, which could be adopted for use in countries with different systems of medical care through community cardiovascular control programmes.

The recommendations of a scientific group on the diagnosis of acute ischaemic heart disease that met in 1969 led to a pilot study in collaborating laboratories in Belgium, Czechoslovakia, Finland, Sweden and Switzerland. The study involved radiological and histochemical examination of the heart, as well as microscopic evaluation of histological slides prepared in a central laboratory in Switzerland. Analysis of the material, completed in 1971, showed that the major predisposing factors were elevated blood lipids, heavy smoking, unhealthy nutritional habits, a sedentary life and mental strain, all of which were found among persons aged 20–30 years or younger, suggesting that prevention programmes should target these age groups. On the basis of this study, a number of measures intended to discourage tobacco smoking, especially among the young, were recommended by the Twenty-fourth World Health Assembly, in May 1971, in its resolution WHA24.48.

Coordination of worldwide activities on smoking and health was reinforced by the adoption by the Health Assembly in 1976 of resolution WHA29.55. In collaboration with other agencies within the United Nations system and nongovernmental and other organizations, WHO was active in such areas as antismoking legislation, antismoking education and disseminating information on the harmful effects of smoking. A WHO expert advisory panel on smoking and health was established in 1977, and plans were made for it to meet in 1978. A network of WHO collaborating centres on smoking and health was also planned.

A double-blind randomized trial in 15 000 men to determine whether the incidence of ischaemic heart disease could be reduced by giving the drug clofibrate to lower blood lipid levels was completed in 1977. This 10-year trial, conducted in four centres in European countries, indicated that the approach had both positive and negative aspects.

Pilot programmes for the control of *hypertension* and the protocol for the establishment of stroke registers were reviewed at a WHO meeting at the end of 1971. A procedure for pilot hypertension control was agreed upon. WHO assumed responsibility for central collection and analysis of data from stroke registers.

A project for community control of hypertension was initiated in 1972. By 1977, it included 18 communities in developed and developing countries, covering approximately 30 000 hypertensive persons, who were registered, followed-up and treated as necessary. The project showed that there were many untreated and previously undetected cases of hypertension in most communities.

Pilot projects for *stroke* control were started in 1971 and were under way in 13 countries within a year. It was soon noted that the incidence of stroke differed significantly among study areas and that not enough was being done at community level to prevent stroke by controlling hypertension. A considerable difference was found in the management of stroke patients: while almost 90% were sent to hospital in some centres, 70% received home treatment in others. It was found that a history of stroke, acute myocardial infarct, hypertension or diabetes mellitus did not markedly affect the prognosis of new stroke cases.

The results of a collaborative project begun in the 1960s on *atherosclerosis* of the aorta and coronary arteries in five towns in Czechoslovakia, Sweden and the USSR were published in 1976. The study showed that some form of atherosclerosis was present in the autopsy findings for nearly all of the 17 287 persons over the age of 10 years studied in five demographically defined populations.

Rheumatic heart disease is readily amenable to prevention, and the need for systematic, wide-scale prophylaxis had been raised repeatedly at meetings convened by WHO. Yet, by 1971, organized, efficient community action remained limited. Two obstacles were recognized: heart disease in children is not easily recognized in the early stages, and the extent of morbidity in the population had seldom been determined; furthermore, it remained to be demonstrated that prophylactic methods that are feasible at community level in developed countries are suitable for use in developing countries. Moreover, investigations were still required into several aspects of the epidemiology of rheumatic fever, such as the role of streptococcal infections in its causation, the development of immunity due to undetected streptococcal infections, and, in particular, possible changes in the clinical pattern of rheumatic fever over time or according to geographical occurrence. In order to facilitate mass screening for rheumatic heart disease, cassette-type tapes with heart sounds and murmurs were prepared for training medical students and nonmedical personnel participating in large-scale screening activities in countries where physicians were scarce.

A WHO consultation on the prevention of rheumatic fever and rheumatic heart disease was held in Cairo, Egypt, in 1972. An operating protocol for the establishment of pilot control programmes, which had been tested intensively during the previous 2 years, was amended and adopted. Pilot studies were initiated in a number of cities in 1973. A review of the experiences of these projects in 1975 led to revision of the operating protocol and preparation of a project specifically in developing countries. An inter-country project of this type was introduced in the Region of the Americas, with the participation of six countries.

Clinical and statistical evidence that *trace elements* may influence cardiovascular function led WHO in late 1967 to set up a collaborative project with the International Atomic Energy Agency (IAEA) to determine which elements are protective and which are detrimental to health. During its first year, the work involved collecting autopsy specimens of the heart and aorta wall from cooperating hospitals in Czechoslovakia and Israel and analysing their mineral content by neutron activation techniques in an IAEA laboratory. In 1969, other institutes joined the project, and testing of samples of tissue, blood, fingernails and hair collected from healthy persons and persons with cardiac disease was initiated.

In 1971, a worldwide survey of cadmium in kidneys and liver was begun to obtain information about the proposed relation between this trace element and hypertension. By 1972, other trace elements were being studied, comprising chromium, cobalt, copper, iodine, iron, lead, manganese, molybdenum, nickel, selenium and zinc; analyses for calcium and magnesium were also made. The studies confirmed the hypothesis that population groups in areas where there is soft, demineralized water have higher mortality rates from cardiovascular diseases than those with hard water, but the nature and biomedical significance of this association remained unknown.

WHO also explored the effects of *high altitude* on cardiovascular function. Studies by collaborating institutes in Peru showed that hypertension is less common among people living at high altitudes than among those living in the lowlands, and that cellular changes play an important part in adaptation to high altitude. Studies were undertaken in collaborating laboratories in Europe of the cellular metabolism and enzymatic action that appear to be responsible for adaptation of the myocardium to high-altitude hypoxia.

Evaluation of the effect of *physical fitness* and physical activity or inactivity on health depends primarily on satisfactory measurement of habitual physical activity. A WHO meeting in 1971 reviewed the available knowledge and advised on suitable measurement techniques. In collaboration with the Federal Polytechnic School, Lausanne, Switzerland, the techniques designed included activity-recall questionnaires, use of pedometers or accelerometers to measure the movement of large muscles, dietary surveys, measurement of deep body temperature and continuous recording of the heart rate.

Cardiovascular status can be measured well in exercise tests, as physical exercise can reveal signs and symptoms of impending cardiovascular disease that would not manifest themselves under everyday sedentary conditions. A WHO publication, *Fundamentals of exercise testing (15)*, published in 1971, described the most commonly used tests, with emphasis on techniques suitable for use under field conditions.

Cardiomyopathy covers conditions of varying, frequently unknown etiology in which the dominant feature is cardiomegaly and cardiac failure. WHO promoted and assisted investigations to clarify the etiology of these conditions and to find effective methods of treatment and prevention. Clinical, experimental and epidemiological studies on ischaemic heart disease and cardiomyopathy showed that more detailed investigations into the functional and morphological changes in the heart muscle were required.

OTHER CHRONIC NONCOMMUNICABLE DISEASES

Other chronic diseases were addressed in a separate programme in the early 1970s, when their impact on health and socioeconomic growth in developed and many developing countries became more marked. The main task of the programme was to achieve uniformity in the terminology used, to elaborate classification and diagnostic criteria and to set up and coordinate training and control programmes through a network of collaborating centres.

The first diseases studied included diabetes mellitus, rheumatoid arthritis and related diseases, chronic nonspecific respiratory disease and chronic renal disease. Chronic liver disease was soon added to the programme.

Diabetes mellitus increases the risks for two types of arterial disease. One, an important cause of disability, is relatively specific and affects the small blood vessels, giving rise to retinopathy and nephropathy. The other, the main cause of mortality in persons with diabetes, is nonspecific, involving atherosclerosis of the large and medium arteries. A collaborative multinational study of vascular disease in persons with diabetes was initiated in 1974 and discussed in 1975 by the Advisory Committee on Medical Research. By the end of

1977, the programme included information on some 5000 patients in 11 countries, focusing on the frequency of large-vessel and small-vessel diseases.

WHO, in close collaboration with the International Diabetes Federation, established an organizing committee during 1977 for a postgraduate course on diabetes mellitus and elaborated a preliminary programme for the course, which was initiated in 1978.

The evidence that *rheumatoid arthritis and related diseases* are associated with immunological abnormalities was reviewed at a meeting of the Arthritis and Rheumatism Council in 1975, in which WHO participated. It was agreed that it would be difficult to conduct an international project, incorporating immunological studies to test etiological hypotheses, and it was suggested that smaller studies should be conducted by individual centres, with internationally accepted clinical and laboratory criteria.

Resolution WHA28.59, adopted in May 1975, highlighted WHO's support of research on rheumatic disease. It recommended that WHO continue to cooperate with the International League against Rheumatism, with a view to intensifying research on the epidemiology, etiopathogenesis, prevention and treatment of rheumatic disease, as well as an information campaign. This direction was reinforced in 1976 by resolution WHA29.66 on the same subject. In that year, a WHO collaborating centre was designated in Mainz, Federal Republic of Germany, to design a standardized method for the histopathological definition and classification of rheumatoid arthritis and allied diseases.

Considerable disagreement on appropriate terminology, methods of diagnosis, identification of probable etiological factors and definition of the principles of prevention blocked progress on *chronic nonspecific respiratory disease*. In 1974, in the European Region, a working group met to review the subject, followed by a meeting of investigators on the epidemiology of these diseases. The available information on the epidemiology of chronic bronchitis, emphysema and generalized airway obstruction was reviewed, and definitions were agreed upon for use in the epidemiological identification of those conditions.

International collaborative research into the pathological aspects of this group of diseases began in 1975, with emphasis on standardizing the method to be used. A group of experts met in 1976 to discuss a definition and classification of what was now called 'chronic lung disease', and their proposals were distributed to pathologists around the world for consideration and comments. A preliminary programme and plan for epidemiological investigation of chronic lung disease in various population groups were drawn up in 1978.

In order to facilitate comparative studies of *chronic renal disease*, a WHO collaborating centre for histological classification was designated in 1974 at the Mount Sinai School of Medicine, New York, United States. Investigators in institutions in different countries that had been formed into a cooperative network by this centre met in 1975 to consider a standardized method for the pathodiagnosis of renal lesions.

A WHO meeting of investigators on *chronic liver disease* met in late 1977 to consider various epidemiological aspects, in an attempt to define the main areas for future investigations in different population groups.

ORAL HEALTH

In 1968, the main work of WHO's dental programme was to define a standard international method for field surveys of major dental and oral diseases. After 2 years of testing, in 1971, a standard method was published as a manual (16), which gave detailed recommendations for planning and organizing surveys, selecting population samples, diagnostic criteria and recording and reporting basic data on the prevalence of major dental and oral diseases and conditions (dental caries, periodontal disease, oral mucosal disease, dentofacial anomalies and some prosthetic needs). It was used in WHO-assisted projects and activities in a number of countries and territories, including Mexico, Papua New Guinea, Viet Nam, Senegal, the United Republic of Tanzania and Western Samoa.

In 1973, a meeting of field investigators resulted in revision of the manual. The meeting also reviewed indices for measuring and recording oral diseases and treatment requirements and outlined the possibility of using patients' treatment records as an additional source of dental epidemiological data. A further review was carried out in 1977, by which time it was recognized that there was dissatisfaction with the basic methods for measuring periodontal disease and treatment requirements. A scientific group, meeting in late 1977, proposed a new method for making surveys, which should be tested against others. They recommended that WHO proceed with such testing as rapidly as possible (17).

Fluoridation of community water supplies was the subject of a resolution adopted by the Twenty-second World Health Assembly (WHA22.30), which recommended that Member States examine the possibility of introducing fluoridation in communities where the fluoride intake from water and other sources was below optimal levels. It requested the Director-General to continue to encourage research into the etiology of dental caries, the fluoride content of diets, the mechanism of action of fluoride at optimal concentrations in drinking-water and the effects of greatly excessive intakes of fluoride from natural sources.

Early in the decade, WHO assisted several countries in organizing dental schools, setting up programmes for training auxiliary dental personnel and establishing dental education services. Assistance was also provided to countries that were introducing fluoridation programmes, especially on the technical aspects. During the decade, more and more countries became involved in the programme, especially as it moved beyond research, into service planning and evaluation.

A WHO scientific group on the etiology and prevention of dental caries that met in 1971 examined which preventive measures should be the subject of further research. They considered fluorides, adhesive sealants, phosphates, antimicrobial agents, enzymes, immunization, oral hygiene and dietary advice. Research on fluoridation was strongly recommended. The mechanism of action of phosphates was not yet understood, and both laboratory research and carefully controlled clinical trials were needed. Research to find better sealant materials was indicated, and studies on antimicrobial agents were judged to be urgent. Enzymes should also be studied in the laboratory. Research on immunization should be pursued, as dental caries induced in monkeys are so similar to those in humans that experiments on nonhuman primates were a useful possibility (18).

Other preventive measures could be taken by individuals; the problem was not only cost but also motivating people to act on advice. The group concluded:

The factors that determine personal and community attitudes to health are complex and incompletely understood. For this reason, dental personnel and behavioural scientists should collaborate in studying factors affecting attitudes to the maintenance of oral health as well as to the application of current or future preventive measures, whether taken individually or at a community level. (*18*)

Six years later, in 1977, another WHO scientific group met to discuss the epidemiology, etiology and prevention of periodontal diseases. In the intervening years, a considerable amount of information had been collected on the prevalence and severity of periodontal diseases and their association with social factors such as age, sex, race and socioeconomic group. Much information had also been collected on local oral and systemic factors and habits. The group concluded that the most important factor was oral cleanliness (*19*). Demographic factors were secondary and were important only as they directly or indirectly affected oral hygiene behaviour. The group proposed that new survey methods be formulated, as noted above, and outlined the research required to test the methods.

Close cooperation was maintained with the International Dental Federation throughout this period. One of their joint activities was field testing of new methods for detecting oral cancer and assessing dentofacial anomalies and periodontal diseases. Another subject of close collaboration was research on organizational patterns for delivering dental care.

The research programme included a project on the etiology of caries, which was carried out in Papua New Guinea, and a project on health-care delivery, which involved designing a comprehensive method for assessing and evaluating oral care delivery. This started as an international collaborative study of dental manpower systems in relation to oral health status in six countries: Australia, the Federal Republic of Germany, Japan, New Zealand, Norway and Poland. In one country, one of the highest prevalences of caries was reduced by one-third over 10–15 years. The project was supported by the United States Public Health Service and participating countries.

The project in Papua New Guinea, which was supported by the United States Institutes of Health, initially explored the presence of trace elements in the food, soil and water used by several population groups with widely differing prevalences of dental caries. The initial results, published in 1970, led to testing of tooth enamel, dental plaque and saliva obtained at oral examinations for microorganisms and trace elements. A final report was published in 1978 (*20*).

The scope of WHO-assisted research was extended in 1972 to include, for example, epidemiological studies on certain oral mucosal conditions in Indonesia and Thailand. In 1974, the emphasis was changed, and a 5-year dental health programme was drawn up, with overall objectives, specific targets and detailed activities for the period 1975–1979. While the existing activities in epidemiology, research and prevention were included and expanded, they were now regarded as services that contributed to projects. The priority was now manpower and services planning and development, to assist governments in training appropriate personnel and to institute, or revise if necessary, national plans for oral health services.

The increase in dental caries brought to light in the WHO global oral data bank resulted in a new programme of prevention of oral diseases in 1976. Financed almost entirely by extrabudgetary funds, the main activity of this programme was to provide direct technical cooperation for planning and implementing preventive programmes within oral health services. By 1977, technical cooperation had been established with 24 countries in four WHO regions.

As part of the new orientation, a second edition of the manual on oral health surveys was published, in 1977 (*21*), which included a section on assessment of treatment needs to ensure more precise manpower planning. A comprehensive manual was completed in 1977 which gave guidance to administrators on choosing dental equipment and materials suitable for different service and staffing situations. It was circulated to 50 dental equipment manufacturers in order to promote the production of robust, easily maintained equipment for all environments. Also in that year, the *World directory of schools for dental auxiliaries* was prepared (*22*), which gave details of courses, entry qualifications and numbers of places available.

RADIATION MEDICINE

WHO's programme in radiation medicine addressed protection against radiation, as a response to the growing use of nuclear energy and of radiation and radioactive materials. It promoted medical uses of radiation, so to obtain the maximum benefit from medical radiology while reducing as far as possible the hazards of exposure. Much of WHO's radiation health programme was developed in collaboration with the IAEA.

Following the request by the Twenty-fourth World Health Assembly, in 1971, to study the optimum use of ionizing radiation in medicine and the risks to health of excessive or improper use of radiation, a joint IAEA/WHO expert committee was convened in October 1971 on the medical uses of ionizing radiation and radioisotopes, to advise on the extent to which radiation medicine should be included in health planning (*23*).

The Committee described three branches of radiation medicine. The objective of diagnostic radiology is to provide information of diagnostic value, by making use of two properties of ionizing radiation, penetration through matter and image formation. Radiotherapy is the treatment of disease with ionizing radiation, making use of biological effects such as the selective destruction of tissue. Nuclear medicine involves application of unsealed radioactive materials for diagnostic and therapeutic purposes, making use of the emission of ionizing radiation from such materials and their distribution within the body. It was noted, however, that a precise definition of nuclear medicine was still under discussion. After an extensive review of each branch, the Committee concluded that radiation medicine is an essential part of preventive medicine and health care, although it recognized that it was not available to a large proportion of the world's population, a situation that should be redressed.

The effectiveness of the methods used in radiation medicine should be evaluated. Regional research projects in developing countries to investigate local disease conditions and to devise measures for combating them should be supported. Diagnostic radiology deserved particular priority because basic examinations are essential for the diagnosis of pathological conditions wherever medicine is practised. It was recognized that the supply of trained personnel was the main limiting factor in planning the use of radiation medicine. Better organization and more training facilities were needed urgently.

The Committee recommended that IAEA and WHO consider a number of actions, which included initiating and supporting training courses; applying techniques of systems analysis to define the need for radiation medicine and to plan its use within health services; encouraging field trials of X-ray diagnostic methods; encouraging use of radiotherapy by promoting regional calibration centres for dosimetry and improving advisory services; and encouraging use of nuclear medicine by promoting training facilities and information services, particularly by establishing reference centres.

Resolution WHA25.57, adopted the following year, requested the Director-General to continue technical assistance to governments in the promotion of radiation medicine; to promote the establishment of reference centres for dosimetry; and to cooperate with UNSCEAR, IAEA and other international organizations in evaluating the world situation as regards the medical use of ionizing radiation and the effects of radiation on populations.

WHO conducted a review in a number of countries in 1973 and confirmed that basic radiological services were generally lacking, particularly in rural areas. In most developing countries, the number of X-ray examinations per capita and per year was less than 1% that in industrialized countries. Furthermore, the review showed that even when equipment was available much of it was inadequately maintained or obsolete; that basic radiation protection requirements were frequently not met; that staff sometimes suffered from overexposure, with, for example, radiation damage to their fingers; and that minimum training was often not obtainable. Advice to improve this situation was given in a number of countries, and assistance was provided in several regions for training radiological technicians, considered to be a key factor in radiation protection.

Several regional projects were initiated to assist in the repair and maintenance of medical equipment, particularly for X-ray diagnosis. WHO issued interim specifications for a basic diagnostic X-ray unit, and manufacturers were asked to produce prototype equipment based on these specifications for testing in a field trial similar to that carried out for general-purpose X-ray units from 1967 to 1971. In 1975, a meeting was held in Washington DC to work out a radiology system that was cheap and easy to operate and could be used in primary health centres under difficult climatic and other adverse conditions.

By 1973, a network of six secondary standard radiation dosimetry laboratories with calibration facilities was established, in Argentina, Iran, Mexico, Romania, Singapore and Thailand; Nigeria was added in 1974. These centres provided facilities for the calibration of dosimeters and radiation sources, which is essential to proper radiation therapy but particularly difficult. They also undertook research on specific problems of dosimetry in their geographical region and organized training programmes for radiologists, medical physicians and health physicists in clinical and radiation protection dosimetry.

In 1974, WHO collaborated with IAEA and UNDP in a seminar on the evaluation of population doses of radiation from all sources and application of radiological safety standards to humans and the environment. The principles of radiation protection in relation to releases of radioactivity in the environment were emphasized, and the main sources of and contributions to the exposure of the population to radiation were reviewed. It became apparent that more information on natural background exposure and from medical and other applications of radiation was needed.

A film badge service for regular monitoring of personnel exposed to ionizing radiation was set up. Badges were supplied monthly free of charge to countries in the European Region by the Central Protection Service against Ionizing Radiation, Le Vésinet, France. Countries in the South-East Asia and Western Pacific regions were given similar services by the Institute for Radiation Protection and Environmental Health, Neuherberg, Federal Republic of Germany.

In the field of nuclear medicine, WHO, in collaboration with IAEA, published a series of atlases of dose distribution, covering typical treatment plans for fixed-field cobalt-60 teletherapy. These gave examples of treatment strategies for cancers at the most common sites. A joint IAEA/WHO expert committee on the use of ionizing radiation and radio-isotopes met in 1975 to examine the most effective ways of using nuclear medicine (*24*). A cost–benefit analysis was made of nuclear medicine procedures and alternatives, and the optimum level and scope of use of nuclear medicine in different circumstances—in particular in countries with medical and public health services at widely differing stages of development—were defined. A pilot cost–benefit analysis was performed in India in 1976–1977.

Five WHO collaborating centres for nuclear medicine were designated in 1976, bringing the total to eight, in Denmark, the Federal Republic of Germany, India, Iran, Japan, Mexico, the United States and the USSR.

A meeting on the organization of services and routine procedures in nuclear medicine was held in Brussels, Belgium, in November 1977. The main topics of discussion were the organization of basic nuclear medicine services and the procedures to be applied; the relation of nuclear medicine to particular disease patterns in a given country; and the requirements as regards premises, equipment, staff and radiopharmaceuticals.

The use of ionizing radiation and radionuclides in medical research, training and for nonmedical purposes was the subject of a WHO expert committee meeting in March 1977. The committee members were asked to evaluate the health risks involved and to recommend measures for controlling them, taking into account the ethical principles laid down by the World Medical Assembly in Helsinki in 1964 and amended in Tokyo in 1975. The report of the meeting (*25*) provided some ideas and guidelines to help decision-makers understand how local conditions and legislation shape decisions.

A scientific group that met later in 1977 addressed the long-term effects of radium and thorium in humans on the basis of studies of the biomedical effects of thorium dioxide, which was used as a radiological contrast medium in the 1930s and 1940s and which caused various types of cancer as a late effect. The group concluded that this unique experience had been essential for forecasting the potential dangers of transuranic isotopes, the public health implications of which are of the greatest importance in view of the growing use of atomic energy.

HUMAN GENETICS

The Organization's programme on human genetics was started in the 1960s in response to growing awareness of the importance of genetics in disease and the prospect of providing practical services through genetic counselling. In the early years of the decade, the programme paid most attention to congenital haemolytic anaemias, such as haemoglobinopathy, thalassaemia and glucose-6-phosphate dehydrogenase (G6PD) deficiency. A number of studies were initiated, most in association with a WHO regional collaborating centre, to determine the prevalences of specific genetic anomalies in a given population and to study these conditions. Thus, surveys were conducted to determine the incidence of sickle-cell haemoglobin in the United Republic of Tanzania and the frequency of the α-thalassaemia gene in Malaysia and Senegal.

For several years, studies were conducted on the relation between malaria and genetic defects, in particular G6PD deficiency. Research carried out at the WHO Regional Reference Centre for G6PD in Ibadan, Nigeria, for example, confirmed that the defective allele is associated with less severe malaria infections, at least in heterozygous females. It was observed that among such persons the malaria parasite attacks normal rather than deficient cells. Further studies confirmed the widespread prevalence of G6PD deficiency in the African Region. The prevalence in Central Africa was found to range from 2% to 25%. Later in the decade, attention turned to the clinical interactions of G6PD deficiency with salmonellosis, lobar pneumonia, viral hepatitis and acute renal failure.

Genetic counselling was addressed by a WHO expert committee on human genetics in 1968, which concluded (*26*) that probably not less than 4% of liveborn infants suffer from some genetic or partly genetic condition that might benefit from genetic counselling. At least 1% of all infants, for example, have a major chromosome abnormality, and much higher rates are found in some areas of the world. Experience at specialized clinics showed that some 90% of enquiries came from couples who had had a child with some disorder and who feared a recurrence. The Committee made suggestions about the organization of genetic counselling services and about suitable medical facilities for afflicted persons. It recommended the establishment of an international register of human chromosome anomalies, and, with WHO support, such a register was established at the Johns Hopkins University School of Medicine, Baltimore, Maryland, United States. By 1977, some 30 countries were involved, and about 25 000 cases of chromosomal abnormalities and variants had been recorded. Three books were published (*27–29*), which were widely used as training manuals.

The Committee also recommended that WHO continue to grant fellowships and training grants to promote training in basic human genetics, human cytogenetics, haematological genetics, human biochemical genetics and other subjects essential for competent counselling. Yearly interregional refresher courses for teachers in medical schools were organized, with the assistance of the Danish International Development Agency. Training for research workers in efficient techniques for analysing data on human genetics was given at the WHO International Reference Centre for the Processing of Human Genetics Data to a number of researchers from around the world.

Scientific groups were convened in the first years of this period to address various subjects related to human genetics:

1968 – Genetic factors in congenital malformations: to discuss the present state of knowledge about the genetic contribution to common malformations, such as pyloric stenosis, cleft lip and cleft palate, anencephalus, spina bifida, dislocation of the hip and talipes equinovarus (*30*);

1970 – Methods for family studies of genetic factors: to advise on the most efficient methods for identifying and characterizing major genetic entities in inherited disease (*31*);

1971 – Treatment of haemoglobinopathy and allied disorders: to review and summarize present knowledge; to review recent findings on the treatment of crises in sickle-cell anaemia; and to outline a procedure for conducting clinical trials of drugs against this disease (*32*);

1971 – Genetic aspects of family planning: to consider the genetic changes likely to occur as a result of family planning and to outline the research required and methods for its conduct;

1971 – Inherited blood-clotting disorders: to evaluate recent studies of the genetic basis of these disorders, their treatment and prevention and carrier detection (*33*);

1971 – Prevention, treatment and rehabilitation in genetic disorders: to review recent advances and consider techniques that might become applicable for prevention and treatment (*34*); and

1972 – Pharmacogenetics: to review current knowledge and consider the most effective ways of preventing the harmful effects of drugs on susceptible phenotypes and to make technical recommendations to encourage coordinated research.

Various studies were carried out during this decade, as summarized briefly below.

Population genetics

Population genetics is the study of the genetic structure of human populations. Consanguineous marriages, for example, have been studied in several populations to assess the number of mutations carried by an average person. In a study in 1974 in Nigeria, with the assistance of the University of Ibadan, the rates of neonatal deaths and congenital abnormalities in the consanguineous group studied were 2.6% and 1.6% as compared with 0.3% and 0, respectively, in the control group.

Population studies of chromosome disorders were supported to determine the rates of spontaneous aberrations in man. The availability of new methods for identifying individual chromosomes of the human karyotype greatly facilitated this work, as even small structural aberrations became identifiable, allowing for their correlation with clinical findings.

Cytogenetics

Cytogenetics is the study of chromosomes and of the disease states caused by numerical and structural chromosome abnormalities. A study in which 2500 unselected newborn infants were compared with 1000 newborns with congenital malformations revealed chromosome abnormalities in 0.8% of the first group and 13.6% of the latter. A further study showed spontaneous chromosome aberrations in somatic cells of 7.4% of premature infants and in 1.3% of unselected full-term newborns. The higher figure in premature infants indicates the extent of environmental effects on embryonic and fetal development.

The relation between leukaemias and chromosomal aberrations was examined in a WHO-assisted study at the Department of Genetics, National Institute of Nutrition, Mexico City, Mexico. Two groups of patients with potential leukaemic myeloid disorders were studied, one of which had chromosomal abnormalities. Leukaemic transformation occurred in the patients of the first group, who maintained a normal karyotype, while leukaemia developed in only one patient in the second group, suggesting that the presence of abnormalities in bone-marrow chromosomes does not necessarily result in imminent leukaemic transformation.

Biochemical genetics

Biochemical genetics is the study of enzymes that are deficient, absent or unstable or have altered activity, which can lead to clinical manifestations in an infant (i.e. birth defects). These types of disorders are usually called 'inborn errors of metabolism', as they are present at birth and affect the body's metabolism.

An investigation into the primary genetic defect in hepatolenticular degeneration conducted by the Institute of Experimental Medicine in Leningrad, USSR, showed that patients homozygous for this disease have a disturbance in the production of ceruloplasmin, the copper-binding protein, which results either in reduced synthesis of ceruloplasmin or in a protein with no copper transfer capacity. Analysis of the structure of the protein showed that it has two amino terminals, suggesting that it is composed of no fewer than two subunits and further indicating that at least two genes are involved.

WHO supported studies at the National Institute of Biology, Mexico City, Mexico, to hybridize cells from mammals of different species to elucidate genetic control of the biosynthesis of some amino acids, by inducing and isolating mutant cell strains.

IMMUNOLOGY

In 1968, the Organization's work in immunology was chiefly for the promotion of research and the provision of training in immunology and immunological research. It was recognized that immunology was a rapidly growing field, with its own techniques and concepts, and should be recognized as a separate discipline. There was a serious shortage of trained personnel, both for research and for teaching, and WHO offered training courses at its immunological research and training centres to partly fill this need. The centre in Ibadan, Nigeria, dealt mainly with the immunology of malaria and trypanosomiasis and with immunoglobulins; that in São Paulo, Brazil, with the characteristics of venoms of local snakes, with a view to preparing better anti-venoms; and the centre in Lausanne, Switzerland, provided advice and training and supplied reagents to the other centres. These and, later, other centres organized annual courses in their areas of specialty.

A series of scientific working groups met to review current knowledge, from which various WHO activities in this field emerged. That on genetics and the immune response, held in October, 1967, noted how little was known about the genetic control of human immune responses, and it was recommended that an organization to facilitate international exchange of information be established. An international cooperative study of patients with immune deficiency syndromes was proposed, which later comprised some 20 centres (35).

The group that met in 1968 on cell-mediated immune response recommended (36) that documents, information and techniques relative to cell-mediated immunity be made available to scientists and clinicians interested in phenomena in which this response plays a role. Training courses in these techniques should be encouraged.

In 1971, the Organization sought to promote applied clinical research in immunology in conjunction with its disease control programmes and to raise the standards of training in this branch of biomedicine, particularly through the immunology research and training centres, which by that time numbered nine: in addition to those in Lausanne, Ibadan and São Paulo, there were now centres in Basel, Switzerland; Beirut, Lebanon; Mexico City, Mexico; New Delhi, India; Rehovot, Israel; and Singapore. Three more centres were added later, in Geneva, Switzerland; Melbourne, Australia; and Nairobi, Kenya.

Other training activities included providing support for participants from all the WHO regions to attend courses organized with the British Society for Immunology in Edinburgh, Scotland, and seminars held in Moscow, USSR, and Copenhagen, Denmark, on the most recent findings on the structure and synthesis of antibodies.

The new data on circulating antibodies and cellular immunity indicated that more effective immunodiagnostic tests were required, with research on effective immunizing procedures and better understanding of the immunopathological lesions that accompany many infectious diseases. The diseases that offer the greatest potential for application of new knowledge in immunological research were considered to be protozoal diseases, such as malaria, trypanosomiasis and leishmaniasis, viral diseases such as dengue haemorrhagic fever, and many bacterial diseases such as leprosy, tuberculosis and enteric infections.

By stimulating and, within limits, carrying out research into the immunological basis of disease, the Organization sought to reach a triple goal: more effective diagnostic tests, more soundly based immunization procedures and, consequently, better control of parasitic and infectious diseases, in particular. Most fundamental immunological research was carried out in developed countries, although the international network of immunological research and training centres facilitated field research and provided the means for increasing the number of immunologists working in developing countries.

Trainees received initial training at a centre located in their country or region, and advanced training was offered at annual courses supported by the Swiss Government in Lausanne, Basel, Rehovot or Melbourne. Visiting immunologists who taught in some of the courses frequently took up research on the immunology of tropical diseases when they returned to their countries, often in collaboration with participants in developing countries.

The growing number of immunological techniques being used in day-to-day patient care led the Organization to start a programme for standardization of immunological reagents and techniques, in 1974, which was established in cooperation with the International Union of Immunological Societies and with the financial support of the Governments of Canada, the Federal Republic of Germany and Sweden. The immunology of tropical diseases was emphasized.

Scientific groups continued to play an important role in setting the international agenda for research in this field. In 1975, the subject of immunological adjuvants was addressed

(*37*). Adjuvants represent an important way of stimulating the immune response; the group addressed the question of how they might be used in preparing vaccines. Suggestions were made for further research.

In 1976, a scientific group discussed the role of immune complexes in disease. Immune complexes are produced when antigens interacts with antibodies. Although their formation is part of the normal immune response, in some situations their formation triggers a sequence of injurious events that lead to disease. The group discussed the mechanisms by which immune complexes can cause disease, their role in human disease and how they can be detected. The recommendations called for improved laboratory diagnostic tests, clinical studies and basic research (*38*).

In 1977, a WHO scientific group addressed the subject of immunodeficiency (*39*). The time was judged to be propitious to extend and apply findings on primary immunodeficiency to better understand secondary immunodeficiency. Primary deficiency is due to some failure in the immune mechanism involving a specific factor, such as an antibody or lymphocytes, or a nonspecific factor, such as a complement component. Secondary deficiency may arise from a variety of pathological conditions and metabolic diseases, as well as from malignancy, malnutrition and cytotoxic drugs. These conditions, which often exist in populations affected by parasitic infestations, are responsible for most immunodeficiency. The group enumerated and described the essential elements of primary immunodeficiency as then understood and explored the factors that lead to the broader problem of secondary immunodeficiency. It concluded that more information was needed about the patterns and incidence of primary immunodeficiency in all countries. The availability of uniform antigens for diagnostic purposes was seen to be critical. Research on histocompatibility assessment and the implications of therapy was encouraged. The influence of parasitic infections, both acute and asymptomatic, of varying degrees of malnutrition and of their combined effects on the immune response also required further study.

With the establishment of the TDR programme in 1976 (see Chapter 5), the immunology programme was reoriented. Technical help was provided for the various scientific working groups that had been established (see Chapter 9), and training activities were increased at all centres. Courses on fundamental and applied immunology continued to be offered in all the centres. Research at the centres continued to focus on problems of public health importance, such as trypanosomiasis and schistosomiasis (Nairobi), trypanosomiasis and leprosy (Geneva), leishmaniasis (Lausanne) and Chagas disease (São Paulo).

A programme for establishing clinical immunology laboratories in the Caribbean area was started, with the financial support of the Government of The Netherlands. The programme had two phases; during the first, scientists in the area were trained in Amsterdam, and during the second phase the trainees were assisted in establishing laboratories on their return home. In 1977, students from Cuba, Jamaica and Surinam attended the first course in Amsterdam.

A collaborating centre for studying the immunopathology of dengue haemorrhagic fever was established in Bangkok, Thailand, in cooperation with the regional offices for South-East Asia, Europe and the Western Pacific. Its first activity was to organize a meeting to identify the research to be conducted. The programme was organized along lines similar to those of the TDR programme.

HEALTH OF WORKING POPULATIONS

WHO's programme on the health of working populations grew steadily during this decade. Many activities were carried out with other agencies, in particular ILO, with whom WHO has had a special relation from its inception, the first meeting of the Joint Committee on Occupational Health having taken place in 1950.

In 1970, the Organization intensified its activities in occupational health in three fields: promotion and establishment of national occupational health programmes, not only for workers in large manufacturing industries but also for those in occupations such as mining, agriculture, small industries and other trades; initiation of a new policy for training and education in occupational health, directed particularly to the demands and conditions in developing countries; and investigation of problems that had barely been touched upon in the past, including exposure of workers to the multiple stresses that cause complex pathological states and that necessitated a review of standards of health and safety.

In 1973, in close collaboration with ILO, the programme was further expanded, to include field investigations of health problems affecting working populations in developing countries, devising guidelines for environmental health monitoring in preventive occupational health practice, and assistance to Member States in building service programmes.

In 1976, following adoption of resolution WHA29.57, activities in all these fields were reoriented to promote occupational health as an integral part of public health services.

National projects in occupational health took various forms, depending on the circumstances of the country involved. In Indonesia, for example, WHO worked with the National Institute of Occupational Health and three regional centres to set up occupational health and industrial hygiene services. The initial phase of this project involved preparation of a national plan covering the type of services, training and research to be undertaken by this Institute during the period 1970–1974. A similar project was established in the Philippines with the cooperation of ILO. In other countries, activities were based on the needs of particular working groups, in particular those in small industries, agriculture and mining. For example, in 1972, national seminars were organized in the Republic of Korea and Singapore, with ILO participation, which led to proposals for the establishment of occupational health centres. By 1972, more than 50 countries were receiving direct assistance from WHO for occupational health and research.

Pilot health centres for seafarers were established in the ports of Auckland, New Zealand, and Gdynia, Poland, with WHO assistance, following a report on the health problems of seafarers and the services available to them, as called for in resolution WHA21.23, in 1968. The Gdynia centre initiated studies on the psychological and mental disturbances of seamen from different countries resulting from their type of work and their limited identification with family and homeland. After several years, the centre began to assist and train marine health personnel from various parts of the world.

A particularly important aspect of occupational health services—monitoring systems that could provide early warning of dangerous working conditions—was the subject of a WHO expert committee meeting in 1973. The committee prepared guidelines for environmental health monitoring schemes at country level, at places of work and for specific occupational risks (40). It asked WHO to help Member States to prepare national inventories of occupational health conditions that could be used in planning and implementing their occupational health programmes.

In 1974, a study group met to discuss early detection of health impairment associated with occupational exposure to health hazards. The group drew up guidelines for occupational health physicians who carry out periodic examinations of industrial workers, and pointed out the gaps in knowledge about early manifestations of diseases affecting working populations.

In response to resolution EB53.R23, the Organization designed a form for collecting and disseminating systematic, uniform information on the health problems prevailing in different occupational sectors in all countries and the kinds of services available. The form also served to collect data on training and research activities. The aim was to make national inventories on occupational health that would be of use, particularly to developing countries, in planning and implementing occupational health programmes and identifying priorities. From the information collected, 76 countries prepared inventories, which formed the background for a discussion by the WHO Regional Committee for Africa in September 1977. The Committee proposed an intercountry and regional programme for providing improved health services for workers and their families and research and training centres in Africa, pooling the resources available to help individual countries (41).

The report of a study group on early detection of health impairment after occupational exposure to health hazards, held in 1975, recommended that a programme be set up to review the available information on methods for biological monitoring of workers exposed to toxic substances and physical hazards and to stimulate research in areas where insufficient information was available. As a follow-up, a meeting was held in late 1975 to consider the early detection of health impairment associated with occupational exposure to industrial solvents that are commonly encountered in industry and are known to induce major occupational diseases. Guidelines were drawn up for detecting early biological changes resulting from exposure to such solvents.

Study of the specific problems faced by workers with various working conditions occupied a major place in the WHO programme throughout the decade. Studies were undertaken by WHO collaborating institutions in occupational health and other institutions cooperating with WHO in this field, the number of which grew to more than 20 by mid-decade.

The Organization supported research programmes in countries in nearly all the WHO regions to investigate health conditions in small industries and to assess their needs. It was found that, in some countries, most of the working population in small industries suffered from a variety of diseases of occupational and nonoccupational origin and had inadequate preventive and curative health care.

In 1971, WHO initiated a long-term study on the epidemiology of toxic hazards in industry in the European Region. Occupational toxicologists were trained to undertake longitudinal surveys of human exposure to industrial toxic substances.

The results of studies undertaken around the world in a variety of small industries were reviewed in 1975. The meeting agreed on approaches to address the health problems of the workers concerned and to provide guidelines for establishing and delivering health care to small industries operating under various organizational, social and economic conditions.

The problems of agricultural societies, such as exposure to pesticides and tobacco and other vegetable dusts, were also addressed.

WHO helped in the preparation of an ILO model code of practice on the safe use of pesticides and gave guidance on the design and effective use of personal respiratory protective devices, especially in developing countries. A study of the effects of simultaneous exposure to heat stress and to certain pesticides in agricultural work began in 1975, with experimental trials in Kiev, USSR, and epidemiological studies in Sudan. Studies were also started that year to investigate exposure of agricultural workers in Algeria to agricultural chemicals and other work hazards.

Studies of respiratory diseases caused by vegetable dusts were undertaken in a number of countries, including Mexico, Thailand and Turkey. Guidelines for epidemiological research in this field were prepared in 1972. Similarly, studies of exposure to toxic dusts in mines were undertaken in many countries. For example, research on the mental and neurological syndromes produced by long-term inhalation of dust containing manganese in mining began in 1972, with assistance from the United States National Institute for Occupational Safety and Health.

In response to resolution WHA23.47, the Organization undertook a preliminary study of health conditions in the mining industry in the African Region and the Region of the Americas, which formed the basis for a joint ILO/WHO consultation on occupational health in miners. In 1976, with ILO and the African–American Labor Center, WHO organized a conference on the health of African miners. One of the conclusions reached was that trained personnel, guidelines and regulations were urgently needed to combat the high incidences of disease and accidents among these workers. In addition, WHO began research on miners' health problems in the Republic of Korea and in Zambia.

Migrant workers were the focus of a number of studies in different regions. In 1975, the occupational health and safety problems of migrant workers and their psychological and social difficulties were considered at the seventh session of the Joint ILO/WHO Committee on Occupational Health. Following this session, a standing committee on the health of migrant workers was established. Information was collected on the state of health of migrant workers in various parts of the world, and guidelines were prepared for protecting the health of these workers, both in their countries of origin and in their host countries.

In 1976, WHO published an *International classification of impairments, disabilities, and handicaps: a manual of classification relating to the consequences of disease (42)*. At the same time, it acknowledged that attempts to draw up guidelines for monitoring the work environment with simplified techniques had not yet been achieved, and that remained a priority for collaborating institutions in different parts of the world.

References

1. *The work of WHO 1968. Official records of the World Health Organization*, No. 172. Geneva, World Health Organization, 1968.
2. *Organization of mental health services in developing countries. Sixteenth report of the WHO Expert Committee on Mental Health* (WHO Technical Report Series, No. 564). Geneva, World Health Organization, 1975.

3. *Prevention of suicide* (WHO Public Health Paper No. 35). Geneva, World Health Organization, 1968.
4. *Suicide and attempted suicide* (WHO Public Health Paper No. 58). Geneva, World Health Organization, 1974.
5. *WHO Expert Committee on Drug Dependence. Nineteenth report* (WHO Technical Report Series, No. 526). Geneva, World Health Organization, 1973.
6. *WHO Expert Committee on Drug Dependence. Twentieth report* (WHO Technical Report Series, No. 551). Geneva, World Health Organization, 1974.
7. *Evaluation of dependence liability and dependence potential of drugs. Report of a WHO scientific group* (WHO Technical Report Series, No. 577). Geneva, World Health Organization, 1975.
8. *Mental health of adolescents and young people* (WHO Public Health Paper No. 41). Geneva, World Health Organization, 1971.
9. *Child mental health and psychosocial development, Report of a WHO expert committee* (WHO Technical Report Series, No. 613). Geneva, World Health Organization, 1977.
10. *The application of advances in neurosciences and the control of neurological disorders. Report of a WHO study group* (WHO Technical Report Series, No. 629). Geneva, World Health Organization, 1978.
11. *Long-term planning of international cooperation in cancer research. Report of the Director-General* (EB55/7). Geneva, World Health Organization, 1975.
12. Olweny CLM, Eckhardt SJ. *The importance and research potentialities of cancer chemotherapy for developing countries* (ACMR19/77.11). Geneva, World Health Organization, 1977.
13. *Report to the Director-General. Advisory Committee on Medical Research, nineteenth session* (ACMR19/77.14). Geneva, World Health Organization, 1977.
14. Brulé SJ et al. *Drug therapy of cancer*. Geneva, World Health Organization, 1973.
15. Andersen KL. *Fundamentals of exercise testing*. Geneva, World Health Organization, 1971.
16. *Oral health surveys: basic methods*. Geneva, World Health Organization, 1971.
17. *Epidemiology, etiology, and prevention of peridontal diseases. Report of a WHO scientific group* (WHO Technical Report Series, No. 621). Geneva, World Health Organization, 1978.
18. *The etiology and prevention of dental caries. Report of a WHO scientific group* (WHO Technical Report Series, No. 494). Geneva, World Health Organization, 1972.
19. *Epidemiology, etiology and prevention of peridontal diseases. Report of a WHO scientific group* (WHO Technical Report Series, No. 621). Geneva, World Health Organization, 1978.
20. *WHO study of dental caries etiology in Papua New Guinea* (WHO Offset Publication No. 40). Geneva, World Health Organization, 1978.
21. *Oral health surveys: basic methods*, 2nd ed., Geneva, World Health Organization, 1977.
22. *World directory of schools for dental auxiliaries*. Geneva, World Health Organization, 1977.
23. *The medical uses of ionizing radiation and radioisotopes. Report of a Joint IAEA/WHO expert committee* (WHO Technical Report Series, No. 492). Geneva, World Health Organization, 1972.
24. *Nuclear medicine. Report of a joint IAEA/WHO expert committee* (WHO Technical Report Series, No. 591). Geneva, World Health Organization, 1976.
25. *Use of ionizing radiation and radionuclides on human beings for medical research, training, and nonmedical purposes. Report of a WHO expert committee* (WHO Technical Report Series, No. 611). Geneva, World Health Organization, 1977.
26. *Genetic counselling. Third report of the WHO Expert Committee on Human Genetics* (WHO Technical Report Series, No. 416). Geneva, World Health Organization, 1969.

27. *Repository of chromosomal variants and anomalies in man. Second listing, April 1976*, Baltimore, Maryland, Johns Hopkins University, 1976.

28. *Repository of chromosomal variants and anomalies in man. Third listing, November 1976*, Baltimore, Maryland, Johns Hopkins University, 1976.

29. *Repository of chromosomal variants and anomalies in man. Fourth listing, April 1977*, Baltimore, Maryland, Johns Hopkins University, 1977.

30. *Genetic factors in congenital malformations. Report of a WHO scientific group* (WHO Technical Report Series, No. 438). Geneva, World Health Organization, 1970.

31. *Methodology for family studies of genetic factors. Report of a WHO scientific group* (WHO Technical Report Series, No. 466). Geneva, World Health Organization, 1971.

32. *Treatment of haemoglobinopathies and allied disorders. Report of a WHO scientific group* (WHO Technical Report Series, No. 509). Geneva, World Health Organization, 1972.

33. *Inherited blood clotting disorders. Report of a WHO scientific group* (WHO Technical Report Series, No. 504). Geneva, World Health Organization, 1972.

34. *Genetic disorders: prevention, treatment, and rehabilitation. Report of a WHO scientific group* (WHO Technical Report Series, No. 497). Geneva, World Health Organization, 1972.

35. *Genetics of the immune response. Report of a WHO scientific group* (WHO Technical Report Series, No. 402). Geneva, World Health Organization, 1968.

36. *Cell-mediated immune responses. Report of a WHO scientific group* (WHO Technical Report Series, No. 423). Geneva, World Health Organization, 1969.

37. *Immunological adjuvants. Report of a WHO scientific group* (WHO Technical Report Series, No. 595). Geneva, World Health Organization, 1976.

38. *The role of immune complexes in disease. Report of a WHO scientific group* (WHO Technical Report Series, No. 606). Geneva, World Health Organization, 1977.

39. *Immunodeficiency. Report of a WHO scientific group* (WHO Technical Report Series, No. 630). Geneva, World Health Organization, 1978.

40. *Environmental and health monitoring in occupational health. Report of a WHO expert committee* (WHO Technical Report Series, No. 535). Geneva, World Health Organization, 1973.

41. *Health of the working populations in the African Region. Report for the twenty-seventh session of the Regional Committee, 7–14 September 1977* (AFR/RC27/7). Brazzaville, Regional Office for Africa, 1977.

42. *International classification of impairments, disabilities, and handicaps: a manual of classification relating to the consequences of disease.* Geneva, World Health Organization, 1980.

CHAPTER 11

Prophylactic, diagnostic and therapeutic substances

In 1968, the topic of drugs was addressed by the department of Biomedical Sciences, Pharmacology and Toxicology, which covered immunology, human genetics, human reproduction, biological standardization, pharmaceutical substances, drug safety, drug dependence and abuse and food additives. As pharmaceutical substances gained in importance, however, some of the programme elements were moved elsewhere: immunology and human genetics to Noncommunicable Disease Control (see Chapter 10), human reproduction to Family Health (see Chapter 7), drug dependence and abuse to Mental Health (see Chapter 10) and food additives to Environmental Health (see Chapter 12). Health Laboratory Services, which had been part of the Organization of Health Services programme in 1968, was moved to this programme and renamed 'health laboratory technology'.

Another significant change, as discussed below, was the establishment, in 1976, of a new programme element on drug policies and management. This programme was considered necessary because drugs were being sold as if they were commodities, often promoted with intensive marketing. Drugs considered essential for human health were not adequately available, especially in developing countries, and health workers in those countries did not know how to use them correctly. Many countries lacked the resources, financial and human, to set policies designed to ensure that safe, effective, cheap drugs were accessible to all who needed them. The grossly uneven distribution of pharmaceutical production between developed and developing countries further complicated the situation.

PHARMACEUTICALS

Quality control of drugs

Although attention had been paid to quality control of pharmaceutical preparations during most of the 1960s, by 1967, as noted in resolution WHA20.34, "desirable results have not yet been reached." One step towards improving the situation, as also expressed in this resolution, was to require that "drugs should not be exported without having been subject to the same quality control as those issued to the home market in the country of origin." The Director-General was requested to formulate principles for quality control procedures to be incorporated into good drug manufacturing practice. Such principles were formulated in 1968 and then revised on the basis of comments received from Member States and the experts to whom they were circulated. They were then issued in the form of WHO good practices in the manufacture and quality control of drugs.

The guidelines were reviewed by several health assemblies and revised on the basis of comments and suggestions received from Member States and expert consultations. A certification scheme was added, which applied to the quality of pharmaceutical products moving in international commerce. Both were adopted by the Health Assembly in 1975, in resolution WHA28.65, which asked Member States to apply the requirements for good practices and to participate in the revised certification scheme. By the end of 1977, 25 Member countries had agreed to participate in the scheme and had designated responsible national authorities.

The guidelines (1) outlined recommended practices for the manufacture of drugs of desired quality, although it was for the manufacturers to assume responsibility for the quality of the drugs they produced. The good practices outlined were presented as general guides, with the proviso that they could be adapted to meet individual needs, provided the established standards of drug quality were still achieved. The certification scheme was designed to ensure that pharmaceutical products circulating in international commerce had been produced in a manner consistent with the guidelines. Issue of certification was subject to the conditions required by the competent authority of the exporting Member State. The scheme allowed the authorities of the importing country to request additional information from the authorities of the exporting country on controls exercised on the product and to communicate serious defects in products imported under the scheme, with a request that enquiries be instituted.

Each time the governing bodies met to discuss this programme in the early 1970s, they made new demands on the Organization and new proposals for consideration. In 1971, the Director-General's report to the Health Assembly addressed three subjects: WHO's role in helping governments with activities in the field of safety and efficacy of drugs, quality control of drugs and cooperation between UNIDO and WHO to establish pharmaceutical production in developing countries, with particular attention to traditional medicines. The discussion reflected the complexity of the subject as well as the difficulty of determining the best course of action for the Organization to follow.

The Swedish delegate, when introducing a draft resolution, noted that "in view of immense difficulties involved in production and control ... WHO would do well to devote even more of its resources to the question." (2) In his statement, he indicated that WHO should help weed out ineffective drugs; it should discourage the abuse of drugs; it should support training in clinical pharmacology; it should extend its activities in international drug monitoring and provide faster service for analysis and information. Other delegates picked up on these points and added new ones.

The original draft resolution confined its request to the Director-General to study "how best the Organization can cope with its obligations in this domain." To this, the delegate from the USSR added two points, which were accepted: to consider creating a system for collecting and disseminating information on the results of safety and effectiveness trials of new drugs and their registration in countries with the necessary facilities, for possible use of these data by the health authorities of countries importing pharmaceutical products, and to publish the list of countries where the state authorities responsible for the quality control of drugs recognized and implemented 'good practices' and used the certification scheme. The delegate of the United States added a request to the first point that the Director-General "report on the feasibility and financial implications of such a system." The final resolution was adopted as WHA24.56.

No new action was taken concerning the establishment of pharmaceutical production in developing countries, despite the fact that the Executive Board, earlier in the year in its resolution EB47.R28, had recommended that the Health Assembly adopt a resolution that invited to Director-General to continue cooperating with UNIDO "in assisting developing countries to establish pharmaceutical production" and to provide, within the limits of available resources, "assistance to the health authorities of Member States to secure that the drugs used are those most appropriate to local circumstances, that they are rationally used and that the requirements for them are assessed as accurately as possible." The subject had been discussed 2 years earlier, at which time the Health Assembly (resolution WHA22.54) had expressed concern about the "widespread use of various traditional medicines in many countries" and the "hazards and economic wastage connected with the empirical use of such drugs as long as their efficacy and safety have not been established."

The Norwegian delegate, Dr Karl Evang, one of the founding fathers of WHO, in his statement, noted that "Norway had always been very interested in the problem of drugs and his delegation was not fully satisfied with the progress made by WHO in relation to standards. It had been anticipated at the International Health Conference in 1946 that Article 21 of the Constitution would be applied but that had not been done." Article 21 (points d and e) gave the Health Assembly the authority to adopt regulations concerning a number of items, including standards for the safety, purity and potency of biological, pharmaceutical and similar products moving in international commerce; and advertising and labelling of biological, pharmaceutical and similar products moving in international commerce.

Dr Evang raised the same point during the Health Assembly in 1972 when this item was discussed. This time his point was incorporated in resolution WHA25.61, which requested the Director-General to report:

(a)   on the feasibility of an international information system providing data on the scientific basis and the conditions of registration of individual drugs;
(b)   on practicable minimum requirements and on other efforts to develop a comprehensive approach to ensuring the quality, safety and efficacy of drugs, including the feasibility of implementing Article 21 (d) and (e) of the WHO Constitution; and
(c)   on the cost of any action foreseen.

Following adoption of resolution WHA24.56, preliminary studies had been made in a number of Member States on the availability of information on the quality, safety and efficacy of drugs for their intended use in humans, before and after market release. With the adoption of resolution WHA25.61, further studies were initiated, but, as indicated to the Executive Board at its fifty-first session, in 1973, "As these studies will necessarily involve a wide range of interrelated aspects of drug control, to which the proposed information systems would contribute, it is envisaged that a longer period of time would be required for their completion." (*3*)

The feasibility study outlined in early 1973 aimed at determining whether the required data on all new drugs could be provided by participating countries. It also examined the possibility of setting up, on a preliminary basis, recording systems for information on new drugs and methods for its retrieval and dissemination in suitable forms. It included a study on the resources required for an operational international system and the basis for assessing the usefulness of the proposed information system. The experts consulted considered the establishment of an information system on drugs "feasible provided that data on new drugs were supplied by the competent national bodies." (4) As the discussions at the Twenty-sixth World Health Assembly in 1973 illustrated, however, WHO could expect to encounter considerable difficulties. The Swedish delegate, for example, indicated that "administrative, legal and other difficulties should not be underestimated." The delegate from the United Kingdom "wished to sound a note of caution, as it seemed to him that some of the suggestions seemed to be difficult of implementation because of the confidentiality and the volume of work involved." The United States delegate suggested "that a careful beginning should be made; and it should not be expected that the international information system would solve all the problems of existing national systems ...." (4)

By the end of 1974, 26 countries had agreed to participate in the feasibility study and to contribute data on newly registered drugs. The envisaged system would provide data on the conditions of registration and withdrawal of drugs, on the basis of the most complete scientific information available. It would also aim to improve the scientific and administrative processes of registration, so as to facilitate the marketing of useful new drugs and prevent the introduction of harmful ones; draw up acceptable criteria for the safety, efficacy and quality of drugs; and reduce the need for repetitive testing in animals while minimizing possible risks in clinical trials.

One step taken by the Director-General, which met with general approval, was to establish an expert advisory panel on drug evaluation. As indicated in his report to the Twenty-fifth World Health Assembly (5):

> To cope effectively with the broad problem that society has to face with the toxic potential of the steadily increasing number of drugs and pollutants, more research is needed to elucidate the basic biochemical mechanisms involved and to supplement it, where feasible, with epidemiological studies in human beings. Continuing review and reappraisal of the relevance of routine tests is also needed to adapt toxicological laboratory testing to the progress of knowledge in order to avoid unnecessary tests and to ensure that requirements for such testing do not give an assurance of safety that may be illusory.

A scientific group was convened in late 1974 to consider all aspects of the evaluation and testing of drugs and to formulate proposals and guidelines for present and future research in this field. The group reviewed reports on evaluation and testing methods used for various categories of drugs and brought these up to date. It proposed (6) that WHO undertake to prepare guidelines for drug evaluation (preclinical and clinical) in specific pharmacological or therapeutic areas, as such guidelines could promote mutual acceptance of the results of testing in different countries. WHO was also asked to initiate and coordinate studies on the ethical problems raised by clinical drug evaluation, and to disseminate the results of post-registration surveillance for safety and efficacy to assist health professional and regulatory bodies in drug evaluation. The group proposed that there should be discussion of the difference in importance attached to effects observed at the highest doses in studies of carcinogenicity and in studies of general toxicity, to determine whether research should be undertaken to establish valid reasons for the difference. WHO was also asked to study the possibility of promoting regional cooperation and the establishment of facilities for drug evaluation, which were inadequate in some parts of the world.

In 1975, the direction of the programme changed, as indicated in the opening paragraphs of this chapter. At the same time, the programme was still grappling with earlier and new demands made upon it. During the discussion of the Executive Board in January 1975 (7), concern was expressed about the pressure exerted on developing countries to purchase drugs. Despite their best efforts, as one African member said, "they were none the less exposed to unscrupulous activities on the part of certain pharmaceutical industries, and he wondered whether WHO could not help in that connexion."

The Director-General, in his reply (7), stressed the problem of sales pressure from drug manufacturers, especially in developing countries. Without unstinting support from the Executive Board and the Health Assembly, the secretariat could do very little to stop that. The Health Assembly would have to consider ways of offering protection that was not merely technical but also political and moral. The global social responsibility that certain members had called for could be exercised only if governments were prepared to limit the activities of the pharmaceutical industry.

In his introduction to the discussions on this item at the Twenty-eighth World Health Assembly, in May later that year, the director of the programme said:

> ... the Director-General considered that the activities of the Organization in relation to drugs should be reoriented and, as regards direct assistance to countries, that a global approach should be developed relating priorities in the matter of drugs to health priorities in general. That global approach was important for developing countries where the people did not have all the drugs they needed. It was necessary that countries should formulate their own national drug policies, setting their own priorities as regards research, production, control, and distribution of drugs. It was clear that those policies would differ in different countries, depending on many factors. Thus WHO could not propose a single model, but rather hoped to stimulate studies and to help countries, on request, to determine their own priorities. For countries that had difficulty in obtaining essential drugs it was also important that WHO should be able to give advice and information and be able to assist with the training of personnel responsible for drug control. (1)

The United States delegate to the Health Assembly noted in his reply that two projects were under way.

> One was the international system of reporting on adverse reactions to drugs [see below]; the other was the international system concerned with information on drug registration [as discussed above]. Programmes of that sort could provide developing countries with the information they needed to develop drug programmes in accordance with their real health needs. That information would be useless, however, in a country that was unable to assess its drug requirements. WHO certainly had a role to play in helping to train personnel in drug evaluation and regulatory control. (1)

Monitoring for adverse drug reactions

The thalidomide disaster in 1961 led health authorities in several countries to collect reports on adverse drug reactions, and various drug monitoring schemes were initiated. WHO was asked to take an active role in ensuring the safety of drugs (resolution WHA15.41, adopted in 1962), and in each subsequent year a new resolution was passed, calling on WHO to continue to collect information on adverse drug reactions and to pursue, with the assistance of the Advisory Committee on Medical Research, discussions on satisfactory methods for monitoring the adverse reactions, especially late toxic effects, of drugs already in use

In 1965, the United States offered to provide facilities for the processing of information on adverse drug reactions under the auspices of WHO. This request was accepted in 1966, and the Twentieth World Health Assembly, in 1967 (resolution WHA20.51), requested the Director-General to initiate a pilot project in this area, the Government of the United States having made available, for a period of 3 years, office space and equipment, computer facilities, advice and financial support. The purposes of the pilot project, in Alexandria, Virginia, were to establish an international system of drug monitoring, devise a system for recording case histories of adverse reactions to drugs, analyse and feed back to national centres data on the types and patterns of adverse reactions to individual drugs and study the contribution of drug monitoring to research in pharmaceutical and therapeutics. Operations began in February 1968, with 10 countries participating, all with national drug monitoring centres. Within 2 years, by which time some 25 000 case reports had been collected, an improved scheme was available, suitable for reporting from national centres and for coding and card-punching by monitoring centres.

The outcome of the pilot phase was welcomed by the Health Assembly in 1970, and the centre was transferred to Geneva. Eight more countries joined the programme. The centre did not publish or report on associations between drugs and adverse reactions, as this was not its responsibility. It did, however, publish papers on methods of drug monitoring, the epidemiology of drug use, the economics of adverse drug reactions and related topics.

The Executive Board, in 1975, in its resolution EB55.R21, expressed its conviction "of the necessity of developing drug policies linking drug research, production and distribution with the real health needs". One of its recommendations was that "the international system for monitoring adverse drugs should be further developed in order to adapt it to national efforts to ensure the safest possible use of drugs."

By the end of 1977, 22 countries were participating in the programme, and steps were taken to transfer the operational aspects of the programme to a WHO collaborating centre in Uppsala, Sweden.

Dissemination of technical information

Several publications in this field are revised regularly to ensure that information on drugs and related substances is as up-to-date as possible. The most fundamental is the *International pharmacopoeia*, a publication that dates back to 1874. It later added a list of international nonproprietary names for new pharmaceutical substances. The *International pharmacopoeia* is compiled in collaboration with members of the WHO Expert Advisory Panel on the International Pharmacopoeia and Pharmaceutical Preparations and specialists from industry and other institutions. The information it contains is collated after consultation and can thus be considered as based on international experience. Each edition is supplemented with monographs on topics of special interest. In 1970, for example, 20 monographs on antituberculosis drugs and radioactive pharmaceuticals were included. The monographs are intended for use in the quality control of drugs in international commerce, and some were used as teaching material in courses organized by WHO with other organizations.

The WHO Expert Committee on Specifications for Pharmaceutical Preparations, meeting in 1974, recommended that the *International pharmacopoeia* concentrate on general methods of testing pharmaceutical products and on specifications for drug substances (pharmaceutical raw materials) rather than on finished products, in order to establish a system in which a steady flow of specifications could be produced (in accordance with resolution WHA20.34) (*8*). Priority was given to drugs that were used widely throughout the world, and high priority was accorded to drugs that were important to WHO health programmes. Since 1979, on the basis of the first report of the WHO Expert Committee on the Selection of Essential Drugs, reference has been made to the list of essential drugs (see below), and specifications have been established for the identification, purity and content of essential drugs appearing in the WHO Model List of Essential Drugs and its updates.

In recognition of the great disparity between developed and developing countries with regard to drug manufacture and distribution, it was proposed that basic tests for well-established drugs used in general health care should be made available at country level when properly equipped and staffed drug control laboratories were not available. The tests would be designed to confirm the identity of pharmaceutical substances and to ensure that gross degradation had not occurred. This recommendation was followed up in revisions of drug quality specifications for new editions of the *International pharmacopoeia*.

An expert committee on nonproprietary names for pharmaceutical substances met periodically to select names for new pharmaceutical substances on the basis of requests received from national authorities or directly from manufacturers. In 1970, *General principles for guidance in devising international nonproprietary names for pharmaceutical pubstances* was published (*9*). The principles were revised in 1975 in the light of new developments. In 1976, a cumulative list of the 3500 international nonproprietary names was published from a computer printout.

BIOLOGICAL STANDARDIZATION

The objective of one of the oldest international health programmes, that for biological standardization, is to ensure the efficacy and safety of biological products used in medicine by setting international standards and making available reference preparations. WHO has a constitutional responsibility and authority for promoting the use of international standards and of requirements for biological substances used in prophylactic and therapeutic substances (Articles 2(u) and 23 of the Constitution).

The work is carried out under the supervision of the WHO Expert Committee on Biological Standardization. Meeting annually, the Committee reviews new requirements on the basis of study results, the availability of new assay techniques and new needs. It is assisted in its work by international laboratories for biological standards, which act as custodians and distributors of the international standards and reference preparations. International reference materials are intended for calibration of national standards used as references in assaying biological products for manufacturing or national control.

The importance of the programme was recognized in resolution WHA25.47, adopted by the Twenty-fifth World Health Assembly in 1972. This led to preparation of a report for the Twenty-seventh World Health Assembly and adoption of resolution WHA27.62, which called on the Director-General to intensify the work of WHO in coordinating standards for chemical and biological diagnostic materials and their use, with emphasis on quality control; to collaborate with both national institutions and nongovernmental scientific organizations in coordinating standardization, including research; and to seek additional resources for the programme outlined in the report as soon as possible, not waiting for their possible inclusion in the regular budget.

New developments, including new techniques, made new standards possible. For example, the existence of radioimmunoassay techniques made it possible to assay hormones accurately. New needs also arose during this period. The increasing use of blood and blood products made available by commercial firms prompted the Twenty-eighth World Health Assembly to take steps to develop good manufacturing practices specifically for blood and blood components (resolution WHA28.72). In that same year, 1975, the Health Assembly addressed the question of the use of laboratory animals for of the quality control of biological products (resolution WHA28.83), and the Twenty-ninth World Health Assembly, in resolution WHA29.67, called on WHO to lead in the preparation of standards, criteria and international guidelines for the supply and use of non-human primates for biomedical purposes and to promote research on replacing non-human primates by other animal species.

Laboratories in developing countries were strengthened by encouraging laboratories in countries with highly developed services to provide not only the collaboration they had freely offered in the past but also testing and other facilities. A guide was drawn up in 1968 (*10*), which outlined the stages that could be followed in building specialized facilities in countries with limited resources. By 1975, the Organization was making available to interested developing countries a design for a control laboratory that could be built up in three stages, thus permitting gradual development as skills and experience were acquired. The programme started with the quality control of vaccines and other biologicals for which only relatively simple facilities are needed.

WHO formulated and published international requirements for use by workers in the production and control of preparations to ensure at least a minimum level of efficacy and safety. Interregional seminars were organized, at which participants from countries with limited facilities for quality control met to discuss principles and practical problems with experts from countries with well-established control organizations.

A research programme to improve existing requirements for various biological substances expanded its activities to address new priorities. Problems associated with testing the potency of pertussis vaccine and in evaluating diphtheria and tetanus toxoids were selected for collaborative research by a number of laboratories in 1970. By 1971, a collaborative group of six laboratories had been established. In 1973, studies were designed to find a new method for titrating the virus of yellow fever vaccines.

The growing interest in setting up expanded programmes for immunization throughout the world (see Chapter 9) led to more emphasis on the production of poliomyelitis vaccine and to studies with combined diphtheria–tetanus–pertussis vaccines, standardized to meet WHO requirements. These studies also addressed the production of an adequate antibody response to different immunization schedules, with only one or two doses of vaccine. With the financial support of UNDP, manuals were prepared on the production and control of diphtheria, tetanus and pertussis vaccines, and staff from developing countries were trained in the production and control of vaccines. Research on the production and testing of more stable measles, poliomyelitis and diphtheria–tetanus–pertussis vaccines was strengthened.

HEALTH LABORATORY SERVICES

At the beginning of this period, the programme for health laboratories was associated with the programme for public health services, at which time 82 countries and territories were receiving assistance from WHO in planning and establishing public health laboratory services, training various categories of laboratory personnel and expanding referral services at national, regional and international levels. The programme cooperated with the International Committee for Standardization in Haematology on questions of international terminology, and with the International Society of Blood Transfusion and the League of Red Cross Societies on principles and practices of blood transfusion.

A review in 1971 broadened the scope of the programme beyond training of personnel to integrating laboratory services into general health services, improving facilities at the intermediate and peripheral levels and promoting quality control with better methods, including standardization of techniques and equipment. An expert committee discussed the planning and organization of health laboratory services in 1971 and recommended that the Organization intensify quality control in laboratories, encourage further studies on international standards in all branches of health laboratory sciences, while continuing to promote the training of different grades of laboratory staff (11).

Resolution WHA25.47 called for WHO to study means for extending its work in setting standards for chemical and biological diagnostic materials and related aspects of laboratory methods and to coordinate research in this field. For this purpose the Centers for Disease Control, Atlanta, Georgia, United States, and WHO held a 4-day international conference in June 1973, which was attended by 154 participants and observers from 27 countries. The participants recommended that the main function of WHO in this field should be to promote and coordinate research, to disseminate technical information, to promote international cooperation and the acceptance of agreed methods and to establish and make available international standards, reference preparations and reference reagents that would be formulated as part of the programme.

Resolution WHA27.62, adopted in 1974, called for intensification of the work of WHO in coordinating the setting of standards for chemical and biological diagnostic materials and their use, with emphasis on quality control. It was at this time that the programme was assimilated into the programme of prophylactic, diagnostic and therapeutic substances. A consultation attended by some 30 experts in laboratory science from 15 countries identified the priorities for WHO's programme in late 1974. Interregional courses were held, which focused on quality control methods.

Three consultations were held in 1975 to further the work of the programme of standardization of diagnostic methods and materials, specifically in clinical chemistry, haematology and microbiology. The experts attending these meetings stressed the need for international guidelines for labelling laboratory reagents and disseminating technical information and reaffirmed the importance of training, particularly in quality control, as an integral part of the programme.

Although the programme continued to provide technical assistance on various aspects of laboratory services, at the end of this period the most important problem remained inadequate or no laboratory services at intermediate and peripheral levels in many developing countries. Furthermore, those services that were available were found to be largely unrelated to the health priorities of communities. It became clear that WHO should reorient its programme in order to provide simple, appropriate techniques for laboratory support for the control of the most important health problems, improve the availability of essential diagnostic reagents and equipment at reasonable cost, and expand the transfer of laboratory technology by organizing training activities.

Accordingly, methods for essential laboratory tests in clinical chemistry that could be used in intermediate laboratories were circulated, including a manual with details of procedures. Similar methods for haematology and bacteriology were sought. Simple guidelines for preparing and evaluating laboratory reagents, including diagnostic kits, were drawn up by the International Federation of Clinical Chemistry on behalf of WHO.

DRUG POLICIES AND MANAGEMENT AND THE ESSENTIAL DRUGS INITIATIVE

By the end of 1974, the issues that had occupied the governing bodies and the secretariat over the previous decade, as described above, made it clear that further progress would depend on the existence of meaningful, realistic national drug policies in countries. Furthermore, those policies must be based on health priorities if they were to serve health interests, as opposed to economic interests, of which there are many in this area.

A background paper prepared for the fifty-fifth session of the Executive Board, in January 1975, described the elements that should be addressed in a national drug policy, including research and development, information, promotion, distribution and legislation for drugs, good manufacturing practice, pharmaceutical inspection and analytical control, registration of drugs, a list of essential drugs, monitoring of marketed drugs and drug use. Although the notion of 'essential drugs' had been expressed on earlier occasions, for example, in the background paper on basic health services written for the forty-ninth session of the Executive Board in January 1972 (*12*), the suggestion of drawing up a list of essential drugs emerged at a meeting of experts who had investigated the difficulties experienced in some developing countries in meeting the cost of the medicines needed for their health programmes (*13*).

The document was slightly revised and then presented to the Twenty-eighth World Health Assembly later that year (*14*). It stressed the urgent need to ensure "that the most essential drugs are available at a reasonable price and to stimulate research and development to produce new drugs adapted to the real health requirements of developing countries". It stated that the Organization had made "a significant contribution towards raising the standard of drugs and assisting countries in improving drug quality, safety and efficacy".

It was now "important to assist countries also in formulating and implementing national drug policies".

The document described what WHO was doing to strengthen each element of drug policies in developing countries, where the need was greatest. Country health programming was seen to be a platform for identifying "drugs most suitable for the functioning of health services and for the implementation of specific programmes and projects". It was pointed out that WHO had been a "forum for discussions of problems associated with pharmaceutical products" over the years. It had instituted activities throughout the world, including: international requirements for the quality control of drugs, specifications for pharmaceutical preparations, guidelines for good manufacturing practice and international nonproprietary names for pharmaceutical substances; guidelines for the scientific evaluation of drugs for safety and efficacy, from preclinical testing to clinical trials, guidelines for drug registration and exchange of information on evaluation of new drugs by national regulatory systems and of data that form the basis for decisions to withdraw drugs from the market; and monitoring of marketed drugs to assess their usefulness in medical practice. It was noted that while international monitoring of adverse reactions for acute toxicity was well advanced, methods for evaluating long-term toxicity, such as carcinogenicity, required further work.

In the future, emphasis was to be placed on assisting countries in further refining and implementing their national policies and programmes in drug research, production, regulatory control, storage, distribution and monitoring of drug use; in procuring, at reasonable cost, essential drugs of established quality for their national health-care systems, particularly programmes for deprived populations, such as primary health care programmes, and in establishing local or regional production of such drugs wherever feasible; in education and training of scientific and technical manpower for drug research, evaluation, quality control and distribution and improving the education of health professions and the public in proper use of drugs. The Health Assembly incorporated each of these directions in resolution WHA28.66.

A group of experts convened in July 1975 to advise WHO on how to assist Member States in formulating national drug policies stressed the importance of the leadership and guidance of WHO in this area. At a meeting held in October 1976, a group of consultants agreed on a provisional list of about 150 categories of essential drugs, by substance rather than actual products, which were considered necessary for first and second levels of health care. The report of this consultation (*15*) was circulated for comments to the WHO regional offices, health administrators, experts and nongovernmental organizations in official relations with WHO.

The desirability of self-reliance in the production of essential drugs in developing countries was stressed on several occasions, in particular at the conference of heads of state of nonaligned and other developing countries, held in Colombo, Sri Lanka, in August 1976. After that conference, a programme of action for economic cooperation was established, with a secretariat and a joint programme on pharmaceuticals provided by WHO, UNCTAD and UNIDO. UNDP funding for this project was obtained in 1977, with WHO acting as the executive agency in association with the other agencies.

The Director-General, commenting on this programme to the fifty-ninth session of the Executive Board, in January 1977 (*16*), noted that "the area under discussion was undergoing a total transformation to become more relevant to Member States, with priority being given once again to the needs of the Third World."

An expert committee on the selection of essential drugs was convened in October 1977 to review the list that had been prepared in 1976 and the comments received. The committee drew up guidelines for establishing a list of essential drugs, applied those guidelines to the list that had been decided upon earlier and came up with its own list. It also outlined information and education activities, indicated how drug use surveys could be used by national authorities to identify which essential drugs they should include and identified areas in which research and development were needed.

The committee recommended that WHO undertake periodic updating of the model list contained in its report, disseminate adequate information on each drug listed and coordinate the transfer of information on practical experience gained in use of the list. It should promote education and training in the proper use of essential drugs and support collaborative clinical and epidemiological research on their use under different conditions in various countries. Finally, for countries in which the need for essential drugs exceeded their financial or technical resources, WHO should consider conducting an action programme of international cooperation to extend the accessibility of these drugs to the largest possible proportion of the population.

References

1. *Official records of the World Health Organization*, No. 227, Annex 12 (WHA28/SR/B/12, WHA28/SR/B/14). Geneva, World Health Organization, 1975.
2. *Official records of the World Health Organization*, No. 194 (WHA24/SR/A/13). Geneva, World Health Organization, 1971.
3. *Quality, safety and efficacy of drugs. Report by the Director-General* (EB51/5). Geneva, World Health Organization, 1975.
4. *Official records of the World Health Organization*, No. 210 (WHA26/SR/A/3). Geneva, World Health Organization, 1973.
5. *The work of WHO 1971. Official records of the World Health Organization*, No. 197. Geneva, World Health Organization, 1972.
6. *Guidelines for evaluation of drugs for use in man. Report of a WHO scientific group* (WHO Technical Report Series, No. 563). Geneva, World Health Organization, 1975.
7. *Official records of the World Health Organization*, No. 224 (EB55/SR/10). Geneva, World Health Organization, 1975.
8. *WHO Expert Committee on Specifications for Pharmaceutical Preparations. Twenty-fifth report* (WHO Technical Report Series, No. 567). Geneva, World Health Organization, 1975.
9. International non-proprietary names for pharmaceutical substances. *WHO Chronicle*, 1970, 24:119–142, 413–433.
10. *WHO Expert Committee on Biological Standardization, twenty-second report*, Annex 3, *Development of a national control laboratory for biological substances (A guide to the provision of technical facilities)* (WHO Technical Report Series, No. 444). Geneva, World Health Organization, 1970.

11. *The planning and organization of a health laboratory service: fifth report of the WHO Expert Committee on Health Laboratory Services* (WHO Technical Report Series, No. 491). Geneva, World Health Organization, 1972.

12. *Organizational study of the Executive Board on methods of promoting the development of basic health services. Background documentation* (EB49/WP/6). Geneva, World Health Organization, 1972.

13. *Work of WHO 1974. Official records of the World Health Organization*, No. 221. Geneva, World Health Organization, 1975.

14. *Prophylactic and therapeutic substances. Report by the Director-General. Official records of the World Health Organization*, No. 226, Annex 13. Geneva, World Health Organization, 1975.

15. *Consultation on the selection of essential drugs, Geneva, 11–13 October 1976* (WHO DPM/ 76.1). Geneva, World Health Organization, 1976.

16. *Official records of the World Health Organization*, No. 239 (EB59/SR/16). Geneva, World Health Organization, 1977.

CHAPTER 12

Environmental health

Item (i) of Article 2 of the WHO Constitution, in which the functions of WHO are described, states that WHO shall "promote, in co-operation with other specialized agencies where necessary, the improvement of nutrition, housing, sanitation, recreation, economic or working conditions and other aspects of environmental hygiene." The First World Health Assembly, in 1947, which discussed this item under the heading 'environmental sanitation', decided that it should be included in the 'top priority' category of the Organization's programme of work.

Despite the high ranking given to this programme, a comprehensive review in 1959 of the work in what was now described as 'environmental health' judged the progress to have been too slow. The Twelfth World Health Assembly recommended (resolution WHA12.48) that national programmes give priority to the "provision of safe and adequate water supplies for communities" and requested the Director-General to invest in this programme "to maintain leadership in a coordinated global programme of community water supply and to provide the necessary technical and advisory services to governments". Although community water supplies were given particular emphasis, other environmental deficiencies that endanger health, such as air and water pollution, sewage and solid wastes and health aspects of housing and physical planning, were also addressed during the second decade.

The programme was expanded in the third decade, as reflected in the aims presented to the Twenty-fourth World Health Assembly in 1971 (1):

- to improve health in all countries through environmental control;
- to enlarge knowledge of the adverse effects on health of components of the environment;
- to determine as rapidly as possible the permissible levels for man of pollutants and other adverse environmental influences; and
- to provide Member States with a system for early warning of the onset of a deterioration in community health or well-being.

Three large international conferences stimulated the growth of the programme. The first was the United Nations Conference on the Human Environment, held in Stockholm in June 1972; the second was the United Nations Conference on Human Settlements, held in Vancouver, Canada, in June 1976; and the third was the United Nations Water Conference held in Mar del Plata, Argentina, in March 1977. Also of importance was the establishment of UNEP in late 1972 as a consequence of the Stockholm Conference (see Chapter 1).

Other general features that characterized this decade were the availability of better statistics on the magnitude of problems of environmental health and a move from individual projects to national plans.

COMMUNITY WATER SUPPLIES AND WASTE DISPOSAL

The first expert committee convened by WHO specifically to consider the problems of community water supplies met in late 1968. It is perhaps of historical interest to note that the meeting was chaired by Professor Abel Wolman, who participated in the interim commission that set up WHO in 1946 and who claims that it was his intervention that led to the inclusion of environmental hygiene in the WHO Constitution (2). The committee reviewed progress and judged that the situation in most developing countries still remained "critical" (3). Population growth in urban communities exceeded the growth of water supplies, and the rate of progress in rural areas was so slow in many developing parts of the world that it would take "more than 100 years to reach a satisfactory level unless present efforts are dramatically accelerated."

The Committee drew some conclusions from the progress made and the experience gained, including the fact that countries should design their programmes in stages; make the water supply an integral component of their development policy; strengthen existing national organizations and define the principal responsibilities of governmental and semi-governmental agencies in the planning, design and health surveillance of water schemes; give engineers in ministries of health the status and authority to allow them to play a responsible role in community water supply programmes and to take part in decision-making at policy level; expand the pilot and demonstration schemes of UNICEF and WHO into programmes that could meet all national needs; and adopt a policy in which water and sewerage schemes were combined.

The committee addressed the complex problem of the economics and financing of community water supply programmes. International and regional banks and other financing agencies should be made "constantly aware of the long-term investment benefits" of such projects. They should be made to realize that deferred repayment of loans, long periods of amortization and low rates of interest were all vital to their success. United Nations funds should not be overlooked for pre-investment surveys and for education and training projects and research and development. The hope was expressed that UNICEF and WHO would continue and, if possible, expand their programmes of joint assistance for rural water supplies.

When the sixteenth session of the Joint UNICEF/WHO Committee on Health Policy met in March 1969 to review progress on environmental sanitation and rural water supply programmes, 73 joint UNICEF/WHO projects were being undertaken, with about 60 WHO sanitary engineers working wholly or partly in the field and in regional offices and headquarters. The general pattern of these projects was that UNICEF provided imported materials and equipment, government funds were used for locally available materials and transport, the villagers themselves supplied labour and such items as sand and gravel, and WHO field staff assisted with the planning, design and supervision of construction. The progress report reviewed by the Committee (4) was based on visits by a WHO consultant to seven of the country projects, on reports by WHO staff and on information supplied by governments.

While the Joint Committee expressed its appreciation for the numbers of supporting staff involved, it considered "that a greater degree of support needs to be given to the planning and implementation of country projects and to the development of environmental sanitation departments in central ministries". It also stated that more data from individual projects should be collected and recorded so that the experience gained could be used for future work. At the same time, there should be more active participation by governments, and early provision of counterpart staff would help to achieve part of the training aspects of the programme.

It was agreed that environmental improvement, particularly in water supplies, was one of the most important means of protecting the health of mothers and children in rural communities. The programmes should be coordinated with activities in the fields of nutrition, community development and education, and would be all the more successful if they were incorporated into national development plans, in cooperation with national health authorities and other government agencies.

The participation of local communities in planning and implementing environmental health improvements should be ensured, especially in the use, operation and maintenance of these facilities. It was observed that there was considerable room for improvement in health education methods and coverage. Sanitation facilities in schools should be used to encourage healthy habits and practices among students and teachers.

The Committee's recommendations reflected these observations and were in line with those of an expert committee that had met several months earlier (see beginning of this chapter). It was stressed that the highest priority should be given to training national personnel. More research was needed on improving the effectiveness of health education. Guidelines should be prepared for governments requesting UNICEF/WHO assistance that would make clear the objectives and limitations of the assistance available. Finally, every endeavour should be made to encourage other international and bilateral agencies to become involved in national programmes for environmental improvement.

The Organization assisted countries in obtaining funds to make pre-investment surveys, the results of which would be needed to prepare requests for loans to finance construction of community water supplies. WHO also initiated research and development to help governments increase community water supplies while at the same time reducing costs and enhancing the efficiency of operation and management.

The Chemical Bacteriological Department of the Institute for Water Supply, The Hague, The Netherlands, was designated in 1968 as the international reference centre on community water supply, responsible for coordinating the work of some 60 collaborating research institutes throughout the world. That same year, a WHO international reference centre on wastes disposal was set up at the Federal Institute for Water Supply, Sewage Purification and Water Pollution Control, Zurich, Switzerland, to conduct an international programme for the collection, storage and distribution of information, with an initial focus on solid wastes. One of its first activities was to devise a simple, cheap process for reducing the volume of domestic solid wastes. By 1970, some 40 institutions in developed and developing countries were collaborating with the centre.

A new element was introduced into the programme in 1970 in India, where, following a joint UNICEF/WHO study, assistance was given for exploiting groundwater to supply water to villages in areas particularly vulnerable to drought.

The cholera epidemic in the early 1970s led to an intensification of WHO's activities in improving water supplies and the sanitary disposal of excreta. WHO field engineers, sanitarians and sanitary chemists participated in cholera control and preventive measures.

New and improved methods for examining drinking-water and changes in the concept of permissible levels led to a third edition of the *International standards for drinking-water*, the second edition of which had been published in 1963 (5). As noted in the annual report for 1971 (6), however, "standards by themselves are of little avail if organizations for applying them do not exist".

In 1971, a formal agreement was concluded with the International Bank for Reconstruction and Development for both international and national investment in a collaborative programme for pre-investment activities, including sector studies, the identification and preparation of pre-investment projects, assistance in the execution of such projects and advice on follow-up.

A detailed survey of water supply conditions in 90 developing countries was carried out in 1971–1972 by WHO, which revealed that progress in making safe water available was not keeping up with population growth, and progress in the provision of sewage disposal facilities lagged even further behind. The major obstacles, in order of importance, were: insufficient internal financing, lack of trained personnel, an inappropriate administrative structure, insufficient external financing, an inappropriate financial framework, insufficient production of local materials and an inadequate or outmoded legal framework.

Basic planning principles and objectives for national programmes and design criteria and technical solutions appropriate for developing countries were discussed by a WHO expert committee on wastes and wastewater disposal that met in the autumn of 1973 (7). The committee also discussed the most suitable types of national organization and methods of financing for planning, implementing and control of community wastewater disposal. It made recommendations on training methods for professional and skilled personnel and on areas requiring further research and investigation, including alternatives to the water-carriage system, reuse of wastewater, removal of deleterious substances, new criteria for the control of effluent quality, manpower and managerial development and low-cost collection and disposal systems.

A new collaborative programme was initiated during 1974 with UNICEF, UNDP, UNEP, the International Bank for Reconstruction and Development, the Organisation for Economic Co-operation and Development (OECD) and the International Development Research Centres of Canada, with the aim of making technological information available at the right time in the right place and emphasizing adaptation of technology to local economic and social conditions, particularly for water supplies and sanitation in rural areas. An ad hoc working group on rural potable water supplies and sanitation was set up, WHO providing the secretariat, which sponsored a study of the technology involved, its application and the social or cultural factors that often hamper application of even tried and proved techniques. A number of activities that could usefully be undertaken were listed, and the institutes in developing countries where they might be carried out were identified.

Proposals were prepared for regional programmes in collaboration with the Pan American Centre for Sanitary Engineering and Environmental Sciences, in Peru, the Pan-African Institute for Development, in the United Republic of Cameroon, and the Inter-African Committee for Hydraulic Studies, in Upper Volta. It was decided that the WHO

Collaborating Centre for Community Water Supply in The Hague should be restructured to serve as an international centre for a network of cooperating centres in other regions.

In the context of the Second United Nations Development Decade (see Chapter 1), a mid-decade review of community water supplies was undertaken for consideration by the Twenty-ninth World Health Assembly, in 1975. Following an extensive discussion, the Health Assembly adopted resolution WHA29.47, which endorsed the regional targets proposed by the Director-General and, inter alia, requested him to continue to accord high priority to collaboration with Member States in this area.

A draft guide on community water supplies and wastewater disposal was distributed to Member States in 1975 as part of the Organization's programme of assistance to national information systems for planning, programming and evaluation in this respect. The guide was tested in a pilot project in India, with the aim of setting up an information system in a selected area (the State of Maharashtra), adapting the WHO guidelines to local conditions and extending aspects to national level.

Country and regional information on community water supply coverage and excreta disposal services and on the investment made during 1971–1975 was published in the *World health statistics report* (*8*) and was used in preparing a strategy and plan of action for consideration by the United Nations Water Conference, which was held in Mar del Plata in March 1977. WHO regional offices made written submissions to the background papers for the Conference and participated in the preparatory meetings organized by regional economic commissions of the United Nations. Strategies and a plan of action to enable countries to achieve the targets set out by the 1976 United Nations Conference on Human Settlements were prepared by WHO in collaboration with the International Bank for Reconstruction and Development and were adopted *in toto* by the Water Conference.

The Conference called on countries to adopt specific, detailed plans for water supplies and sanitation services suited to their conditions and recommended that the international community adopt a more effective approach in supporting, financially and in other ways, the increased national commitments of developing countries. The decade 1980–1990 was designated 'International Drinking-water Supply and Sanitation Decade', for implementation of the plan of action. The positive outcome of this Conference, from WHO's perspective, was "contrary to expectations", as expressed by the WHO secretariat to the Thirtieth World Health Assembly, in May 1977 (*9*).

On the basis of the recommendations of the Conference, the Health Assembly in May 1977 urged Member States to act upon resolution II of the Conference immediately, by proceeding with a rapid assessment of their existing programmes and the extent to which they could usefully be expanded. The Health Assembly (resolution WHA30.33) also requested the Director-General to ensure WHO's fullest participation in implementing the plan of action, to reinforce WHO's longstanding leadership in community water supplies and sanitation in cooperation with other relevant United Nations organizations and to strengthen collaboration with multilateral and bilateral agencies and other donors for the provision of resources to Member States in implementing their programmes.

In response to a decision of the twenty-first session of the Joint UNICEF/WHO Committee on Health Policy, in January 1977, a study was initiated to focus on issues in coordinated approaches for planning and implementing accelerated programmes for community water supplies and sanitation in the context of overall development plans and policies of which primary health care is a part. The issues included political will and national commitment, community motivation and participation, manpower development, appropriate technology, financial requirements and issues relating to planning, operating and maintaining these services and facilities (*10*).

HUMAN SETTLEMENTS AND HEALTH

From 1956, WHO's work on housing was linked with urban development and was carried out in association with programmes of other international agencies concerned with housing, building and regional planning. The results of a study, begun in 1964, were published in 1968 under the title *The physiological basis of health standards for dwellings* (*11*). The publication reviewed the present state of knowledge and research in various countries on basic human requirements for housing, including temperature regulation, lighting and other factors affecting health and comfort in the home. A new study, started that year, was directed to establishing environmental health criteria for use by persons responsible for urban and regional planning.

WHO continued to cooperate in related activities of the Economic Commission for Africa by providing a sanitary engineer, who participated in planning and conducting courses for building contractors and a course in cooperative and self-help housing.

A study of the environmental health aspects of urban planning was undertaken in 1970 by a physician, a sanitary engineer and an architect–urban planner, who reviewed planning criteria on the basis of experience in different parts of the world and ways in which they could be applied at local, national and regional levels. Their report was used as the basis for a scientific group meeting held in 1971 on environmental health criteria for urban planning (*12*).

A WHO expert committee on the epidemiological aspects of housing and the environment, which met in the autumn of 1972, reviewed statistical and epidemiological data on communicable diseases, mental illness and home accidents in relation to the residential environment in various parts of the world. The committee assessed their epidemiological significance and implications for housing programmes and considered the physical and biological aspects of the environment, man-made changes in environmental factors and social and economic circumstances of populations, including their beliefs, culture and relationships. The committee recommended (*13*) further study and research and emphasized that planning authorities should have an understanding of the social and epidemiological aspects of housing. As a consequence of this recommendation, a study of the literature was initiated, which led in 1976 to publication of a 118-page annotated bibliography on housing, the housing environment and health (*14*).

Following the Stockholm Conference on the Human Environment, which drew attention to the influence of dwellings and the residential environment on human health, WHO's programmes in this field were extended, notably with financial assistance from UNEP. Four new projects were initiated in 1974: to draft guidelines for preventing health hazards in transitional settlements, to formulate minimum requirements for basic sanitary services in human settlements in developing countries, to establish health criteria for planning residential environments and housing, and to draw up guidelines for hygienic water supplies and waste disposal in buildings.

Work continued in the pilot project initiated by the Inter-agency Committee on Housing and Urban Development to rehabilitate slums on the outskirts of cities in Colombia, Ecuador, El Salvador, Mexico, Peru and Venezuela. Through the Pan American Centre for Sanitary Engineering and Environmental Sciences, the Organization assisted several countries in formulating physical planning programmes, including the colonization of several underdeveloped areas in eastern and western Peru and a multisectoral plan for rural development in the Dominican Republic.

The Organization took an active part in the preparatory work for Habitat, the United Nations Conference on Human Settlements, held in June 1976. A WHO report, *Health and environment in human settlements*, assessed the interaction between humans and their settlements in terms of health. Also as part of the preparations for the Conference, the technical discussions held during the Twenty-ninth World Health Assembly addressed the health aspects of human settlements. A review based on these discussions was published in 1977 (*15*). The report of the technical discussions and other inputs of the Organization, including contributions from the regional offices, ensured that health was prominently mentioned in the Declaration of Principles of the Conference. They also influenced the adoption of three recommendations for national action that related particularly to health: one calling for targets for the provision of safe water and hygienic waste disposal, the second related to the control of pollution, and the third urging that health, nutrition and other social services receive priority in national development planning and in the allocation of resources.

ENVIRONMENTAL HEALTH CRITERIA AND MONITORING

In 1968, the report of five WHO scientific groups on research into environmental pollution was published (*16*), which reviewed recent trends in environmental pollution and the problems of air, water and soil pollution. Areas in which research was recommended were environmental pollution in general, standardization of observations, experiments in animals, enzymes, the metabolism of absorbed pollutants, carcinogenicity and mutagenicity and long-term effects of pollutants on ageing.

At the end of 1967, an expert committee met to discuss water pollution control in developing countries. In view of widespread, severe water pollution in recent years, the committee was asked to review the subject and make recommendations for planning water use and pollution control in urban areas, agriculture and industry; to formulate general principles for the prevention of water pollution in relation to the management of water quality; to make recommendations for the training of personnel in water resource management and the control of water pollution; and to point out areas in which further research was necessary.

The committee observed that the effect of pollution had generally not been realized until the damage was done, although most of the 16 reporting countries were beginning to take legal, administrative and technical measures to deal with the situation. It discussed the main health aspects of water pollution on the basis of reports received from countries. It addressed the technical requirements for planning, surveying and quality management of water resources. The need for public support was highlighted, as the success of a system for water pollution control was seen to depend to a great extent on a national sense of responsibility. It was suggested, in this regard, that WHO might make films on water pollution and its control, which could be supplied, with accompanying texts, to schools in developing countries. In addition to recommendations on the basic principles to be applied by developing countries, the committee recommended that WHO render further assistance to Member countries in establishing training institutions and using them to promote studies of the potential uses of wastes, particularly for crop production. The committee further recommended that WHO investigate the possibility of assisting Member countries to improve and extend services for information retrieval (*17*).

Assistance from WHO for the development of water pollution control programmes included the preparation of requests to UNDP for aid from the Special Fund component, the provision of technical assistance in the control of pollution caused by industrial wastes, and assessment of the water pollution situation in various parts of the world. In the European Region, a study was undertaken on trends and developments in water pollution.

An expert committee on urban air pollution, with particular reference to motor vehicles, which met in July 1968, drew attention to the need for periodic appraisals of individual pollutants, especially carbon monoxide, lead, hydrocarbons, nitrogen oxides and other oxidants, and for less costly, simpler sampling methods.

As part of its research programme, WHO established, at the end of 1967, an international reference centre on air pollution at the Air Pollution Research Unit of the Medical Research Council, London, England, and a number of regional and national reference centres and collaborating laboratories. The functions of the international reference centre included giving advice and coordinating research on such subjects as the effects of air pollution, organization of air pollution surveys, identification and measurement of air pollutants and control methods. As its first task, the centre undertook a critical review of a number of methods for measuring air pollutants.

A meeting of directors of reference laboratories was convened in October 1969 to coordinate the programmes of the WHO international reference centres, regional reference centres and collaborating laboratories. International collaborative research into the various effects of air pollution on health was discussed, the highest priority being given to studies of the effects on children and, with regard to the effects of single pollutants, to the effects of exposure to carbon monoxide, lead, arsenic and cadmium. The need for training epidemiologists and statisticians to work in this field was also stressed.

By 1970, the results of a long-term study undertaken by the centre in London showed a striking association between estimated exposure to pollution and the incidence of lower respiratory tract infections, even in children as young as 9 months. These effects persisted up to school-leaving age, which suggested that pollution may cause some damage early in life that can have lasting effects. With the assistance of the centre, methods for routine measurement of sulfuric acid aerosol, sulfur dioxide, suspended particulate matter, carbon monoxide and oxides of nitrogen were tested and, after review, issued as a series of WHO documents. These provided a critical appraisal of most of the methods available and singled out a number as suitable for specific types of work. The methods were intended for routine use in the field by people unfamiliar with air pollution monitoring, and most required only simple equipment.

A 5-year study on the long-term effects of pesticides on health, carried out in Italy with support from WHO, was completed in 1969. One of the main conclusions was that high levels of chlorinated hydrocarbons in fruit, vegetables, water and soil were associated with increased general morbidity. No association appeared to exist, however, between the levels of pesticides in the environment and the amounts stored in fatty tissues.

The work of the Pan American Sanitary Engineering and Environmental Sciences Centre, established in Lima, Peru, in 1968, was referred to in Chapter 4. An important related development was a decision taken in 1970 at the request of a number of Latin American countries to expand the existing Pan American Air Pollution Surveillance Network (comprising numerous stations, financed by PAHO or by governments in 15 countries) to include the monitoring of water quality, pesticide levels and other changes in the environment that might adversely affect human health.

WHO's participation in the International Hydrological Decade, a programme under UNESCO auspices designed to stimulate national research on water resources, was intensified in 1970, following the decision that WHO should provide the technical secretariat for a working group on hydrological aspects of natural and artificial changes in water quality. One of the group's first tasks was to prepare a practical handbook on the hydrological measurements required in water quality surveys.

One of the main recommendations of the 1972 United Nations Conference on the Human Environment was that monitoring and epidemiological and experimental research programmes be set up to provide data for early warning and prevention of the deleterious effects of environmental agents and for assessing their potential effects on human health. WHO was asked to coordinate the organization and use of an appropriate international collection and dissemination system and to assist governments in coordinated monitoring in areas where pollution might pose a risk to health. The establishment of working limits for environmental pollution was suggested, and WHO was called on to set primary standards for the protection of the human organism, especially from pollutants that are common to air, water and food. The proposals made in Stockholm were not new to WHO, as the Twenty-fifth World Health Assembly, meeting just before the Conference, had already confirmed, in resolution WHA25.58 the importance of most of the measures later advocated by the Conference.

Following the Stockholm Conference, the Organization embarked on an expanded programme for assessing the effects of biological, chemical and physical agents in the environment, including new and potentially hazardous substances used in the home, in industrial production and in agriculture, with the aim of setting environmental health criteria and standards. The Twenty-sixth World Health Assembly (resolution WHA26.58) requested the Director-General to accord high priority to the early identification of environmental health hazards and to the prevention of their effects.

The major objective of the WHO environmental health criteria programme was to prepare critical reviews of the available information on exposure to specific environmental pollutants and hazards and of the effects of exposure to these substances on health. The programme stressed the need for an integrated approach to the assessment of health effects, taking into account all pathways of exposure.

A pilot study was initiated in 1973 for monitoring a few important pollutants in urban air. Programmes were prepared for monitoring selected contaminants in food, water and the working environment, as part of a coordinated international programme for monitoring the environment within the United Nations system's Earthwatch Programme. WHO and UNEP collaborated in this activity.

A WHO scientific group on environmental health criteria met in April 1973 to identify the research needed to improve the basis for criteria and guidance on exposure limits. The list of priorities suggested by the group comprised some 70 substances and physical factors, the highest priority being accorded to nitrogen oxides, nitrates, nitrites and nitrosamines; cadmium; lead; mercury; manganese and its compounds; polychlorinated biphenyls; mycotoxins; and noise.

The Advisory Committee on Medical Research, at its fifteenth session in June 1973, pointed out that information on human toxicity was the best basis for estimating risks from environmental exposure. Every effort should be made to improve the database by careful epidemiological studies. Similarly, although this was a difficult and costly task, the predictive value of animal experiments should be improved.

A WHO expert committee on the planning and administration of national programmes for controlling adverse effects of pollutants met in October 1973. After reviewing the role of health authorities in establishing national and environmental quality standards, enforcing legislation, surveillance and inspection of services, the committee set out general principles for the prevention and abatement of pollution, outlined the function of health authorities in this field and provided practical guidelines for planning and implementing national programmes for the control of adverse effects of pollutants on human health and well-being. The recommendations called on WHO to expedite the preparation of criteria documents, pay particular attention to promoting acceptable, comparable methods of measurement and programmes for inter-laboratory data quality control and compile scientific and technical information on environmental pollution and disseminate this information to national institutions (18).

Preliminary reviews were prepared in 1974 on a number of potential pollutants, such as tellurium, selenium, germanium, titanium and tin and their compounds and selected petroleum products. These substances were also covered in a programme on health and environmental monitoring that was being set up at that time.

In order to advance knowledge on this subject, a WHO study group on health hazards from new environmental pollutants was convened in autumn 1974 to assess existing methods of forecasting health hazards from such pollutants, to review some important problems and to provide guidance on initiation of national programmes in this field (19). Forecasting was considered to be important on the basis of several incidents, including mercury poisoning among people living in the Minamata Bay area of Japan. In that tragic episode, inorganic mercury used in a local acetaldehyde manufacturing plant was converted to methylmercury in the environment. Fish and shellfish became polluted, and people who ate large quantities were severely affected by mercury poisoning. Better knowledge of possible methylation reactions could have prevented this tragedy.

The group recognized that setting up information and warning systems for adverse health effects from the environment was complex and that "no satisfactory solution" had yet been found. Methods for obtaining information on the health hazards associated with chemicals were reviewed, including registration of new chemicals, the creation of toxicological data banks, rapid laboratory bioassay systems and warning systems. The priorities identified were the environmental health impact of power production and use and the technology of chemicals and materials, including plastics and plasticizers, fire retardants, metals, photosensitizers and pesticides.

With regard to forecasting in environmental health, the study group recommended that WHO draw up detailed guidelines on the type of information needed to assess possible health risks associated with new chemicals and with new uses of existing chemicals. Test systems were needed for assessing the fate of chemicals in the environment. The study group called on Member States of WHO to establish systems for evaluating new chemicals that are introduced into commerce, regulating their use where appropriate, and establishing, strengthening and consolidating toxicological data banks, with particular attention to the ready accessibility of the data by the international scientific community. WHO should encourage research into rapid bioassay systems and should ensure the comparability of methods.

With respect to the environmental health impact of energy production and use, the group recommended that WHO, in cooperation with other interested international organizations, should encourage comparative cost–risk–benefit studies of the health consequences of the use of conventional and nuclear sources of energy.

The study group concluded its report with a series of recommendations on developments in the technology of materials and chemicals. The introduction of new materials should not be permitted until their adverse effects, if any, have been adequately assessed. Known toxic chemicals and particularly certain metals that accumulate in the biosphere should not be used in new products if their use or disposal would result in the release of these chemicals into the environment. A greater proportion of national and international research activities on environmental pollution should be directed to identifying and assessing new problems associated with chemicals.

A meeting on the WHO environmental health monitoring programme was held in July 1974, at which its scope and content were reviewed and suggestions made for its implementation through international collaboration. Past WHO activities in this area had emphasized different environmental media and conditions (air, water, food and work environment); now, integrated monitoring systems were proposed to determine total exposure and to assess whether the populations at highest risk are exposed to concentrations that are sufficiently high or of sufficient duration to induce prompt, delayed or long-term adverse effects. The meeting stressed that the primary objectives of the programme were to advise and assist Member States in setting up national monitoring systems, to document the effects on health of changes in environmental quality and to evaluate the effectiveness of control programmes and progress towards achieving improved environmental quality.

Six task group meetings were convened in 1975 to evaluate the health risks of exposure of both the general population and specific occupational groups to mercury, lead, cadmium, manganese, polychlorinated biphenyls, and nitrates, nitrites and nitrosamines. Draft documents were prepared for several other compounds, and the final documents were published in subsequent years.

In order to promote harmonization of toxicological testing techniques, a book outlining the principles and methods for evaluating the toxicity of chemicals was prepared in 1975 (*20*), in collaboration with 50 experts from 13 countries and financial support from UNEP. A revised draft was reviewed by a WHO scientific group that met at IARC in December of that year. That group also discussed current problems and needs in the methodology of toxicity testing, chemobiokinetics and metabolism, studies of organ function, neurological and behavioural tests, carcinogenesis, mutagenesis and teratogenesis, exposure by inhalation and ecotoxicology.

A new Pan American centre for human ecology and health was established in Mexico in 1975, the main purpose of which was to formulate methods for the identification, definition and control of human health problems related to environmental change. The centre assisted countries of the Region by direct technical cooperation, by distributing technical information and by collaborating in research and training programmes. High priority was given to assessing the effects of development projects on health and the environment.

A scientific group that met in December 1976 reviewed the possibility of using existing health information systems for assessing health effects related to changes in environmental conditions. They concluded that it was premature to undertake routine monitoring of health effects before health information systems had been improved. Such monitoring could be undertaken, however, in specific populations, such as infants and children, an example being epidemiological studies on the effects of air pollution on child health carried out by the Regional Office for Europe.

The Thirtieth World Health Assembly, in resolution WHA30.47, requested WHO to study long-term strategies to prevent acute, chronic and combined toxic effects that can result from exposure to chemicals in air, water, food, consumer products and workplaces, particularly if combined with exposure to other chemicals, infectious agents and physical factors. WHO was also asked, in collaboration with appropriate national institutions and international organizations, to examine the options for international cooperation, including the financial and organizational implications.

As part of UNEP's Global Environmental Monitoring System, WHO and other relevant international organizations initiated global projects on monitoring air and water quality. The objectives of these projects were to strengthen national environmental quality monitoring programmes for the protection of human health and to collect data for global assessment of the environment. By 1977, some 60 Member States were participating in the air quality monitoring project, based in national centres and involving all the WHO regional offices. The preparatory phase of a similar global water quality monitoring project was completed by the end of 1977, and sampling locations were selected in about 70 Member States. Technical cooperation for these projects included the provision of equipment, training and technical advice and the organization of interlaboratory data quality control studies.

FOOD SAFETY

The basis for food legislation was established in the nineteenth century, with the introduction of food technology, leading to a revision of legislation. The need for internationally acceptable food standards led to the establishment in 1963 of the joint FAO/WHO Food Standards Programme, the principal organ of which is the Codex Alimentarius Commission. By 1968, the Commission had 93 member countries and had prepared some 200 standards for foodstuffs. The Commission also formulates advisory codes of hygienic practice. Two important subsidiary bodies are its committees on food additives and on pesticide residues, which work in conjunction with the Joint FAO/WHO Expert Committee on Food Additives and the FAO/WHO Joint Meeting on Pesticide Residues. These bodies met at various times during the decade to review the results of studies, to determine whether additional studies were needed before standards could be set and to agree on new standards when sufficient data were available.

In the joint FAO/WHO work on standards of food hygiene, undertaken in cooperation with the Codex Alimentarius Commission, research was promoted on formulating standard procedures for microbiological examination of foodstuffs, the detection and enumeration of pathogenic viral agents in various foods and the effects of different technical processes on microbiological flora in food products. Emphasis was laid on specialized training in the field of food hygiene, particularly for developing countries.

At the Commission's sixth session, in 1969, it decided that once standards had been adopted they should be published as 'recommended Codex standards'. If they were accepted by governments, the Commission would then decide to publish the standards in the *Codex Alimentarius*. In giving final approval to Codex standards, the Commission gave priority to the health aspects, especially in respect of food additives.

In 1970, the first four of a series of recommended international standards, formulated and adopted by the Codex Alimentarius Commission, were sent to members and associate members of FAO and WHO for acceptance. The standards, which are compatible with the norms considered to best guarantee the promotion and protection of health, took a number of years to elaborate. Each year during the decade, several such standards were established.

The Twenty-third World Health Assembly, in 1970, expressed concern about the potential health hazards of food additives and adopted resolution WHA23.50, in which it agreed that the results of research on the toxicity of food additives should be disseminated rapidly. They asked the Director-General to take expeditious steps to evaluate any significant new evidence for the toxicity of a specific food additive, including, if necessary, convening a meeting of experts, where appropriate in consultation with FAO. In effect, this resolution introduced an information service on food additives similar to that already in operation on drugs.

The Twenty-fifth World Health Assembly, in 1972, recognizing the need for a comprehensive evaluation of the hazards related to unwholesome food and the need for internationally agreed standards for food hygiene, adopted resolution WHA25.59, which requested the Director-General:

- to promote research on the effects on human health of modern food technology and especially of the effect of residues, additives and food contaminants;
- to promote international agreement on criteria and acceptability levels for biological, physical and chemical contaminants in food;
- to intensify the participation of WHO in the Joint FAO/WHO Codex Alimentarius Commission with a view to protecting the health of consumers;
- to prepare, in close collaboration with the Codex Alimentarius Commission, guidelines and codes of practice for the hygienic production, processing, storage and handling of food; and
- to make coordinated efforts in this field, taking into account the multiplicity of aspects involved.

In 1972, WHO initiated systematic collection of existing toxicological and related data on food additives, pesticide residues and contaminants and started publishing a new WHO Food Additive Series. The ninth session of the Commission adopted general principles for the use of food additives and decided that they should be included in the third edition of the *Codex Alimentarius* procedural manual (*21*).

In 1973, a joint FAO/WHO conference on food additives and contaminants addressed both biological and chemical food contaminants and proposed that an international, coordinated monitoring programme be established, covering a number of important chemical and biological agents in food. The proposal included the preparation of guidelines for establishing or strengthening national monitoring systems, undertaking national food consumption surveys to calculate the intakes of contaminants in food, training to assist governments in conducting monitoring studies and international exchange of information between countries where food contaminants were already being monitored and the rest of the world.

In 1973, proposals made jointly by FAO and WHO for assisting developing countries in food control, in keeping with Recommendation No. 82 of the Stockholm Conference, were accepted by UNEP for financial support. These proposals concerned preparatory work for establishing microbiological standards and standards regarding pollutants in foods as well as the preparation of a 'food control manual'. UNEP also agreed to provide financial support for pre-programme activities related to the proposed programme for monitoring food contaminants.

In 1974, concerned about the deficiencies in food control activities in many countries, the Joint FAO/WHO Food Standards programme conducted a survey of codes and ordinances pertaining to catering establishments and prepared a draft model code for such establishments.

In the same year, the first session of the Coordinating Committee for Africa was held under the umbrella of the Codex Alimentarius Commission. The Committee stated that the main problem in acceptance of food standards by the countries of the African Region was lack of appropriate, modern food legislation, regulations and the means for enforcement.

In 1975, a joint FAO/WHO expert committee finalized two draft documents. The first provided guidelines for an effective national food control system in developing countries, outlining the infrastructure and methods required. The second document, on food hygiene in catering establishments and the role of legislation, included model legislation.

The Joint FAO/WHO Expert Committee on Food Additives at its meeting in 1977 indicated that annual meetings were inadequate to evaluate the increasing amount of toxicological data and the large number of food additives, flavours, processing aids, packaging materials and contaminants (22). In May 1977, the Health Assembly asked (resolution WHA30.47) the Director-General to find ways of overcoming this problem.

During 1976–1977, the Codex Alimentarius Committee reappraised its programme of work and its priorities, and decided to pay more attention to the needs of developing countries. Codex coordinating committees were established for Africa, Latin America and Asia to devise a concerted approach to instituting modern food law and regulations and other aspects of food control.

The Organization continued to encourage the establishment in Member States of the necessary infrastructure for maintaining the safety, nutritional value and quality of foods and to promote national food control programmes and training. A food control strategy was set out by a working group convened in late 1977.

ENVIRONMENTAL HEALTH PLANNING

WHO assistance to national health agencies in planning, organizing and managing environmental programmes emphasized the necessity of undertaking studies of factors that hinder the setting up of such programmes, the measures required for achieving realistic objectives and integration of environmental programmes into national health and socio-economic development plans.

An expert committee on planning, organization and administration of national environmental health programmes, which met in June 1969, pointed out that WHO could "provide significant assistance with the development and evaluation of national programmes, and with the development of criteria, manpower, and research" (23). To this end, in 1971, WHO started work on an environmental health planning guide, which was to identify the factors that contribute to a healthy environment, the steps involved in achieving and maintaining it, the resources needed and the appropriate timing of activities to bring about the required result gradually. It was also to include the information needed for planning in various environmental health fields. Although early versions of such a guide were prepared, the increasing complexity of the subject resulted in it emerging in different forms in different contexts, beginning with one based on the systems approach.

Application of the systems approach led to the publication in 1974 of a 242-page guideline on administration of environmental health programmes (24). Part 1 of this paper introduced general systems theory as applied to administration and outlined a systems view of environmental health. Part 2 began with an overview of administration and then addressed planning, decision-making and evaluation; programme planning; management planning; design and implementation; management operations; communications and information; control and evaluation of management operations; and prospects for administrative and technical development in environmental health programmes.

An interregional seminar on human ecology in environmental health, held in the summer of 1972, addressed the sociocultural and technical aspects of community acceptance of and response to environmental health planning. The participants stressed the need for better understanding of the influence of environmental change on human well-being and of the social changes necessary to reap the benefits of planning. They reviewed the epidemiological, biological, physical and socioeconomic aspects of the ecology of human settlements and considered social, cultural and psychological influences, to ensure that planning was not limited to the technical aspects. These topics were covered again in 1974 in technical discussions on the role of the health services in preserving or restoring the full effectiveness of the human environment in the promotion of health (see Chapter 10).

WHO convened an interregional symposium on environmental health planning and management in the summer of 1974 to discuss modern concepts and methods. The participants, who were drawn from five WHO regions, reviewed recent experience in some Latin American countries in preparing their first national environmental plans and advised on the elaboration of guides on environmental health planning. They stressed that such planning was necessitated by the interdependence of the many environmental and other activities that affect health and by the fact that they compete for resources. Following this symposium, steps were taken to prepare another series of guidelines on planning national environmental health services. Actual cases and experience were reviewed, such as the results of a study conducted in 1975 in Colombia and Ecuador.

A study carried out in 1974 by WHO dealt with environmental health activities and services provided as a component of basic health services. The purposes of this study were to examine the objectives of this component; to review the methods of planning, organizing, implementing and evaluating environmental health activities and services; and to determine the effect of these activities on improving basic health and the environment. The study showed that, while successes had been achieved in some cases, far too often the potential role and participation of health administrations in environmental health were limited, while the power, initiative and resources resided in other ministries, particularly with respect to water supplies and waste disposal. The findings pointed to the value of establishing departments of public health engineering in health ministries and, as appropriate, in other ministries, such as those for public works, which are involved in large programmes for water supplies, waste disposal and other environmental problems. Concern was expressed about the tendency to move health-oriented engineers from health organizations to agencies in which the interest in health may be minimal.

These and related findings led the Twenty-seventh World Health Assembly, in 1974, to adopt resolution WHA27.50, which recommended to Member States that health agencies participate fully in planning and implementing national environment programmes and any other national programmes that might affect health, and recommended that health authorities be authorized and equipped, both technically and administratively, to perform this role. The Twenty-eighth World Health Assembly added the recommendation (resolution WHA28.63) that Member States establish adequate coordination at national level to ensure that improvement and protection of human health became an important objective in planning and implementing environmental programmes and that the capacity of WHO be used towards attaining that objective.

The delegate from Finland to the Twenty-ninth World Health Assembly, meeting in May 1976, expressed

> uneasiness at the way in which WHO and its Member States were dealing with health and environmental issues. Just as the concepts of 'hygiene' and 'environmental health' had not been taken seriously in the past, so nowadays was the programme for 'human health and environment' receiving only lip service from many people who thought it was not proper to be against environmental health. Some of the reasons for that situation were that the health field as a whole was still dominated by physicians and nurses conditioned by their traditional medical thinking and training; the complex field of environmental health was not well understood; and those in technical, social, economic, and medical professions were still not able to collaborate across their professional boundaries as true equals. As a result, the health authorities sometimes tried to concentrate everything in their own hands; or 'pure' environmental authorities, with a very weak health input, were established. (25)

The secretariat, in its reply, agreed:

> With a few exceptions, the situation was bleak, and in a number of countries, personnel formerly available in ministries of health had moved to other ministries. Ministries of health should pay more attention to creating environmental health programmes, to staffing them with specialists, and to giving them a status that would allow them to command the respect of others and to attract the necessary resources. At the same time ministries of health should introduce health aspects into other environmental programmes such as programmes for water resources development and housing, but that, too, depended on the availability within health ministries of technical expertise at a high level of authority. (25)

Throughout this period, assistance was provided to countries in planning their environmental health services. The assistance took different forms in each region. Thus, in the South-East Asia Region, seminars were organized to give planners and administrators an opportunity to exchange views and experiences on the subject and to consider proposals for overall environmental health programmes within their national health plans. In the Eastern Mediterranean Region, a number of projects were initiated. For example, in Iran in 1975, projects were financed by UNDP for undertaking nationwide surveys of the extent of industrial and agricultural pollution. Similar studies were carried out in Libya and Syria. General advisory services in environmental health were organized in several countries of the Western Pacific Region and on an intercountry basis in the South Pacific area; a Western Pacific Regional Centre for Promotion of Environmental Planning and Applied Studies was authorized in 1977, with the objectives of promoting and facilitating collaboration among institutions and scientific and technical personnel of Member States in the Region, and promoting national self-reliance in environmental health and environmental protection.

An interregional symposium was convened in the summer of 1977 to review the problems and factors involved in environmental quality planning and policy in developing countries. Attended by nationals from 20 countries and by representatives of United Nations economic commissions and specialized agencies, the symposium proposed a strategy for setting up national environmental quality programmes and means for improvement, including the enactment of legislation, organizational arrangements, changes in planning, and information and education. It also suggested that each country establish a high-level national coordinating body for overall environmental policy and planning and for approval of standards, as the traditional approach involving uncoordinated actions taken by separate ministries was no longer sufficient.

References

1. *Official records of the World Health Organization*, No. 194 (WHA24/SR/A/4). Geneva, World Health Organization, 1971.
2. Hollander W Jr. *Abel Wolman: his life and philosophy. An oral history*. Chapel Hill, North Carolina, Universal Printing and Publishing Co., 1981:771–775.
3. *Community water supply. Report of a WHO expert committee* (WHO Technical Report Series, No. 420). Geneva, World Health Organization, 1969.
4. *Joint UNICEF/WHO Committee on Health Policy. Report on the sixteenth session, 5–6 March, 1976* (JC16/UNICEF-WHO/69.4). Geneva, World Health Organization, 1969.
5. *International standards for drinking-water*. Geneva, World Health Organization, 1971.
6. *Work of WHO 1971. Official records of the World Health Organization*, No. 197. Geneva, World Health Organization, 1971.
7. *Disposal of community wastewater. Report of a WHO expert committee* (WHO Technical Report Series, No. 541). Geneva, World Health Organization, 1974.
8. *World health statistics report*, Vol. 29, No. 10, 1976.
9. *Official records of the World Health Organization*, No. 241 (WHA30/SR/A/7). Geneva, World Health Organization, 1977.
10. *UNICEF/WHO joint study on water supply and sanitation components of primary health care (JC22/UNICEF-WHO/79)*. Geneva, World Health Organization, 1979.
11. *The physiological basis of health standards for dwellings* (WHO Public Health Paper No. 33). Geneva, World Health Organization, 1968.
12. *Development of environmental health criteria for urban planning. Report of a WHO scientific group* (WHO Technical Report Series, No. 511). Geneva, World Health Organization, 1972.
13. *Use of epidemiology in housing programmes and in planning human settlements. Report of a WHO expert committee on housing and health* (WHO Technical Report Series, No. 544). Geneva, World Health Organization, 1974.
14. *Housing, the housing environment, and health; an annotated bibliography* (WHO Offset Publication No. 27). Geneva, World Health Organization, 1976.
15. *Health aspects of human settlements* (WHO Public Health Paper No. 66). Geneva, World Health Organization, 1977.
16. *Research into environmental pollution. Report of five WHO scientific groups* (WHO Technical Report Series, No. 406). Geneva, World Health Organization, 1968.
17. *Water pollution control in developing countries. Report of a WHO expert committee* (WHO Technical Report Series, No. 404). Geneva, World Health Organization, 1968.
18. *Health aspects of environmental pollution control: planning and implementation of national programmes. Report of a WHO expert committee* (WHO Technical Report Series, No. 554). Geneva, World Health Organization, 1974.
19. *Health hazards from new environmental pollutants. Report of a WHO scientific group* (WHO Technical Report Series, No. 586). Geneva, World Health Organization, 1976.
20. *Principles and methods for evaluating the toxicity of chemicals*. Geneva, World Health Organization, 1978.
21. *Codex Alimentarius Commission: procedural manual*, 3rd ed. Rome, Joint FAO/WHO Codex Alimentarius Commission, 1973.

22. *Evaluation of certain food additives. Twenty-first report of the Joint FAO/WHO Expert Committee on Food Additives* (WHO Technical Report Series, No. 617). Geneva, World Health Organization, 1978.

23. *National environmental health programmes; their planning, organization, and administration. Report of a WHO expert committee* (WHO Technical Report Series, No. 439). Geneva, World Health Organization, 1970.

24. *Administration of environmental health programmes: a systems view* (WHO Public Health Paper No. 59). Geneva, World Health Organization, 1974.

25. *Official records of the World Health Organization*, No. 234 (WHA29/SR/B/11, WHA29/SR/B/12). Geneva, World Health Organization, 1976.

CHAPTER 13

Health statistics

International cooperation in health statistics has a history as long as that of the Sanitary Conventions, as exemplified by the publication of an international list of diseases and causes of death (see below). Epidemiological research performed in the early decades of WHO's existence drew attention to the importance of collecting data and to WHO's central role in assisting governments in improving their health statistics and improving the techniques used for data collection and analysis.

Although, in principle, the aim of assisting governments to improve the use of statistics was for planning, management and evaluation, at the beginning of the decade health statistics were based mainly on information that required statistical handling. By mid-decade, however, WHO had clearly indicated its intention to change health statistics from routine collection and treatment of individual components, in a more or less isolated way, to an integrated approach that met the information needs of health planning and evaluation in all its ramifications.

Restricted availability of computer power in the early years meant that data were processed centrally at headquarters in Geneva. Only as computers became more readily available did decentralization of health statistical services begin.

HEALTH STATISTICS METHODS

This element of the programme was responsible for ensuring that sound statistical methods were used in the Organization's research and technical programmes. Many programmes were served during the decade, with various statistical methods. Below, a small sample of the activities is described.

In the field of communicable diseases, the main statistical problems were monitoring disease incidence, evaluation of disease control programmes in longitudinal or repeated surveys, the statistical design and evaluation of controlled trials of prophylactic and therapeutic procedures and operations research, involving mathematical models and computer simulation of disease dynamics. Statistical support was also provided for vaccine trials, such as of BCG vaccination against leprosy in Burma and of Japanese encephalitis vaccine in the Republic of Korea.

With regard to noncommunicable diseases, emphasis was placed on measuring the magnitude of problems in the community, elucidating the natural history of diseases, analysing a wide range of etiological factors and evaluating intervention measures. Use was made of multivariate analysis, discriminant and cluster analysis and regression methods to handle the large numbers of variables involved. These methods were applied to studies of the risk factors for cardiovascular disease in selected subpopulations; to analysing data from the melanoma register at the WHO Collaborating Centre for Evaluation of Methods of Diagnosis and Treatment of Melanoma, Milan, Italy; and to analysing data from the register at the WHO International Reference Centre for the Study of Connective Tissue Disease, Paris, France, and especially the problems of automatic classification for diagnosis. Epidemiological studies were carried out on trachoma in six countries and on schizophrenia in nine.

Judging that the statistical principles in public health field studies were inadequately defined, scattered throughout the literature and known only to experimentalists, the WHO Expert Committee on Health Statistics, at its fifteenth session, in 1972, issued a report on the general principles of research design for field studies, developments in sampling and measurement, the experimental approach in field studies, nonexperimental studies on etiology or interventions, application of field studies in public health services and data handling and analysis (1). The Committee recommended that manuals be prepared on sampling and on certain statistical problems. It also recommended that research on statistical principles and methods for public health field studies be encouraged and the statistical aspects and practical utility of mathematical models in planning and administering health services be explored further.

A variety of mathematical models were developed during the early years of this decade. In 1968, for example, a model was found to describe the dynamics of the transmission of typhoid fever, making it possible to analyse the effect of mass vaccination programmes on the incidence of the disease. In the same year, a linear programming decision model was created to determine the optimum use of medical and financial resources in tuberculosis control and to determine the optimal size of control groups in BCG vaccination trials. This model was further developed in 1969, with the addition of calculation of health benefits.

Mathematical models and computer simulations were devised to identify the most efficient intervention strategies for malaria control. Data-based studies in northern Nigeria were designed not only for validation of the models but also for evaluation of actual control programmes (see Chapter 5).

Many of WHO's activities on the statistical aspects of population dynamics and family health were supported by UNFPA. These included the collection and processing of data on the influence of various socioeconomic and biological factors on perinatal mortality, protocols for studies of infant mortality and a study on the influence of changing mortality on the life cycle of the family, starting with marriage and ending with the death of spouses. Statistical evaluation of the impact of family planning on health was the subject of a consultation in 1972, at which the main requirements for statistical information in this field were defined. In addition, guidelines were formulated for the collection and analysis of relevant data, and suggestions were made for future work in this field. A consultation was held early in the decade on the statistical aspects of the family as a unit in health statistics. Four approaches were reviewed: epidemiological (medical), social, economic and demographic. The social approach, for example, considered different types of family structure and their stages of development, and characteristic crises that might be experienced (2). The statistical aspects of family health and family health care were also discussed at a consultation on family health in late 1973 (see Chapter 7) and again by a study group that met in early 1975 (3). All three meetings made recommendations designed to encourage the formulation of suitable indices for studying family health. The complexity of the methodological and substantive questions involved in using the family as a statistical unit in health studies was acknowledged. WHO was called on to continue its activities in this area, including holding further meetings and conducting specific studies of family health.

Contact was established in 1974 with the recently formed International Institute for Applied Systems Analysis, Vienna, Austria. Studies of multisectoral systems were promoted to provide greater integration between the technical and policy levels of WHO's overall programme of work.

Most of the projects described above involved the collaboration of investigators in different countries, and considerable attention was therefore paid to appropriate working protocols, including standard record forms, in order to ensure satisfactory uniformity in data collection and evaluation. The data obtained in these international studies were processed and analysed centrally at WHO, maximum use being made of the computer facilities at the International Computing Centre in the WHO headquarters building.

DISSEMINATION OF STATISTICAL INFORMATION

In 1965, the title of the Organization's annual statistical publication was changed from *Annual epidemiological and vital statistics* (under which it had been issued since 1948) to the *World health statistics annual*. The publication was issued in three parts: the first volume covered vital statistics and causes of death; the second, data on infectious diseases; and the third, statistics on health personnel and health establishments. Monthly reports were also issued, which contained recent data received from individual countries and detailed information on selected subjects of current interest.

The third volume, published in 1968, included for the first time charts showing the percentage distribution of populations, health personnel and hospital beds in urban and rural areas. From the beginning of that year, the most recent data on health personnel and hospital establishments were published in the monthly report.

The use of computers for data processing considerably facilitated preparation of the *World health statistics annual*. Contact was established with other members of the United Nations system to supplement the information in its data banks, to bring together all health-related statistical information. The availability of electronic data processing also made it possible to bring together morbidity and mortality statistics that had been collected over the previous 20 or so years. Requests for information from research workers and others could be answered more promptly. Similarly, data banks were set up on health personnel and hospital establishments.

Statistics on specific aspects of health were also addressed, in order to improve how statistics were gathered and to determine which statistics deserved closer attention. Thus, for example, at a meeting organized jointly in 1968 by the United Nations and WHO on the quality, sources and use of mortality statistics, recommendations were made for a detailed programme of research on such subjects as mortality trends in relation to demographic, economic and social characteristics, and differences in mortality rates in urban and rural areas.

In 1969, a special statistical study was carried out on the distribution and extent of schistosomiasis and helminthic infections on the basis of information derived from reports, surveys and the medical literature to provide a measure of the magnitude of these health problems. The results were published in the *World health statistics* report. Similar studies were conducted throughout the decade and reported in the annual or the monthly version of the *World health statistics* report.

The Organization's information services were reorganized in 1974 in order to provide quantitative information for identifying major health problems, defining and evaluating health policy, planning health programmes and managing health services efficiently; to bring producers and users of statistical information into constant contact, as an integral part of a systematic effort to improve health statistical information systems and adjust them to changing needs; to contribute to wider, more rapid dissemination of information to users, whether research or health administration workers; to promote critical appraisal, analysis and feedback on the use of health data in decision-making; and to generate better understanding of the limitations imposed upon international comparability by national practices and to define more precisely their effect on comparative studies.

The Twenty-seventh World Health Assembly in resolution WHA27.60 requested the Executive Board to consider rationalizing the collection and summarizing of information on the health situation in various countries and to determine the frequency with which information should be published. At the same time, the Director-General was requested to continue his work on preparation of a sixth report on the world health situation.

Periodic issuance of a report on the world health situation began with a request from the Ninth World Health Assembly to the Director-General to prepare such a report covering the period 1954–1956 (resolution WHA9.27) for the Eleventh World Health Assembly. The second, third, fourth and fifth reports each covered a period of 4 years and were published in the *Official records* of WHO, while supplements were issued as mimeographed documents.

A critical review of the Organization's statistical publications was undertaken in 1975 on the basis of comments and suggestions made in response to a questionnaire addressed to the users of these publications. Beginning in 1975, all requests to countries for national statistical data on health were routed through the regional offices as part of the Organization's effort to coordinate and rationalize the use of questionnaires by WHO for collecting health information.

HEALTH STATISTICAL SERVICES

During WHO's first decade, its assistance to governments was largely meant to improve their ability to collect sound data on diseases, injuries and causes of death, primarily for the purpose of facilitating international comparisons of statistics. Towards the end of the first decade, WHO began to provide consultants to advise countries on health statistics and epidemiology in planning their health programmes. Fellowships were given to provide advance training for the increasing number of nationals involved in statistical work in the health services of their countries. This trend continued in the second decade; by 1967, some 40 WHO-assisted projects on various aspects of vital and health statistics were in operation, as compared with 18 in 1958.

Each region recognized the importance of strengthening national health statistical services, as reflected in the brief summary of regional trends in Chapter 4. The role of headquarters was essentially to provide guidelines that could be used in training programmes and directly by health administrators responsible for health statistical systems at all levels.

To this end, the thirteenth session of the WHO Expert Committee on Health Statistics, in late 1968, concentrated on the statistics required for the organization and administration of health services (4). Earlier sessions had dealt with problems of hospital and morbidity statistics in general. It had become evident, however, that the scope and content of existing statistics from health services required adjustment so that they responded to the requirements of modern health administrations. Beginning with an outline of why health statistics were needed, the Committee addressed the question of statistics as they applied to resources, to activities and to the use of health services, including special services. Evaluation of the efficiency and effectiveness of health services was addressed, as were the organizational requirements for statistical services. With regard to the last point, the Committee recommended that WHO pay further attention to specialized training in health service statistics and consider organizing courses on this subject for health administrators and statistical technicians.

Training programmes for all categories of health statistical personnel were thus set up by WHO. In addition to formal and informal courses given as part of WHO-assisted projects on health statistics, WHO provided staff to lecture on special topics at national and international training centres. Training in health statistics for holders of international fellowships and other university graduates was organized in three European training institutes, the London School of Hygiene and Tropical Medicine, London, England, the Free University of Brussels, Belgium, and the Institute for Postgraduate Medical Education in Bratislava, Czechoslovakia, for students speaking English, French and Russian, respectively. Similar training in Spanish was made available in the Region of the Americas.

In 1969, a study group met to draw up guidance on establishing medical record systems and the standardization of medical records. The group made recommendations on methods of collection, recording, storage and retrieval of medical information, the organization of a medical records department, basic medical records, training of personnel, research and future development in this field.

By 1970, it was judged that the rapid increase in the use of computers in national health statistical services and corresponding developments in WHO's work were hindering the improvement of health statistics in developing countries (5). While advanced automated systems were being used in some countries for processing data, many lacked the organization and personnel required to provide even basic health statistics. Furthermore, the statistics had actually been used in only a few countries, even those with the most modern statistical services and equipment, and action had been taken on the basis of an evaluation of the information collected. The inadequate use of statistics, even where available, was considered to be due partly to a lack of coordination between statisticians, health programmers and health administrators.

These problems were addressed at the fourteenth session of the Expert Committee on Health Statistics in late 1970, which recommended a critical examination of existing national statistical systems and of the use made of the information they provided in planning. It considered that countries should develop their information systems with the needs of health planners in mind and gradually introduce the full range of components needed for producing integrated national, regional and local statistics. Particular stress was laid on the training of health and statistical personnel in the use of health statistics for health planning. Each country should establish a national commission that would include representatives of agencies concerned with health planning and health statistics and other bodies requiring social, economic and other data with a bearing on health and health services.

The Committee also indicated that WHO should stimulate and support research into scientific methods for the study of health, health services, health manpower, health facilities, health planning and health systems from the point of view of their effect on populations (6). Such research should include methods based on the techniques of health statistics, biostatistics, epidemiology, demography, the behavioural sciences, operational research, systems analysis and economic analysis. The Committee went on to propose that WHO set up a model health information system for health planning, a formal information exchange system for rapid communication of reports on methods, systems, policies and data from one country to another, and formal arrangements for reviewing current health statistical systems and their use in health planning in each country.

The increased attention given to the subject of health statistics and health planning led to more requests for assistance in this area around the world. In the South-East Asia Region, for example, assistance was provided to Ceylon for a comprehensive study of health manpower (see Chapter 8) and to Thailand for health planning and the evaluation of health programmes.

The need for a multidisciplinary approach was emphasized at a UNICEF/WHO meeting held in 1973 to discuss problems in the collection, processing, interpretation and use of information on the health status of schoolchildren. Stress was laid on the need for a minimal set of information, consisting of data on educational and socioeconomic aspects and on the school environment, as well as on health.

A consultation was held in 1972 to discuss means of improving assistance to countries. It was considered that feasibility missions should be sent to selected countries to investigate ways of improving existing services and to assess the need for external aid. WHO was asked to encourage communication between offices in developed and developing countries and to provide help in selected statistical offices that could act as demonstration and development centres for neighbouring countries. The Organization arranged for teams to visit nine countries in the African and Eastern Mediterranean regions in 1973, to study the structure of their health statistics information systems, evaluate their adequacy and assess their impact on health services. Data on training facilities, particularly with regard to family health programmes, were also collected. The teams tested various methods of assessing the need for statistical information and suggested ways of improving the health statistical services in the countries visited.

The assessment carried out in 1973 formed the basis for a model health statistics information system to be set up in Tunisia under an agreement, signed in 1974, between the Tunisian Government, the United States Government and WHO. The systems approach in planning and evaluation of health statistical information systems was also used in a model for a health information system in relation to schoolchildren, which was set up on a trial basis in the same country. Another pilot project was established in Pakistan in 1975. In both, emphasis was placed not only on the reorganization and extension of central health statistics services, but also on the establishment of peripheral statistical services that were properly coordinated with services at national level. Following the projects initiated in Tunisia and Pakistan, systems analyses of vital statistics services were conducted in Honduras, Jamaica, Mexico, Philippines and Thailand.

In the Region of the Americas, the Regional Advisory Committee on Health Statistics, at its meeting in January 1975, discussed the role and relations of health information and health statistical systems. The Committee recommended that a study be conducted on health information systems and the organizational problems involved, including improvement of existing vital and health statistics programmes; standard definitions and methods for determining data components and indicators; research into priority setting and cost–benefit analysis; and preparation of a series of manuals on computer use, basic statistics and data sets.

Other activities undertaken in the last biennium of the decade included a regional working group on measuring levels of health, held jointly with the International Epidemiological Association, in Poland, in March 1977, to be followed by preparation of a publication (7); a joint working group with the International Federation for Information Processing on health data banks, held in Prague, Czechoslovakia, in August 1976; a regional seminar on civil registration, in Washington DC, United States, in October 1977; a working group on primary health records and their use in developing countries, organized jointly with the Faculty of Medicine and Health Centre, Rijeka, Yugoslavia, in October 1977; a regional seminar on medical records, in Montevideo, Uruguay, in November 1977; preparation of an outline for an information system for analysing national health expenditure and cost; and a meeting held in Geneva in November 1977 on the statistical principles of monitoring and surveillance in public health.

The last of these activities focused comprehensively on the multitude of problems for which monitoring and surveillance were being used, e.g. drug monitoring (see Chapter 11), epidemiological surveillance of communicable diseases (see Chapter 9) and monitoring of food contaminants (see chapters 10 and 12) (8). The meeting reviewed the critical components of monitoring and surveillance and, while recognizing that monitoring and surveillance of any health activity or programme was primarily the responsibility of national governments, concluded that WHO could play a vital role in this area. It should advise on standards, methods and parameters for assessment, and sponsor training programmes in monitoring practices. The usefulness and adaptation of various standard branches of statistical sciences for monitoring systems should be examined. WHO could assist Member States by setting out a framework in which alternative monitoring and surveillance systems could be clearly seen, so that opportunities for choice would be promoted.

At the end of the decade, technical cooperation for promoting and strengthening national health information systems continued, particularly as regards the statistical component. The programme covered about 50 developing countries and was designed to improve information services for decision-making in health.

INTERNATIONAL CLASSIFICATION OF DISEASES

The interim commission that met between 1946 and 1948 to establish WHO, at its third session, in spring 1947, set up an expert committee to prepare the sixth decennial revision of international lists of diseases and causes of death. The first such list had been prepared at the end of the nineteenth century; the idea of decennial revisions came from the American Public Health Association in 1898.

By the 1960s, the *International statistical classification of diseases, injuries and causes of death* (ICD) had become firmly established and was used by many countries, not only for statistics on cause of death but also for information on morbidity and as a basis for diagnostic indexing of hospital clinical records. The seventh revision, which was in use from 1958 to 1967, had been limited to the correction of inconsistencies and to small but essential amendments; however, the eighth revision, adopted by the Nineteenth World Health Assembly, in 1966, introduced major changes and was the outcome of prolonged, intensive work at national and international level. The English version of the *Manual of the international statistical classification of diseases, injuries and causes of death* was issued in late 1967; the French, Spanish and Russian editions were published in 1968.

When adopting the eighth revision, the Nineteenth World Health Assembly requested the Director-General (resolution WHA19.45) to prepare a compendium of recommendations, definitions and standards that would be useful to Member States in preparing health statistics and would improve their international comparability. An outline of this compendium was first prepared in 1968 in collaboration with the WHO Centre for Classification of Diseases in London, England. This was sent to interested Member States for comment and was subsequently reviewed by a study group that met in 1969, by which time the ninth revision of the ICD had begun.

Other developments in the early years of the decade included confirmation of the rules for selection of causes of death for primary tabulation of mortality; formulation of a statistical classification for surgical operations; preparation of lists of pharmaceutical products on national markets; drafting rules for the classification and tabulation of mortality from multiple causes; building up a thesaurus of diagnostic terms to allow coding by computer; and a more sophisticated (full three-digit code) classification of radiological procedures

The first step in the ninth revision of the ICD was taken in October 1969, when a study group met to consider the structure that was best suited for the wide variety of purposes for which the classification was being used. The group agreed that the next revision should provide for multiple-condition coding and analysis in order to enable use of additional categories of information. In 1970, a questionnaire was sent to all Member States about the use they made of the current classification, and the replies were used to prepare draft proposals for changes. These were reviewed by a study group in late 1971, which recommended that those chapters for which considerable changes had been proposed (particularly cardiovascular, maternal and perinatal conditions) should be subjected to trials in parallel with the existing classifications to test their validity and to justify the extent of the amendments.

The end of 1972 was the closing date for the submission of proposals for the ninth revision. A meeting of the heads of the four WHO international reference centres recommended that double coding be introduced to allow identification of both elements in cases for which a single diagnostic statement contained two elements of information, e.g. 'diabetic cataract', so that records could be retrieved according to either element.

The large volume of proposals received from Member States and international professional bodies for the ninth revision of the ICD, ranging from isolated comments on single categories to fully worked-out proposals for whole sections or chapters, was reviewed in Geneva by a study group early in 1973. Whereas the eighth revision classified conditions according to their underlying causes, many of the proposed revisions called for a classification based on the particular manifestation for which medical care was being provided. It was stated that such a classification would be more appropriate for use by clinicians and more informative in medical care statistics, and in the planning and evaluation of health services. Wishing to preserve the continuity of medical statistics, the study group proposed a classification that would contain elements of information about both etiology and clinical manifestation. This proposal was endorsed at a meeting of the heads of the four WHO international reference centres for the classification of diseases in April 1973. As a result of this recommendation and others made at these two meetings, the Organization was able to complete the first draft of the ninth revision soon after mid-1973, and this was circulated for comments.

Another consultation, held late in 1973, reviewed the results of field trials of alternative drafts of an international certificate of cause of perinatal death. It concluded that a special form for stillbirths and deaths in the first week of life was desirable, and that there should be separate notifications of conditions in fetuses or infants and in mothers. Field trials of a method for lay reporting of perinatal and maternal morbidity and mortality were undertaken with UNFPA support in several countries in Africa and Asia. Comparison and evaluation of the results contributed to the solution of a number of practical and methodological difficulties. A system of application that could be adapted to local conditions was then formulated.

Comments on the first draft of the ninth revision of the ICD began to be received in 1974 and showed that opinions were mixed. The subject was discussed by the Twenty-seventh World Health Assembly that year, which adopted resolution WHA27.55, in which delegates expressed their concern that the increasing demand for relevant data for evaluating clinical activities might be met by a diversity of systems in different countries, with a consequent lack of international communication. The Director-General was asked to ensure that the next revision included the means of meeting these needs, without prejudice to continuing use of the classification for its usual purposes.

The WHO Expert Committee on Health Statistics reviewed the subject at its meeting in June of that year. It endorsed the principle of dual classification and considered that it should be implemented more fully than in the first draft proposals. The second draft incorporated the changes suggested and was circulated to members and associate members in the spring of 1975, in preparation for the International Conference for the Ninth Revision of the International Classification of Diseases, which was held in Geneva in October. This Conference was attended by 95 delegates from 46 Member States and by representatives from the United Nations, ILO and 11 nongovernmental organizations. The Conference approved the proposals for the ninth revision, subject to consideration of a number of minor modifications proposed by delegates. The Conference recommended that the revised classification come into effect as of 1 January 1979 and that classifications of procedures in medicine and of impairments and handicaps be published as supplements to, and not as integral parts of, the ninth revision. The Conference approved, with some amendments, a series of proposed definitions and recommendations for perinatal and maternal mortality, including a certificate of cause of perinatal death that was different from the international form then recommended for use for persons of all ages. It recognized that many countries might have difficulty in introducing the certificate but urged that it should be used wherever possible.

Attention was given to the question of securing badly needed morbidity and mortality statistics in countries that still lacked sufficiently qualified personnel, and it was recommended that WHO should assist developing countries in that respect.

The biennium 1976–1977 saw culmination of the programme for decennial revision of the ICD, when the draft proposals for the ninth revision recommended by the International Revision Conference in 1975 were adopted by the Health Assembly in 1976 (resolution WHA29.34). The new revision would come into effect on 1 January 1979.

The Health Assembly also approved publication of supplementary classifications, for trial purposes, of impairments and handicaps and of procedures in medicine, endorsed recommendations of the Conference for the collection of morbidity and mortality statistics by lay personnel in developing countries, and proposed that an international nomenclature of diseases be prepared to improve the 10th revision of the ICD (resolution WHA29.35).

References

1. *Statistical principles in public health field studies. Fifteenth report of the WHO Expert Committee on Health Statistics* (WHO Technical Report Series, No. 510). Geneva, World Health Organization, 1972.
2. *Report on consultation on the statistical aspects of the family as a unit in health studies, Geneva, 14–20 December 1971* (DSI/72.6). Geneva, World Health Organization, 1972.
3. *Report of WHO study group on statistical indices of family health, Geneva, 17–21 February 1975* (DSI/75.5). Geneva, World Health Organization, 1975.
4. *Statistics of health services and of their activities. Thirteenth report of the WHO Expert Committee on Health Statistics* (WHO Technical Report Series, No. 429). Geneva, World Health Organization, 1969.
5. *Work of WHO 1970. Official records of the World Health Organization*, No. 188. Geneva, World Health Organization, 1970.
6. *Statistical indicators for the planning and evaluation of public health programmes. Fourteenth report of the WHO Expert Committee on Health Statistics* (WHO Technical Report Series, No. 472). Geneva, World Health Organization, 1971.
7. *Measurement of levels of health.* Copenhagen, WHO Regional Office for Europe, 1979.
8. *Statistical principles of monitoring and surveillance in public health. Report of a WHO meeting, Geneva, 15–19 November 1977* (HSM/MS/77.11). Geneva, World Health Organization, 1977.

CHAPTER 14

Health and biomedical information

In the review of work carried out by WHO during its second decade, two information-related activities were described. The first concerned information for health authorities and the medical and other health professions, and the second was information for the general public. This distinction remained during the third decade; however, library services, which also featured in earlier decades, took on greater importance as computer access to information gained ground, making the services offered by the Organization more accessible than before.

Resolution WHA25.26, adopted in 1972 by the Twenty-fifth World Health Assembly, stated that WHO should assume a leading role in preparing, coordinating and improving biomedical communications, particularly in fields of major concern to national health services and that were subjects of international cooperation. This conclusion emerged from an Executive Board organizational study on medical literature services that had been undertaken between 1970 and 1972. The resolution called upon the Organization to:

- give more prominence in the publications programme to the social and behavioural sciences and to the economic aspects of health;
- find means of improving both the free distribution and the sales of WHO scientific and technical publications;
- undertake a feasibility study on whether the Organization should prepare and publish medical textbooks;
- consider the importance of improving medical library services for effective use of published biomedical information and particularly setting up regional medical libraries; and,
- organize a study by an international group of experts on the role of WHO in modern biomedical communications.

In 1976, a health and biomedical information programme was formed, linking the WHO publications programme, which maintained a flow of biomedical information from the Organization to the outside world, with the library and health literature services, which are concerned with the flow of biomedical information from the outside world into the Organization. A third component of the programme was transmitting health information to the public. The aim of this reorganization was to enable WHO to deal more responsively and coherently with its widely varied target audiences. At the same time, in response to resolution WHA29.48, these services suffered substantial cuts in funds and manpower, with reallocation of regular budget funds to increase technical cooperation during 1977–1980. Further actions taken in response to resolution WHA25.26 are described below.

HEALTH LITERATURE SERVICES

The need for an adequate library and reference service, as an essential adjunct to the technical work of the Organization, was recognized from the earliest days: the first books and periodicals were acquired in December 1946. The WHO library grew rapidly, and by the end of the first decade, thanks in part to inheritance of the library of the Office International d'Hygiène Publique, Paris, France, it contained over 35 000 volumes.

The WHO library is responsible for collecting, maintaining and monitoring all the documents and printed publications issued by WHO, in both Geneva and the regional offices. The regional structure of WHO led to the establishment of small libraries in each regional office, the WHO library in Geneva functioning as a central library, providing central acquisition and cataloguing services and supplementing local resources with loans, photocopies and assistance with reference enquiries. A reference service on medical and public health subjects was made available on request, not only to WHO staff but to the medical and health departments and institutions of WHO Member States and to the United Nations and specialized agencies.

The WHO library also administers a scheme for international exchange of duplicate medical literature, by which medical libraries notify WHO of surplus medical literature that they are prepared to donate to another library. A distinguishing feature of the WHO library is its use as a training centre. WHO fellowships have been awarded for training on study tours for medical librarians, who often spend a considerable part of their period of study in the WHO library.

In 1967, a computerized bibliographical retrieval system was proposed, based on magnetic tapes provided without cost by the Medical Literature Analysis and Retrieval System (MEDLARS) of the National Library of Medicine of the United States. Delays prevented the WHO MEDLARS search centre from becoming operational until the beginning of 1972, by which time MEDLARS had gone online with the introduction of MEDLINE, an interactive searchable base of data from the 1966 *Index medicus*. In 1976, however, it was decided to phase out the WHO MEDLINE centre, as the MEDLARS–MEDLINE database was considered insufficiently oriented to public health in developing countries. In cooperation with the regional offices, other arrangements were made for Member States in need of MEDLINE services to gain access. For example, to make current medical literature available to developing countries at minimum cost, arrangements were made for shipments of journals and other literature from libraries in developed countries to countries in need, the cost of shipment being borne wherever possible by the donor institutions.

During 1974, a global WHO health literature programme was initiated, with the establishment of a series of health literature 'centres of excellence' in developing countries in Africa, Asia and the Pacific. Each centre brought a variety of health literature and information services within easier reach of neighbouring countries and facilitated access to a wide range of books, periodicals and audiovisual materials on health. To further the idea of a network of regional medical and public health libraries and documentation centres that would bring health literature closer to users in Member States, arrangements were made by the Regional Office for the Eastern Mediterranean with the Pahlavi Library of Medicine and the Biomedical Communications Centre in Teheran, Iran, to make their facilities available on a regional basis from January 1978.

WHO PUBLICATIONS

The WHO publishing programme was not conceived as an end in itself. In general, WHO publications are the vehicles for making the products of WHO activities or programmes available to the governments of Member countries and their health workers. WHO publications can be grouped as follows:

- Periodicals:
  Original scientific and technical articles: *Bulletin of the World Health Organization*
  News of WHO activities: *WHO chronicle*
  Legislation: *International digest of health legislation*
  Statistics: *World health statistics report*
  Epidemiology: *Weekly epidemiological record*
  Popular: *World health*
- Technical Report Series
- Monograph series
- *Public health papers*
- *Official records*
- Reference works
- Directories
- Bibliographies
- Statistical publications
- Non-serial publications

Over the years, various WHO programmes started producing, at regular or irregular intervals, what were known as 'recurrent informational documents'. Examples included *Mental health news*, the *Human genetics newsletter* and the *Information circular on vector control*. These contained technical information and varied in both presentation and distribution pattern. In 1969 it was decided to discontinue these publications, with the exception of four publications, mostly related to vector control, and to use the *WHO chronicle* to provide accounts of WHO activities and WHO-assisted activities that had previously been described in the recurrent documents (information circular No. 49, 2 June 1969). Epidemiological and other technical information that had been published in these documents was now published in ordinary technical documents, with the appropriate symbols and numbers and the usual disclaimer.

The governing bodies occasionally decided that particular publications should be prepared. For instance, resolution WHA28.52, adopted in May 1975 by the Twenty-eighth World Health Assembly, deemed it necessary "to summarize and describe in a major publication the experience of smallpox eradication throughout the world...." The result was a book of nearly 1500 pages, published in 1988 (*1*).

Towards the end of the decade, the content of certain periodicals and publications pro-duced at headquarters was modified to reflect the Organization's emphasis on meeting the problems and needs of the developing world.

With the agreement of the Member States concerned, two new working languages, Arabic and Chinese, were introduced, selectively, in the documentation for the Health Assembly and the Executive Board, and, in the case of Arabic, in publications, to provide a service to persons using these languages, with minimum diversion of funds from technical cooperation. Limited programmes were established in close cooperation with the Regional Office for the Eastern Mediterranean and the Council of Arab Ministers of Health in the case of Arabic and with the appropriate national authorities in the case of Chinese.

Budget cuts arising from resolution WHA29.48 led to a reduction in the number and volume of some headquarters publications, particularly the *Official records*. To reduce the volume of documentation for the Health Assembly, the Assembly agreed (resolution WHA30.30) to a 50% cut in the Director-General's comprehensive report to the Health Assembly and the United Nations on the work of WHO, that the proposed programme budget be presented biennially and that the financial report be presented annually.

The necessary groundwork was laid for complete reorientation of the *Bulletin*, beginning with the first issue of 1978, to enable it to respond more closely to the technical needs of Member States. This reorientation reduced the proportion of specialized knowledge, so that readers, particularly those in developing countries without access to such information, could keep abreast of new developments in fields of concern to WHO.

Efforts were made to improve the effectiveness of the *Chronicle* as a vehicle of infor-mation transfer, by including livelier, more topical articles, greater use of illustrations and emphasis on regional activities.

In 1977, responsibility for publication of the *International digest of health legislation* passed from the Legal Division to the Health and Biomedical Information Programme. As the Health Assembly showed renewed interest in health legislation in technical cooperation, in resolution WHA30.44, the role of the *Digest* and other health legislation activities came under study. Resolution WHA30.44 called on the Director-General to strengthen WHO's programme on health legislation, as new demands were being made on the Organization. For example, the delegate from Finland proposed that WHO's role in health legislation "should not only be to promote cooperation between different countries, but also to enable the peoples of those countries to share in the political and social processes that were even-tually expressed in the form of legislation." (*2*) Nevertheless, as pointed out by the secretariat, the programme had been reduced by the abolition of two permanent posts at headquarters and a cut in the number of pages of the *International digest*. The Director-General and the secretariat would try to interpret the wishes of the Health Assembly so as to "determine whether or not a completely revised programme of health legislation would respond fully to what the Health Assembly had called 'a strengthened programme' with more limited means, or whether the strengthening of the programme would also call for a strengthening of support activities." (*2*)

Non-periodical technical publications were limited to material of direct value to Member States, and in particular to developing countries. One result of this policy was that infor-mation on activities of interest to only a limited audience was increasingly offered for publication in non-WHO media. Another was that duplicate publication of the same material by two or more international agencies was discouraged, and the principle of one agency being the sole publisher was introduced.

New sales promotion measures to bring WHO publications to the attention of a wider range of potential readers throughout the world were applied during the 1976–1977 biennium. In 1976, for example, WHO publications were shown at 87 international and national conferences and book fairs, covering about 30 subject areas. They were also advertised in scientific and technical journals and were sent to a large number of such journals for review.

One indication of the success of these promotional activities was that sales reached record levels, despite the worldwide recession, which had seriously reduced library acquisition budgets in certain countries.

PUBLIC INFORMATION

One of the constitutional functions of the Organization is to ensure informed public opinion on matters of health. The health information programme of WHO seeks to fulfil this function by acquainting the lay public and its opinion-makers with the facts about general health and on specific topics of current interest or importance and by promoting awareness of what the Organization does and why. These purposes are achieved by mass communication through the media and in other ways, such as information sessions and exhibitions in educational institutions.

World Health Day on 7 April each year marks the coming into force of WHO's Constitution in 1948. It provides an annual opportunity to focus on a major health theme. Events are organized around the world involving all the media and institutions and personalities appropriate to the chosen theme. Each country organizes the celebration of this event; e.g. Greece had an official policy to celebrate World Health Day in a different provincial town each year. In Uganda, in 1975, for example, all assistant health visitors in the country were asked to give talks in primary schools in their areas on the subject of immunization, and essay competitions were held in all secondary schools on the effect of vaccination on common diseases.

The scope of the themes chosen to celebrate the twentieth and twenty-fifth anniversaries of the Organization was wide: that of 1968 was 'Health in the world of tomorrow', and that of 1973 was 'Health begins at home'. In 1969, the theme chosen was 'Health, labour and productivity', in recognition of the fiftieth anniversary of ILO. The theme for 1971, 'A full life despite diabetes', marked the fiftieth anniversary of the discovery of insulin. In other years, the World Health Day theme was chosen to mark programme developments, as was the case in 1975, when it was 'Smallpox—the point of no return'.

Television stations were offered two films for programmes on the twentieth anniversary: 'Man alive', a film on WHO made by the United Nations, and a short cartoon illustrating the aims of WHO, which was made in Prague, Czechoslovakia, for this occasion, entitled 'The fight continues'. Two other films won prizes in film festivals that year: 'Smallpox—merciless traveller' received the first prize in the cartoons category at the second international festival of films on prevention, held in Lisbon, Portugal, in April; and

'False friends', a colour cartoon on drug-taking, was awarded a gold medal at the annual festival of the British Industrial and Scientific Film Association in June. WHO produced two films on the occasion of its twenty-fifth anniversary in 1973: a 10-minute history of WHO and a 10-minute animated cartoon entitled 'Health begins at home'. The former was made in Romania by Studio Beureşti, and the latter was produced in Moscow, USSR, by Soiuzmultfilm.

In order to make WHO better known to the public in the United States before the start of the Twenty-second World Health Assembly, 10 fact sheets describing the structure and functions of WHO and the Health Assembly and a number of programme activities were distributed in Boston, Massachusetts, in 1969. Twenty-three short radio announcements were recorded by well-known personalities in the United States: an astronaut, a baseball champion and prominent actors and actresses.

A new radio series was started in 1969: 'WHO around the world'. Each programme ran for about 15 minutes and was produced in English, French and Spanish. Tapes of the programmes were distributed with an accompanying script to radio networks on request. That same year, in cooperation with UNDP, efforts were made to interest public information media in health and other development projects in Ceylon, Niger and Senegal. In Ceylon, a group of four journalists from different countries visited a variety of projects, including some assisted by WHO. In 1970, as part of its continuing collaboration with the UNDP programme 'Development support information', a coordinated interagency plan was drawn up to ensure wider use of material and to avoid duplication.

'Health, community and development' was the title of a radio series initiated in 1973 in the Americas in response to a call by the Regional Committee to emphasize community participation in health programmes. This series of 15-minute interviews or round-table discussions aimed to show that communities can and were promoting health. The programmes were sent to over 100 stations in Latin America.

Each year, tens of thousands of photographs were produced and distributed, and photographic feature stories were made on various issues, such as education and training (1971) and malaria control (1973). WHO publications and photographs were regularly exhibited at various international congresses and fairs.

About twice the volume of press cuttings were received in 1972 as in 1971, and comments continued to be largely favourable. Such criticism as there was related to the attitude of the Health Assembly with regard to the German Democratic Republic, its application of membership being deferred, until it was admitted in 1973, and WHO's position on DDT. On the latter issue, efforts were made to counteract criticism. In the United States, for example, one programme in a television series entitled 'The Advocate', carried by a national network, showed a live 'prosecution and defense' debate on whether DDT should be banned entirely; the outcome was wide approval for continued use of DDT in the developing world until suitable substitutes could be found.

The circulation of *World health*, WHO's illustrated magazine, rose steadily throughout the decade. In 1972, all editions in different languages exceeded 220 000 copies. In 1974, Italian and Farsi were added to Arabic, English, French, German, Portuguese, Russian and Spanish.

The name of the quarterly *Gazette*, published by the Regional Office for the Americas, was changed to *Pan American health* in 1975, and steps were taken to enliven it by revising its presentation. In the same year, in the European Region, a newsletter, *Euro information*, was launched for governments and cooperating organizations, summarizing the main WHO activities in the Region during the year.

The series of 25 fact sheets on public health problems issued during 1973 proved so successful that another series on similar lines was started in 1974. Each month, these 'In point of fact' leaflets offered information about a variety of health topics.

Public interest in the dramatic progress being made towards eradication of smallpox was notable in 1974 and stimulated many press inquiries, particularly in the South-East Asia Region. Press, radio and television teams were briefed on the smallpox eradication campaign, and film material on smallpox was included in a scientific programme prepared by a television network in the United States. WHO's work in eradication was filmed in India by British, German and Swedish television teams, and a film about the eradication activities in Uttar Pradesh, India, was made in Hindi and English in collaboration with the television services of All-India Radio.

As already noted, the theme for World Health Day in 1975 was 'Smallpox—the point of no return'. On this occasion, WHO distributed some 30 000 information kits and posters and about 5000 photographs, mostly at the request of the regions and various national bodies. Daily newspapers throughout the world carried editorial comment on the significance of smallpox eradication, most of the articles being based on, and illustrated with, material supplied by WHO.

References

1. *Smallpox and its eradication*. Geneva, World Health Organization, 1988.
2. *Official records of the World Health Organization*, No. 241 (WHA27/SR/A/7). Geneva, World Health Organization, 1977.

Alma-Ata: The International Conference on Primary Health Care

Alma-Ata would not have taken place without the insistence of the USSR, whose delegation drafted a resolution during the 1974 Health Assembly that included a proposal for "an international conference under WHO auspices for the exchange of experiences as regards the development of national health services" (*1*). That proposal was not, however, included in the final resolution adopted (WHA27.44), nor at the fifty-fifth session of the Executive Board in January of the following year. Finally, although the WHO secretariat indicated that the Director-General did not want such a conference, the Twenty-eighth World Health Assembly passed resolution WHA28.88, which considered an international meeting or conference "desirable".

More than 3 years would pass from the time resolution WHA28.88 was adopted (May 1975) to the time the conference took place (September 1978). During that period, many parallel events took place, and the concept of primary health care was refined.

ORGANIZATION OF THE CONFERENCE

Resolution WHA28.88, adopted in May 1975, instructed the Executive Board to consider and determine at its fifty-seventh session the date, place and concrete programme for the Conference. The secretariat prepared a background paper in which it noted that "the Director-General questions whether it is opportune to hold a large international meeting or conference on the subject at the present time". Indicating that "attention should be given to enabling relevant persons from interested countries to acquire experience in functioning national and field settings, and to providing concrete assistance in planning and implementing a series of national programmes", two alternative courses of action were presented (*2*). The first proposed that the WHO/UNICEF joint study on alternative approaches (see Chapter 6) be extended and its results discussed in a "series of technical meetings", followed by a series of regional meetings and, then, an international conference. The second alternative (assuming that the Conference was "retained" by the Executive Board) was creation of a conference committee in 1976, after which the Director-General would approach "a group of countries, preferably in the developing world, which might be prepared to act as host to such a conference" and "a number of countries and donor agencies to inquire whether they would be prepared to assist with the cost or act as co-sponsors", as no budgetary provision had been made for a conference.

The introduction of this subject to the Board (*3*) again indicated that the Director-General "was not convinced that the time was opportune". It also reported that a formal offer had been received from the Minister of Health of Egypt, "welcoming the convening of a conference in Cairo".

The delegate of the USSR to the Executive Board expressed "surprise" at the way in which the subject had been introduced, as the secretariat's report did not mention that his Government had proposed that the conference be held in 1977 "in any of the Republics of the Soviet Union, and that the Government was willing to make substantial financial resources available in that connexion—in particular to cover the costs of participants from developing countries". Furthermore, he continued, the initiative of the Government of the USSR was driven by

> a desire to give participants the opportunity of voicing their various opinions on the development of primary health care. It did not matter if the conference failed to make recommendations: what was important was that the discussions should be recorded for the use of all who were interested. The Soviet Government was prepared to show participants what had been done in that connexion in its country over the past fifty years. (3)

The Director-General apologized if the presentation of the subject had been "misleading". It was up to the Board, he continued, "to consider the most appropriate time for such a conference and that it might be useful to sensitize the regions and countries before it was held". In the discussion that followed, the Chinese member of the Board indicated that, if the conference was to be held, "it should be held in a developing country and would favour Egypt as the venue". Other alternatives, he indicated, were available for exchanging experiences and information, such as visits, study tours and meetings. The developing countries that had "been the subject of imperialist, colonialist and hegemonic oppression" shared the same health problems and could learn from each other in order to compensate for their respective deficiencies (3).

The Board member from the United States expressed the opinion that the main issue was "to decide on the time, place and programme for the conference", but he had found it difficult to do so without a clear understanding of its objectives. He had identified four: to exchange and analyse experiences, to examine the different systems in order to ascertain how they operated under WHO's sponsorship, to draw up guidelines for WHO's programme, and to sensitize opinion. He suggested that a committee be established "to draw up an outline for the conference which could then be submitted to the Health Assembly". He also noted the tendency to view the primary health care programme as a kind of "competitive ideological effort", no doubt triggered by the insistence of the Chinese delegate that the conference be held in a developing country rather than the USSR, a position that possibly explains the Chinese Government's eventual decision not to attend the conference.[1]

An ad hoc committee of the Executive Board was established, which met in March 1976, when it decided that the objectives of the Conference should be to exchange experiences and information on setting up primary health care in the framework of comprehensive national health systems and services; to promote the concept of primary health care in Member States and to prepare a report and recommendations to be submitted to the World Health Assembly. It was also agreed, after consideration of various options, that the conference should be governmental, with participants appointed by governments, as well as technical and intersectoral. The latter point was to be "stressed in the invitation in order to provide guidance on the types of expertise desired".

---

[1] China was one of some 10 countries that did not attend the Conference.

During the discussion, considerable concern was expressed about the contradiction between extensive review and reporting of national experiences and the associated costs, the huge volume of paper required and the feasibility of handling the material effectively. It was decided that preparatory discussions should take place at national level in appropriate venues, such as workshops and seminars, and that the secretariat would prepare a "set of critical questions related to a set of topics" as a guide for the discussions. Regional reports would serve as "the prime mechanism for reporting to the international conference the different national experiences and approaches" and would be used as background documents for the discussions at the conference. Limits were set on both conference and preconference documentation.

While it was considered premature to fix the details of the topics to be discussed, it was agreed that the programme would consist of plenary sessions and three committees of the whole. The main areas of the agenda were seen to be the conceptual aspect of primary health care, its relation to national health services and overall socioeconomic development, and operational and technical aspects. A programme of five and one-half days was outlined, not counting time for field visits.

By the time of the meeting of the ad hoc committee of the Executive Board, Egypt had withdrawn its offer, and a new offer had been received from Costa Rica. At the time, it was rumoured that the Government of the USSR had pressured Egypt to withdraw its offer. Geneva was proposed as well, but was quickly ruled out. When Costa Rica indicated that it was not in a position to offer significant financial support towards the costs, it was unanimously resolved that "the Soviet Union would be the host country" and that the Conference should be held in late August or early September 1978.

Possible UNICEF participation in the Conference was discussed and agreed to by their Executive Board in early May 1976, at which time the Executive Director estimated financial requirements in the order of US$ 400 000 to US$ 500 000, half of which would be required for UNICEF's own preparatory activities and the other half as a contribution to the costs of the conference. The Twenty-ninth World Health Assembly, in its resolution WHA29.29, welcomed "the possibility of UNICEF co-sponsoring the International Conference on Primary Health Care", in addition to "noting with appreciation the arrangements made for the International Conference on Primary Health Care which will be held in the Union of Soviet Socialist Republics during the second half of 1978". It is perhaps of interest to note that the Steering Committee on Primary Health Care, during a meeting earlier that year, had considered that co-sponsorship of the conference by UNICEF or by any other group was "not appropriate" but that UNICEF's cooperation "would be invaluable" (minutes of a meeting of the Steering Committee on Primary Health Care, 20 February 1976). The USSR, however, favoured cosponsorship by UNICEF (minutes of a meeting of the Steering Committee on Primary Health Care, 22 April 1976).

In addition to a multitude of activities to promote primary health care and to clarify its meaning (see below), planning was undertaken for the various logistical, financial and legal aspects of the organization of such a large-scale event. Visits were made to the USSR to decide upon the most favourable venue; Alma-Ata was chosen in early September 1976. It had been agreed by then that the conference would last 7 days, 5–5.5 of which would be working days, with the possibility of an additional working day to be considered later. Field visits were optional and would be fully the responsibility of the USSR Government.

A budget was prepared, which amounted to some US$ 2.2 million. UNICEF's contribution was US$ 100 000 for the conference itself and US$ 250 000 for its preparation. The contribution of the USSR was first suggested to be of the order of US$ 400 000–500 000 (minutes of a meeting of the Steering Committee on Primary Health Care, 31 March 1976). The offer included making available the best hall in Alma-Ata, in the V.I. Lenin Palace of Culture, which held over 2000 people and the premises needed for sectional and working meetings, all properly equipped for simultaneous interpretation into the working languages of the conference; payment for the accommodation of delegates representing WHO Member States and members of the WHO secretariat involved in the conference; local transport; a 30% reduction on air fares; and transport for participants wishing to study the Soviet experience in health services and primary health care in Alma-Ata and in other Soviet national republics.

Three phases had to be planned: preparatory steps, the conference and follow-up. The plans were presented to the Executive Board at its fifty-ninth session, in January 1977 (4). The Board passed resolution EB59/R.16, which confirmed that the conference would be held in Alma-Ata and asked the Director-General to explore all possible means of obtaining extrabudgetary funds to reduce the regular budget allocation for the conference.

The idea of having three committees of a whole was retained. The first would address the broad issue of primary health care and development; the second, technical operational aspects; and the third, national strategies and international support. If the delegates from a country included a person from a ministry of planning (or equivalent), that person would be a member of Committee A. The director-general of health (or equivalent) would be a member of Committee C, and the technical delegate would participate in Committee B.

It was foreseen that the follow-up phase would begin with a debate at the 1979 Health Assembly on the recommendations of the Conference and on actions to support the establishment of primary health care in countries identified in the first phase (and others). Follow-up would continue indefinitely, it was hoped, as part of the programmes of both WHO and UNICEF.

An initial list of "critical topics" for discussion at the Conference was prepared. The following items were identified: the concept of primary health care as an integral part of national health services; basic conditions for planning and establishing primary health care; primary health care within national health services; primary health care as part of the socioeconomic development of the community; other health services at intermediate level; alternative organization of primary health care (country experiences); primary health care personnel as part of the health team: selection and training; activities (vital statistical information, preventive measures, promotion of health, curative measures, rehabilitation, case reference); manuals for routine daily work; activities in fields other than health; periodic information on primary health care activities; evaluation of services; supervision; progressive improvement of primary health care personnel; use of traditional medicine in primary health care (opportunities and constraints); and international aspects of health care.

A working paper prepared for the meeting of the Director-General with the regional directors in January 1977 indicated that the conference could assist "wider political and technical needs at national and global levels". The debate at the conference itself "will involve other sectors of government in addition to the ministries of health and could present clearly the relationships of health and development and highlight some of the national and international actions which could be used to move forward along such a developmental path". These objectives were consistent with the decision that Committee A of the conference would deal with primary health care as part of national development.

More detailed annotated agendas for the three committees were prepared in January 1977, comprising a list of subjects as well as questions. Thus, for example, one item on the agenda for Committee A (primary health care as a part of national development) was "relationship of health with poverty, other sectors (education, etc) and development", and another was "primary health care as part of a national health service system and both as part of overall national development", under which several questions were presented, including "Is a new type of first referral level required for primary health care? What are the essential qualities of a second referral level? Does a separate village health committee result in decreased inter-sectoral actions?" The agenda for Committee B (technical operational questions) included an item on "Possible methods of defining and measuring objectives and results of actions in development, health service coverage, health status, effectiveness, costs" and included questions such as "Can poverty groups be defined on purely economic criteria? Are registration systems for births, deaths, morbidity, etc., needed initially? How can you compare costs of different alternatives when one is purposely using a labour intensive system?" The agenda for Committee C (useful steps in furthering primary health care activities in countries) was largely composed of a series of questions, the first of which were "On what basis can a country decide that change is required in a health system? By information on health status? Economic criteria? Coverage? Cost?" The last was "What are some of the ways in which WHO, UNICEF, international and bilateral agencies and nongovernmental organizations could best help countries in health development?"

The annotated agenda received mixed reactions. While the Regional Office for the Eastern Mediterranean considered that it was "quite comprehensive and elaborate, perhaps to the extent that it might not be fully covered during the Conference" (memorandum from Regional Director EMRO to secretary for Steering Committee on Primary Health Care, HQ 17 February 1977), the Regional Office for Africa found it "too lengthy and and directive for one week conference", adding, in their telegram, that it "would greatly appreciate avoidance highly conceptualized academic jargon. Stop. Primary health care subject should remain clear, simple, concise as possible if successful conference output wished for African countries." (telegram from Regional Director AFRO to Dr Tejada de Rivero, 28 February 1977).

UNICEF contributed its preliminary suggestions in July 1977. In commenting on the purpose of the Conference, it noted that "the interaction of various programmes affecting health needs to be understood and deliberately reinforced. The fact that the policy and approach to primary health care that is being promoted depends on population participation has important implications for the health sector, and requires far-reaching reorientation of current approaches to the delivery of health services" (Preliminary UNICEF suggestions about major issues for the conference agenda and the basic report to the conference, attached to letter from Newton Bowles to Dr Tejada de Rivero, 19 July 1977). Regarding

Committee A, for which UNICEF envisaged three 'perspectives'—communities, development planners and health administrators—communities were listed first because services at the community level are an important part of any anti-poverty programme and for achieving greater equity; they use idle or partially idle resources (community management resources, community level workers, community contributions to costs) and thus increase gross national product; and sectoral differences between ministries are not relevant to the communities' views of needs and services to which they are willing to contribute. "This has an important implication for the organization of the delivery of supporting services."

UNICEF proposed that the word 'technical' be dropped from the tasks of Committee B, which would address operational and organization problems and issues in the political and policy context. It should not be asked to deal with specific technical matters. In fact, at Alma-Ata, Committee B was asked to consider both technical and operational aspects of primary health care; however, the background paper addressed only operational aspects. Community involvement was seen as one of the issues that this Committee would address. In this regard, UNICEF envisioned such questions as how to encourage and achieve two-way interaction and information flow between community and governmental services.

The reactions of UNICEF and the WHO regions led to simplification of the draft annotated agendas in the months that followed. For example, instead of a list of issues and questions, the annotated agenda for Committee A (primary health care and development) now consisted of three sections: health as an integral part of overall development, primary health care as part of community development, and primary health care as part of a national health-care system. Five sub-issues were described in a short paragraph, at the end of which one question was posed. Thus, for example, meeting basic human needs ended with the question: "What are the ways and means for ensuring intersectoral cooperation to meet basic human needs?" Community participation in health ended with "What approaches are being developed to actively solicit community participation and intervention in the delivery of health care?"

At this point, UNICEF decided that it would engage four consultants to address the items to be covered by Committee A, i.e. those concerned with general planning. It was also decided that the conference would issue a 'Declaration of Alma-Ata', which would endorse and recommend primary health care to governments and external aid agencies, both United Nations and bilateral. For a while, the idea of a "world plan of action" was entertained, but it was dropped owing to insufficient time.

At the same time, the "information component" of the Conference began to be formulated. The audiences identified were decision-makers, health professionals, health institutions, the lay public and affluent countries. The working group established for this component reviewed earlier information activities and judged that "the message of primary health care had not come through to the public in a comprehensive way ... too much emphasis on primary health care being linked with rural development which was causing confusion, giving the impression that the idea of primary health care is only for rural populations" (minutes of a meeting of the Steering Committee on Primary Health Care, 27 April 1977). Similarly, an in-house survey showed that understanding of primary health care ranged from "first-aid to disease prevention and vaccination in developing countries. No-one connected primary health care with affluent countries or with self-care. The common denominator of present understanding appears to be that of the organization of health care services at the lowest echelon including delivery of health care by personnel trained in the field".

It was decided that a film would be shot, from which slides could be made.[2] Short radio interviews with people involved in primary health care in various countries would be distributed as widely as possible to stress the approach. The need for an information kit was agreed to, while a proposed seminar for key editors in various parts of the world was deleted.

In July 1977, it was agreed that all invitations to the conference should be sent jointly by the Director-General of WHO and the Executive Director of UNICEF. On the question of to whom the invitations should be addressed, UNICEF considered that, in order to ensure the intersectoral nature of the conference, "they should be addressed to the ministry of foreign affairs or to the national planning body" (minutes of the meeting of the Steering Committee on Primary Health Care, 7 July 1977). This led to the decision that two letters of invitation should be issued to each Government, one to the ministry of health and the other to the ministry of foreign affairs. It was also agreed that all United Nations agencies would be invited and that WHO and UNICEF would draw up a list of nongovernmental organizations that each wished to invite.

Detailed planning of each day of the conference began in late 1977. In the final account of the conference, its aims and objectives had been revised to read:

- to promote the concept of primary health care in all countries;
- to exchange experiences and information on establishing primary health care in the framework of comprehensive national health systems and services;
- to evaluate the present health and health-care situation throughout the world as it relates to, and can be improved by, primary health care;
- to define the principles of primary health care as well as the operational means of overcoming practical problems in establishing it;
- to define the roles of governments and national and international organizations in technical cooperation and support for establishing primary health care; and
- to formulate recommendations for establishing primary health care.

A joint letter sent on 20 February 1978 and signed by Dr Mahler, Director-General of WHO, and Mr Henry Labouisse, Executive Director of UNICEF, stated:

> The Conference is intended to stimulate a discussion among national planning and health authorities on effective ways of promoting health as an important factor in the achievement of development goals and the improvement of the well-being of all peoples. The Conference will be organized into a plenary and three committees of the whole, addressing themselves to the topics of primary health care and development, technical and operational aspects of primary health care, and national strategies for primary health care and international support.

The Conference was attended by delegations from 134 countries and by representatives of 67 United Nations organizations, specialized agencies and nongovernmental organizations in official relations with WHO and UNICEF. The Declaration of Alma-Ata was adopted in the final plenary session before closure of the Conference. Only one change to

---

[2] This proved impossible within the funds available; however, some 15 films were selected to be shown, mostly contributed by national governments.

the Declaration was proposed from the floor, which was addition of "traditional practitioners" to the list of health workers in paragraph 7 of section VII. This was accepted, with the addition of the phrase "as needed".

PREPARATORY EVENTS

Already in late 1975, some of the regional offices had taken steps to organize national discussions or debates on primary health care and to plan regional meetings on the subject, in accordance with the recommendations of the ad hoc committee of the Executive Board. The report of the ad hoc committee, sent to the regional directors in July 1976, indicated that the "critical topics" (see above) could be used to "guide the analysis of country situations and preparation of the required reports" (memorandum from the secretary of the Steering Committee on Primary Health Care to regional directors, 23 July 1976). They should be used as guidance, to be adopted by each region and each country as considered necessary. It further proposed that selected, relevant countries in each region be encouraged to conduct national dialogues or debates, supported by WHO and UNICEF when necessary. The major topics to be considered were: the development status of the country, the health status of the population, government policies, health sector planning, health service programmes, intersectoral programmes and international aspects of health care. Critical questions were added for each topic. The debate was expected to involve the government health ministry, other sectors, including planning, rural development and education, nongovernmental organizations, health professionals and representatives of consumers and villages. The purpose of the debates was to examine the present national health system, make proposals for change and consider new objectives and alternatives, taking into account the principles of promotion of national health services and primary health care. Reports of each such dialogue or debate were to be made available for presentation at a regional meeting.

The contributions from each region were expected to differ in either balance or content. Not only were the problems different in each region, but the successes of the past decade were different in strength and relevance. It was nevertheless considered useful for each report to be structured in such a way that it would reflect that of the conference: conceptual difficulties for the plenary session and for the three committees of the whole, as described above. Each region therefore approached the preparatory phase differently.

In the African Region, WHO representatives were asked to organize a meeting, workshop or round table on the subject of primary health care, addressing the "critical questions". Workshops were held in a number of countries, including three organized jointly for the Sahel countries by nationals, WHO, UNICEF and the United States Agency for International Development. The results of these efforts were analysed, and a summary was prepared as a working paper for a regional expert committee meeting on primary health care in March 1977. One outcome of the meeting was identification of means of promoting and strengthening the implementation of primary health care.

In the Region of the Americas, three international working groups were organized in 1976: one in Mexico to discuss formal and informal health systems; one in Central America to discuss technology; and one in Washington DC, United States, to discuss administration and organization. National working groups defined their governments' positions. On the basis of the conclusions of these activities, PAHO prepared a document entitled *Extension of health services coverage using primary care and community participation strategies* (5). A special meeting of ministers was convened in September 1977 to analyse the concepts and the factors affecting extension of primary health care coverage as well as the results of the country reviews.

In the Eastern Mediterranean Region, "major events" relevant to the subject were used to prepare the report. These events included the 1975 technical discussions, the Sudan experience with its primary health care programme, a travelling seminar on primary health care in Iran, an interagency meeting on primary health care held in October 1977 and a regional seminar on primary health care in February 1978. The latter was organized in collaboration with UNICEF and the League of Arab States. Also taken into account in the Regional report were the results of workshops on primary health care held in 1976, such as one in Ethiopia in August and another in Sudan in November. The major topics suggested by headquarters were not used owing to their "complex terminology".

In the European Region, an outline was prepared consisting of three elements: a country position paper on progress in primary health care and proposals for the future, a description of national projects and major problem areas. Studies were conducted on, for example, the health centre concept in various countries. Another activity was a working group on consumer responsibility for and participation in primary medical care delivery, held in September 1977 in Finland. Two reports were issued by the working groups: *Definition of parameters of efficiency in primary health care* and *The role of nursing in primary health care*.

In the South-East Asia Region, countries were invited to organize workshops, seminars or debates on primary health care. Six agreed to hold national dialogues, and a regional meeting was held in October 1977. The regional background paper also contained the results of a regional seminar on traditional medicine, held in April 1977.

In the Western Pacific Region, national seminars, debates and conferences on primary health care were held, followed by a regional conference. Reports of seven national dialogues were discussed, with contributions from other countries in the Region, at a Regional meeting held in September 1977. The Regional background paper also included the results of a Regional seminar on delivery of maternal and child health and family planning within primary health care, held in September 1976, and the report of the first Regional working group on basic health services, which followed the seminar.

In parallel with the activities of the WHO regions, UNICEF asked their field staff to support national activities contributing to pre-conference promotion of primary health care. The note that went out to their officers stated:

> UNICEF is in a unique position to ensure that the primary health care policy is seen in a broad perspective, i.e. in the context of overall basic services (see Chapter 1) and not simply from the sectoral health point of view. We should use our influence to involve national planning departments and other concerned ministries in whatever way seems most appropriate in each country's review of policies, needs and the formulation of a programme/plan of action (letter to UNICEF field officers from Newton Bowles, 6 April 1977).

The World Federation of Public Health Associations was invited in May 1977 to write a position paper representing the views of nongovernmental organizations on primary health care, for presentation at Alma-Ata. In cooperation with the Canadian Public Health Association and cosponsored by WHO, the Federation held its second international congress in Halifax, Nova Scotia, in May 1978, with the theme 'Primary health care: a global perspective'. The focus of discussions was the future role and responsibility of the private nongovernmental sector in providing primary health care in underdeveloped areas. The objectives of the congress were to review the primary health care concept; identify key issues in primary health care, especially with regard to public health; define alternative approaches for increasing private sector support for key primary health care issues; and propose a strategy and national goals to achieve national primary health care.

The report of the congress (unpublished) presented the concerns and involvement of nongovernmental organizations in issues of health and development, as discussed below. It endorsed the WHO and UNICEF concept of primary health care and described the historical role of nongovernmental organizations and ideas on "what nongovernmental organizations can do". It pointed out that they can work for greater understanding of and positive attitudes to primary health care, assist national policy formulation, establish means for greater collaboration and coordination of primary health care activities, and contribute to programme implementation.

Another contribution to the Alma-Ata Conference was the publication *Primary health care in industrialized nations*, which was the outcome of a meeting held in December 1977 in New York City (6), organized by the New York Academy of Sciences and cosponsored by the Sandoz Foundation, the United States Public Health Services and WHO.

UNICEF dedicated the June 1978 issue of its journal *Les carnets de l'enfance* (*Assignment children*) to primary health care. The issue contained articles written by consultants who had participated in preparing the conference background paper.

THE CONCEPT OF PRIMARY HEALTH CARE

The basic principles of primary health care were defined in 1975 (see Chapter 6). In the background paper prepared for the meeting of the Director-General and the regional directors in early 1977, primary health care was presented as a "code word describing a health related response to the international and national cry for social equality and justice with equal emphasis upon the developing world and the underserved groups of many countries" (working paper on the International Conference on Primary Health Care for meeting of Director-General with regional directors, January 1977). Furthermore, primary health care was "not only a health concern because it is improbable that any organizational health service response *by itself* will be sufficient to significantly alter the poverty syndrome to the vast mass of rural populations". Despite this and other statements that portrayed primary health care in broad, developmental terms, there was a tendency in many circles to limit it to health services at community level, with little attention to the broader question of health as part of community and national development. When, for example, in January 1977, the question of whether the Executive Board might be asked to adopt another resolution on primary health care was raised, Dr Mahler responded, "no, the resolution would reflect their health service obsession" (personal notes of one participant in the meeting). Part of the problem was seen to derive from the fact that in many developed countries 'primary care' was the first contact of a patient with a physician. More work was needed "to infuse the full understanding of what was intended by the concept of primary health care" (minutes of meeting of the WHO/CMC Standing Committee, 2 February 1977).

Following the discussions of the ad hoc committee of the Executive Board, it was envisaged that the Director-General's report to the Conference would be "no more than 200 pages in length", would draw on both the regional reports and previous documentation, and would cover "the nature and extent of the problem, the conceptual basis of the primary health care approach, its technical/operational aspects, its relationships with socio/economic development, and possible lines for future action on the part of the Member States, WHO and other organizations" (notes on International Conference on Primary Health Care, role of the agenda, 23 November 1976).

A consultant was engaged to prepare the first draft of the Director-General's report, which was now (spring 1977) seen to be more likely to consist of 50–100 pages rather than the 200 pages agreed upon earlier. By July 1977, it had been decided that the report would be the only working document for the conference, that it should be a joint report by the heads of WHO and UNICEF and that it would be sent out in April 1978.

The first draft was received in June 1977. It followed and built upon earlier descriptions of the failures of the basic health services approach (see Chapter 6). It was composed as if it were a speech by the Director-General (frequent use of "I", phrases beginning "Let me ..."). Its first section was entitled 'Introduction: statement of the problem'. The next section, entitled 'What can primary health care mean?', began with a subsection on social poverty and health, a theme that Dr Mahler had proposed in 1975 when he first introduced the idea of health for all by the year 2000 (see Chapter 1).

The draft was circulated widely among WHO and UNICEF staff. UNICEF, while recognizing that much of the paper would have to be re-cast, noted "it is much to be desired that the freshness and vigour of the writing is retained. It will add greatly to the tone of the Conference to have as its central working document a paper which is so free from jargon and which carries with it the ring of conviction" (comments on Dr Newell's preliminary draft for the global paper for the International Conference on Primary Health Care, attached to letter from Newton Bowles to Dr Tejada de Rivero, 19 July 1977). At the same time, UNICEF indicated that the draft devoted "too much space to re-arguing the case for the primary health care policy". It could, instead, start with the fact that this policy "had the endorsement of both the World Health Assembly and the Executive Board".

Indicating a need to strengthen the chapter on primary health care as part of national development, UNICEF proposed that the chapter include: 'Will an anti-poverty programme without specific health components solve major health problems?', 'How can dealing with health problems contribute to an anti-poverty programme?', 'What are the major linkages to other sectors, e.g. agriculture, nutrition and water supply?' and 'How can development programmes be designed to reflect and support community priorities in various sectors (i.e. not only within the health sector, which is the only application discussed)?' It was noted that health planning should be adapted to this reality.

WHO staff, too, commented that the draft overemphasized the need for primary health care, "given that there already exists a general acceptance of the concept" (summary of the major comments of WHO staff on the preliminary first draft). The emphasis on social poverty was considered to ignore the fact that variation in health status, rising costs, maldistribution of services, nonacceptance of services and misuse of technology were "not solely confined to the socially poor in developing countries. The accent that has been put on the primary health care approach to alleviate social poverty detracts from the concept of 'health for all' in rural and urban settings, developed and developing countries. Thus, the primary health care approach ought to be presented as one which is relevant to the health-related problems of all people." Furthermore, the paper could be shortened, and the language should be simplified.

An important building block for the post-Alma-Ata plan of action was put in place during the Thirtieth World Health Assembly, in May 1977, when it approved a resolution proposed by the Director-General (resolution WHA30.43) that WHO's main social target for the coming decades should be the attainment by all citizens of the world by the year 2000 a level of health that would permit them to lead socially and economically productive lives. Several months later, in his *Blueprint for health for all* (*7*), the Director-General indicated that primary health care was

> a front-line activity that is the corner-stone to ensure essential health for all in any society. It contained a proper blend of all essential health promoting elements: adequate food and housing, with protection of houses against insects and rodents; water adequate to permit cleanliness and safe drinking; suitable waste disposal; services for the provision of ante-natal, natal and post-natal care, including family planning; infant and childhood care, including nutritional support; immunization against the major infectious diseases of childhood; prevention and control of locally endemic diseases; elementary care of all age groups for injury and diseases; and easy access to sound and useful information on prevailing health problems and the methods of preventing and controlling them.

The first draft had not specified what in time would be considered the "essential elements of primary health care". Instead, like earlier statements, it was based on principles and policy directives. The demand for more precision led to the introduction of such elements into subsequent statements, until it emerged in the Alma-Ata Declaration (see below).

Each of the regional papers approached the subject differently. For example, the final report of the ministers of health of the Americas defined primary health care as

> a systematized combination of multisectoral activities applied to man and his environment and designed to produce an increasingly higher level of health for the community and to satisfy the health needs of its members. The resources are largely to be found in the community itself. These resources, which provide services without the benefit of technology, make up what may be called the community or traditional system. Carefully selected, they can be developed and mobilized with the support of the institutional system of health services; articulated with it, they can ensure that the communities have access to all levels of care for solving both their own problems and those of their individual members. The scope and the form of the primary care being provided varies from country to country. There is no single model that is applicable in all the countries; but, whatever the model used, it must be dynamic if adjustments and advances consistent with the development of the communities are to be made. (*8*)

The statement from the African Region summarized primary health care as

a health approach which integrates at the community level all elements necessary to make an impact on the health of the people through a series of measures that are simple, effective in terms of costs, technique and organization; are acceptable to the people in need and which help to improve their living conditions. Primary health care is the responsibility of each country and should be fully integrated into other community programmes of agriculture, education, public works, housing and communications with community participation in decision-making; primary health care and appropriate technology must go hand-in-hand in order to reduce as much as possible, the current dependence on imported costly technology which benefit few people and contribute little to rural populations.

The report of the seminar held in the Eastern Mediterranean Region indicated that primary health care was

a concept applicable to all countries, irrespective of the form of government or stage of development. It did not signify 'second-class medicine'. While it might lack the glamour of large modern hospital services, it was not necessarily less expensive but was relevant to the health needs of communities, aimed realistically at total population coverage, and was markedly advantageous in terms of cost-effectiveness. (9)

Despite the extensive discussion on the importance of poverty in the conception of primary health care, in the final version that went to Alma-Ata, references to poverty were reduced to two points:

- In developing countries in particular, economic development, antipoverty measures, food production, water, sanitation, housing, environmental protection and education all contribute to health and have the same goal of human development.
- The other levels of the country's health system can also assist development on condition that they are attuned to providing support to the full range of primary health care activities. For example, they can concentrate selectively on combating health risks which directly or indirectly influence poverty.

The links between primary health care and human development were not as sharply drawn in the official background paper as they had been in the nongovernmental organization position paper, which affirmed:

It is not enough, for example, to disseminate health and nutrition education if land tenure and utilization preclude the production of adequate food for local consumption. It is futile to promote a health insurance scheme if employment opportunities are so limited that participation is beyond the reach of many. Provision of a source of clean water to a community will have an impact on water-borne diseases only in so far as the community is educated in its use and management.

In the joint report (10), the role of the agricultural sector was "to ensure that production of food for family consumption becomes an integral part of agricultural policy and that food actually reaches those who produce it, which in some countries may require changes in the pattern of land tenure." The joint report did not make any reference either to employment or to health insurance, nor is there any specific point on the importance of an educated community concerning waterborne diseases. Instead, the general role of the educational sector is outlined. In this regard, it is of note that a key UNICEF officer expressed

UNICEF's "disagreement" over the fact that the report had not recommended that a "country's primary health care organization would be most effectively attached to the Prime Minister's office or another organ with intersectoral responsibility, rather than leaving health, a ministry often low on the totem pole, to seek the participation of the other ministries that should be concerned." (memorandum from EJR Heyward, July 2000).

Another issue that received less emphasis in the background paper than might have been expected, given the Director-General's statements in other contexts, was the degree to which the medical establishment had contributed to the very problems that primary health care was to address.

In a paper in which the Director-General documented the resemblance between primary health care and the outcome of a meeting held in Indonesia in 1937 and organized by the Health Organization of the League of Nations, he commented on why the earlier recommendations had not been implemented:

> The progress that has resulted [since 1937] has yielded benefits for only a relatively small proportion of the world's population. The more serious scourges of mankind have not been the focus of attention of the 'facilities and opportunities for research'. Exotic, rare diseases and degenerative conditions have received attention disproportionate to their importance. No one can deny that such conditions need attention, but the health profession has been derelict in its duty to recognize that available resources are limited and that they should be applied in a manner to obtain the greatest improvement in health of all the people, not just a select few. (*11*)

In a meeting organized by the Rockefeller Foundation that Dr Mahler attended in June 1977, the opposition to his "crusade to build a new health system" was described as being "the massed phalanxes of the world's medical professions—in industrial and developing countries alike—who will oppose that idea with all their power and prestige."

In the final report for Alma-Ata (*12*), a section entitled 'Ways of overcoming obstacles' indicates:

> Resistance to such change is only to be expected; for instance, attempts to ensure a more equitable distribution of health resources could well meet with resistance from political and professional pressure groups .... Obstacles such as these can be overcome if they are prepared for in advance ... it may be possible to influence those health professionals not already convinced of the importance of primary health care by involving them in its development.

In regard to community participation, one of the UNICEF representatives to the Conference later wrote:

> a number of delegates said that they found the statements about community participation and delegation of authority to intermediate and community levels too weak. They found that the tone of the report stresses too much the handing down of services, and not enough dialogue with the community, accountability to the people, and community management and evaluation of services being received. (memorandum from EJR Heyward to UNICEF regional directors and representatives, 12 September 1978)

Had the background paper overly diluted the issues that had led to the re-birth of primary health care? Or was the grossly inequitable situation in the world such common knowledge that what was of paramount importance was a consensus that primary health care was needed, rather than seeking a deeper understanding of what primary health care might mean in practice or a debate on the causes of the situation? There are no doubt still a great diversity of replies to these questions. What cannot be denied, however, is that the Declaration of Alma-Ata, with its supporting background paper, strongly resonated with the progressive public health forces that were then operating. Furthermore, the subsequent slow and sometimes painful progress no doubt explains why the results of the Conference are receiving renewed attention some 30 years later.

References

1. *Official records of the World Health Organization*, No. 218 (WHA27/SR/A/7). Geneva, World Health Organization, 1974.
2. *Promotion of national health services relating to primary health care* (EB57/20). Geneva, World Health Organization, 1976.
3. *Official records of the World Health Organization*, No. 232 (EB57/SR/14, EB57/SR/15). Geneva, World Health Organization, 1976.
4. *Progress report on the International Conference on the Promotion of National Health Services and Primary Health Care* (EB59/INF.DOC. No. 4). Geneva, World Health Organization, 1977.
5. *Extension of health services coverage using primary care and community participation strategies. Summary of the situation in the Region of the Americas* (Official document No. 156). Washington DC, Pan American Health Organization, 1978.
6. Burrell CD, Sheps CG, eds. Primary health care in industrialized nations. *Annals of the New York Academy of Sciences*, 1978, 310.
7. Mahler H. Blueprint for health for all. *WHO Chronicle*, 1977, 31:491–498.
8. *Final report of the IV special meeting of ministers of health of the Americas* (REMSA4/FR). Washington DC, Pan American Health Organization, 1977.
9. *Document EM/WHO-UNICEF/IA.CONS.PHS/15*. Alexandria, Regional Office for the Eastern Mediterranean, 1977.
10. *Alma-Ata 1978 primary health care*. Geneva, World Health Organization, 1978.
11. Mahler H. Promotion of primary health care in member countries of WHO. *Public Health Reports*, 1978, 93:107–113.
12. *Primary health care. Report of the International Conference on Primary Health Care, Alma-Ata, USSR, 6–12 September 1978* ("Health for all" series, No. 1). Geneva, World Health Organization, 1978.

DECLARATION OF ALMA-ATA

The International Conference on Primary Health Care, meeting in Alma-Ata this twelfth day of September in the year Nineteen hundred and seventy-eight (Alma-Ata 1978), expressing the need for urgent action by all governments, all health and development workers, and the world community to protect and promote the health of all the people of the world, *hereby makes the following Declaration:*

I

The Conference strongly reaffirms that health, which is a state of complete physical, mental and social well-being, and not merely the absence of disease or infirmity, is a fundamental human right and that the attainment of the highest possible level of health is a most important world-wide social goal whose realization requires the action of many other social and economic sectors in addition to the health sector.

II

The existing inequality in the health status of people particularly between developed and developing countries as well as within countries is politically, socially and economically unacceptable and is, therefore, of common concern to all countries.

III

Economic and social development, based on a New International Economic Order, is of basic importance to the fullest attainment of health for all and to the reduction of the gap between the health status of the developing and developed countries. The promotion and protection of the health of the people is essential to sustained economic and social development and contributes to a better quality of life and to world peace.

IV

The people have the right and duty to participate individually and collectively in the planning and implementation of their health care.

V

Governments have a responsibility for the health of their people which can be fulfilled only by the provision of adequate health and social measures. A main social target of governments, international organizations and the whole world community in the coming decades should be the attainment by all peoples of the world by the year 2000 of a level of health that will permit them to lead a socially and economically productive life. Primary health care is the key to attaining this target as part of development in the spirit of social justice.

VI

Primary health care is essential health care based on practical, scientifically sound and socially acceptable methods and technology made universally accessible to individuals and families in the community through their full participation and at a cost that the community and country can afford to maintain at every stage of their development in the spirit of self-reliance and self-determination. It forms an integral part both of the country's health system, of which it is the central function and main focus, and of the overall social and economic development of the community. It is the first level of contact of individuals, the family and community with the national health system bringing health care as close as possible to where the people live and work, and constitutes the first element of a continuing health care process.

VII

Primary health care:

1. reflects and evolves from the economic conditions and socio-cultural and political characteristics of the country and its communities and is based on the applications of the relevant results of social, biomedical and health services research and public health experience;

2. addresses the main health problems in the community, providing promotive, preventive, curative and rehabilitative services accordingly.

3. includes at least: education concerning prevailing health problems and the methods of preventing and controlling them; promotion of food supply and proper nutrition; an adequate supply of safe water and basic sanitation; maternal and child health care, including family planning, immunization against the major infectious diseases; prevention and control of locally endemic diseases; appropriate treatment of common diseases and injuries; and provision of essential drugs;

4. involves, in addition to the health sector, all related sectors and aspects of national and community development, in particular agriculture, animal husbandry, food, industry, education, housing, public works, communications and other sectors, and demands the co-ordinated efforts of all those sectors.

5. requires and promotes maximum community and individual self-reliance and participation in the planning, organization, operation and control of primary health care, making the fullest use of local, national, and other available resources; and to this end develops through appropriate education the ability of communities to participate;

6. should be sustained by integrated, functional and mutually-supportive referral systems, leading to the progressive improvement of comprehensive health care for all, and giving priority to those most in need;

7. relies, at local and referral levels, on health workers, including physicians, nurses, midwives, auxiliaries and community workers as applicable, as well as traditional practitioners as needed, suitably trained socially and technically to work as a health team and to respond to the expressed health needs of the community.

VIII

All governments should formulate national policies, strategies and plans of action to launch and sustain primary health care as part of a comprehensive national health system and in coordination with other sectors. To this end, it will be necessary to exercise political will, to mobilize the country's resources and to use available external resources rationally.

IX

All countries should cooperate in a spirit of partnership and service to ensure primary health care for all people since the attainment of health by people in any one country directly concerns and benefits every other country. In this context the joint WHO/UNICEF report on primary health care constitutes a solid basis for the further development and operation of primary health care throughout the world.

X

An acceptable level of health for all people of the world by the year 2000 can be attained through a fuller and better use of the world's resources, a considerable part of which is now spend on armaments and military conflicts. A genuine policy of independence, peace, détente and disarmament could and should release additional resources that could be devoted to peaceful aims and in particular to the acceleration of social and economic development of which primary health care, as an essential part, should be allotted its proper share.

The International Conference on Primary Health Care calls for urgent and effective national and international action to develop and implement primary health care throughout the world and particularly in developing countries in a spirit of technical cooperation and in keeping with a New International Economic Order. It urges governments, WHO and UNICEF, and other international organizations, as well as multilateral and bilateral agencies, nongovernmental organizations, funding agencies, all health workers and the whole world community to support national and international commitment to primary health care and to channel increased technical and financial support to it, particularly in developing countries. The Conference calls on all the aforementioned to collaborate in introducing, developing and maintaining primary health care in accordance with the spirit and content of this Declaration.

Index

in the Eastern Mediterranean Region, 79
in the Region of the Americas, 64
in the South-East Asia Region, 69–70
in the Western Pacific Region, 83
mental, 216
research on, 106, 155, 163, 165–6, 257
training in, 59, 60, 64, 69, 70, 76, 81,
151, 153, 160
Health laboratory services, 61, 84, 106,
241, **249–50**
Health literature services, **286–7**
Health manpower (see also 'Auxiliaries,
health' and 'Community, health
workers')
appropriate, 2, 118, 130
categories of, 69, 167, 170, 215
development of, 54, 111, 121, **159–74**,
280
integration of into health services,
168–72
in the African Region, 58–9
in the Eastern Mediterranean Region,
72, 76
in the European Region, 72–4
in the Region of the Americas, 64
in the South-East Asia Region, 72, 73
in the Western Pacific Region, 81
environmental, 164
indigenous, 151
in health education, 150, 152
in smallpox eradication, 179
integrated, 166, 170, 171, 172
migration of, **161–2**, 170, 172
model of, 2
planning of, 59, 64, 81, 130
shortages of, 65, 67, 75–6, 84, 117, 159,
233
training of, 69, 72, 76, 89, 124, 126, 132,
133, 142, 154, **159–74**, 219
village, 83, 154, 166, 168, 215
voluntary, 70
Health planning
approaches to, 130
assistance in, 9, 127, 172

environmental, **269–72**
health statistics in, 275, 280
in socioeconomic development, 13, 54
in the African Region, 58, 59
in the Eastern Mediterranean Region, 76,
79, 94
in the European Region, 73–4
in the Region of the Americas, 63, 64
in the South-East Asia Region, 67, 68,
69, 72, 131
in the Western Pacific Region, 81
primary health care in, 303
radiation medicine in, 228
research on, 63, 73, 79, 89, 93, 107, 130,
169
training in, 12, 63, 68, 88, 159, 160
Health promotion, 9, 20, 33, 47, 54, 109,
112, 117, 128, 216, 267
communities' role in, 117, 121
effectiveness of the human environment
in, 33, 216, 270
in primary health care, 168, 296, 301, 308
in rural areas, 168
in the African Region, 60
in the South-East Asia Region, 72
in the Western Pacific Region, 80
voluntary fund for, 47, 50, 100, 106,
178, 191
Health services
administration of (see also 'Public health,
administration'), 33, 276, 278, 279
basic, 9, 25, 58, 61, 63, **117–20**, 125,
128, 144, 167, 178, 181, 183, 197,
213, 250, 270, 301, 303
communications in, 285
community involvement in, 64, 81, 94,
106, 152, 166, 168
coverage by, 63, 64, 66, 72, 80, 83
delivery of, 7, 60, 71, 82, 109, 297
development of, 33, 54, 62, 64, 67, 78,
82, 92, 293
drugs for, 251
environmental health in, 164, 271
health education in, 74, 150, 152, 153,
155